Psychopharmacology Series 3

Clinical Pharmacology in Psychiatry

Selectivity in Psychotropic Drug Action – Promises or Problems?

Editors

S. G. Dahl L. F. Gram S. M. Paul W. Z. Potter

With 79 Figures

Springer-Verlag Berlin Heidelberg New York
London Paris Tokyo

Svein G. Dahl, Cand Real, Dr. Philos.
Professor of Pharmacology, Department of Pharmacology, Institute of Medical Biology, University of Tromsø School of Medicine, N-9001 Tromsø, Norway

Lars F. Gram, MD
Professor of Clinical Pharmacology, Department of Clinical Pharmacology, School of Medicine, Odense University, DK-5000 Odense C, Denmark

Steven M. Paul, MD
Chief, Clinical Neuroscience Branch, National Institute of Mental Health, Building 10, Room 4N214, Bethesda, MD 20205, USA

William Z. Potter, MD, PhD
Chief, Section on Clinical Psychopharmacology, Laboratory of Clinical Science, Building 10, National Institute of Mental Health, Bethesda, MD 20205, USA

Vols. 1 and 2 of this series appeared under the title "Psychopharmacology Supplementum"

The figure on the front cover, showing the molecular structure and the solvent-accessible surface of the chlorpromazine molecule, was produced by Dr. S.G. Dahl during a period (1985/86) as visiting professor at UCSF, San Francisco. The colouring of the surface indicates the electrostatic charge of the molecule: blue – negative, white – positive. The structure was derived by molecular mechanics calculations using the Assisted Model Building with Energy Refinement (AMBER) programs, and the illustration was produced by the Molecular Interactive Display And Simulation (MIDAS) programs at the Computer Graphics Laboratory, Department of Pharmaceutical Chemistry, University of California, San Francisco.

ISBN-13:978-3-642-71290-6 e-ISBN-13:978-3-642-71288-3
DOI: 10.1007/978-3-642-71288-3

Library of Congress Cataloging-in-Publication Data. Clinical pharmacology in psychiatry. (Psychopharmacology series; 3) Based on papers presented at the Fourth International Meeting on Clinical Pharmacology in Psychiatry, held in Bethesda, Md., Sept. 5–8, 1985 and dedicated to the memory of Earl Usdin. Includes bibliographies and index. 1. Psychotropic drugs – Congresses. 2. Neuropsychopharmacology – Congresses. 3. Usdin, Earl. I. Dahl, S. (Svein), 1942– . II. Usdin, Earl. III. International Meeting on Clinical Pharmacology in Psychiatry (4th: 1985: Bethesda, Md.). IV. Series [DNLM: 1. Mental Disorders – drug therapy congresses. 2. Psychotropic Drugs – pharmacodynamics – congresses. 3. Psychotropic Drugs – therapeutic use – congresses. WM 402 C6405 1985] RM315.C5496 1986 616.89'18 86-27880
ISBN-13:978-3-642-71290-6 (U.S.)

Softcover reprint of the hardcover 1st edition 1987

2125/3130-543210

Preface

The Fourth International Meeting on Clinical Pharmacology in Psychiatry was held in Bethesda, Maryland on 5–8 September 1985 and was dedicated to the memory of Dr. Earl Usdin. Earl was one of the organizers of the three previous meetings held in Chicago (1979), Tromsø (1980), and Odense (1982). During the organization of the fourth meeting Earl became ill and had to relinquish his role as one of the principal organizers. It is safe to conclude that there was no better, or more professional, or more efficient an organizer of scientific meetings in the field of neuropharmacology and psychiatry than Earl Usdin, and it was quite a task for the remaining organizers to fill the void left when he withdrew from this one. Those of us who have organized previous meetings with Earl were struck by how much more difficult our work became without him. This obviously speaks well for his subtle (and at times not so subtle) organizational skills. Nevertheless, in Earl's memory the organizers proceeded to invite a group of internationally renowned neuropsychopharmacologists to address the problem of selectivity in psychotropic drug action and to try to reconcile the amazing advances in basic preclinical neuropsychopharmacology with the problem of clinical specificity encountered by the psychiatrist. In addition, the meeting attempted to address whether or not an understanding of the neurochemical actions of a given class of psychotropic drugs could be applied to the prediction of selectivity in neuropsychiatric patients; and (or) how such information might be useful in predicting novel psychotropic agents. The scientific conclusions of the meeting are contained in this volume, which is divided into four sections, including our section on molecular pharmacology and drug development and a section each on anxiolytics, antidepressants, and neuroleptics. The organizers want to thank the invited participants, the pharmaceutical companies who graciously supported travel and lodging for the participants, and the National Institute of Mental Health and the National Institutes of Health for helping to host the meeting on the NIH campus in Bethesda, Maryland.

San Francisco, Odense, Bethesda, 1986

Svein G. Dahl
Lars F. Gram
Steven M. Paul
William Z. Potter

Contents

Antidepressants

Neuroleptics

List of Contributors

You will find the addresses at the beginning of the respective contribution

Ator, N.A. 83
Aulakh, C.S. 135
Blier, P. 127
Brady, E.J. 12
Brady, S.F. 12
Breier, A. 248
Brøsen, K. 184
Bunney, B.S. 225
Cascieri, M.A. 12
Casey, D.E. 243
Christensen, P. 184, 193
Coble, P.A. 167
Cohen, R.M. 135
Colton, C.D. 12
Cowen, P.J. 72
Dahl, S.G. 266
De Montigny, C 127
De Vane, C.L. 174
Doran, A.R. 248
Dorow, R. 37
Duka, T. 37
Ellinwood Jr., E.H. 77
Fork, P. 20
Freeman, A.S. 225
Freidinger, R.M. 12
Friedman, H.L. 62
Garrick, N.A. 135
Gerlach, J. 236
Goldman, M.E. 201
Gommeren, W. 214
van Gompel, P. 214
Gram, L.F. 147, 184
Greenblatt, D.J. 62
Griffiths, R.R. 83
Hals, P.-A. 266
Havoundjian, H. 29
Heatherly, D.G. 77
Höller, L. 37
Hommer, D.W. 52
Honoré, P. le Fèvre 147
James, D. 179
Kebabian, J.W. 201
Kellar, K.J. 99
Kistrup, K. 236
Korsgaard, S. 236
Kragh-Sørensen, P. 147, 184
Kupfer, D.J. 167
Labarca, R. 248
Laduron, P.M. 214
Lamb, R.J. 83
Leysen, J.E. 214
Linnoila, M. 157
Lloyd, K.G. 113
Marshall, G.R. 3
Martino, A.M. 99
Matsuo, V. 52
Meltzer, H.Y. 255
Montgomery, D.B. 179
Montgomery, S.A. 179
Murphy, D.L. 135
Nikaido, A.M. 77
Nutt, D.J. 72
Paleveda, W.J. 12
Paul, S.M. 29, 52, 248
Perel, J.M. 167
Perlow, D.S. 12
Pichat, P. 113
Pickar, D. 248
Pinder, R.M. 107
Pollock, B. 167
Potter, W.Z. 157
Rickels, K. 88
Roache, J.D. 83
Rudorfer, M.V. 157

Molecular Pharmacology in Drug Development

Molecular Modeling in Drug Design

G. R. MARSHALL[1]

1 Introduction

Molecular recognition plays a central role in biological systems and is the basis of the specificity seen in antigen-antibody, substrate-enzyme, hormone-receptor, and drug-receptor interactions. The importance of this problem had been recognized by scientists like Pasteur and Ehrlich at the end of the nineteenth century. Structure-activity relations in which one probes the basis of recognition by chemically modifying one of the partners form a significant segment of medicinal chemistry. Attempts to correlate activity with physical properties such as solubility, refractive index, etc., are a reasonable approach to defining the characteristic properties associated with activity in a given biological assay (Hansch 1966). In most systems, these correlations reflect the effective concentration of the drug in the critical biophase rather than the critical features necessary for bimolecular recognition. We would like to concentrate on what can be deduced regarding bimolecular recognition from structure-activity data.

A major dichotomy between quantitative structure–activity relations (QSAR) and molecular recognition exists on two levels. First, potency is the primary raison d'etre of QSAR and depends on a multitude of parameters, such as distribution, metabolism, transport, recognition, and affinity. On the other hand, good pharmacological data implying recognition at a common receptor site are the criterion for inclusion in studies of molecular recognition regardless of the relative potency if one can be convinced the activity lies in the compound tested and not in some contaminant, for example. The purpose is to deduce the minimal recognition requirements as a basis for understanding how a diverse set of chemical structures can activate the same receptor. Secondly, recognition is critically dependent on the three-dimensional arrangement of electron density in a molecule, and the determination of the receptor-bound conformation is a logical goal in attempts to deduce recognition requirements.

Since the primary concerns in drug-receptor interaction are the bound conformation of the drug and those interactions with the receptor that are responsible for activity, one must ignore information which is unlikely to be relevant. This includes most of the studies focusing on the minimum energy conformation, whether one is speaking of theoretical in vacuo calculations, solution conformations from NMR, or crystal structures of small molecules. Because of the binding

[1] Department of Pharmacology, Washington University Medical School, St. Louis, MO 63110, USA.

Clinical Pharmacology in Psychiatry
Editors: Dahl, Gram, Paul, Potter
(Psychopharmacology Series 3)

process, a significant amount of interaction between the receptor and the drug must occur. The receptor is asymmetric and presents a potentially dominant perturbation to the conformational equilibrium in the adjacent solution. Affinities of receptors for natural transmitters are under evolutionary control, as exemplified in the large differences in affinity of pre- and postsynaptic receptors for neurotransmitters such as dopamine. One mechanism by which the affinity can be modulated is binding of a higher energy form of the transmitter.

In the absence of the three-dimensional structure of the receptor, one can only rely on measurements of the response of the receptor to ligand binding as a measure of successful recognition and activation. By varying the structure of the ligand, one can probe the receptor and attempt to separate the variables which lead to recognition and activation of the particular receptor under study. This approach requires numerous assumptions, some of which are often tacit, and can lead to erroneous concepts if the particular assumptions are invalid. Only by consistency with the set of observations and by prediction of new and testable results can any model derive credibility. Continued refinement of the hypothetical receptor model in the face of new data is obligatory, and emotional attachment to any particular model must be firmly resisted, as most are underdetermined.

2 Pharmacophore Hypothesis

One oversimplification which is, nevertheless, a good starting point is the traditional concept of pharmacophore, normally credited to Ehrlich at the turn of the century. In more modern terms, the pharmacophore is the critical part of the key which interacts with the tumblers necessary to unlock the appropriate events leading to receptor activation (Fig. 1). In other words, it is unique three-dimensional pattern of electron density in the ligand which activates the receptor. One basic

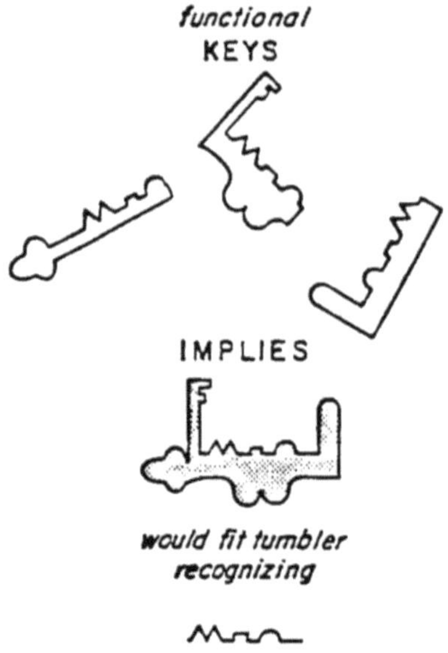

Fig. 1. Schematic view of pharmacophore and volume requirements

problem facing medicinal chemists is the absence of information regarding their target, the receptor. Since they must design new compounds, they often modify known active structures as the most likely strategy to retain the desired activity. Only by insight into the nature of the drug-receptor interaction can they transcend the constraints of known structures and design truly novel compounds with sufficient probability of activity. The basis for this insight is the concept of pharmacophore, i.e., those features common to a set of drugs acting at the same receptor which are responsible for recognition and transduction of the appropriate response.

With this simplifying assumption, a basis (Marshall et al. 1979) for computer-assisted drug design is established, the "active analogue approach." The first problem is to determine possible three-dimensional arrangements of features common to the set of active drugs. Each of these common arrangements becomes a candidate pharmacophore, which can be rejected because of incompatibility with other observations (inconsistency) or because of lack of predictability of activity of new compounds. What are the features that should be considered? These can be the traditional concepts of medicinal chemistry; heteroatoms, lone pairs, pi centers, aromatic planar groups, hydrogen-bonding functions, etc.; or more sophisticated physical chemical concepts, such as fragment dipole moments, electrostatic potential properties, lipophilicity. If one makes the further assumption that the receptor-bound conformation is the one of lowest energy, then the problem becomes straightforward. For each analogue, one determines the appropriate conformer and simply looks for common three-dimensional features present in the set of active analogues. Programs for detecting such common features have been described by Gund (1979). Unfortunately, efforts to correlate activity with conformers seen in crystal structures, in solution by NMR, or derived by theoretical calculation have been disappointing. The physical chemical basis for this lack of correlation should be clear: *These procedures ignore the perturbation caused by interaction between the drug and the asymmetric force field represented by the receptor.* In other words, there are no a priori reasons to assume that a receptor binds the low-energy conformer of a drug, and considerable evidence exists to suggest just the opposite in several well-documented cases, such as dehydrofolate reductase (DHFR) (Mathews et al. 1985), ribonuclease S (Bierzynsk et al. 1982), and NAD (Parthasarathy and Fridey 1984). It is, therefore, imperative to consider the ensemble of conformers accessible by perturbation of the solution ensemble upon binding to the receptor.

In the active analogue approach (Marshall et al. 1979), a single pharmacophore is assumed to exist for a set of compounds active at a given drug receptor, and a logical approach is used to help determine whether such a simplified concept is consistent with the observed data. For example, inhibitors of angiotensin converting enzyme all seem to have a C-terminal carboxylate, an amide bond, and a group capable of binding to zinc. One could examine the possible three-dimensional arrangements of these three groups available to each analogue to see whether a common pattern were accessible. One approach would be to link each of the groups together across the series of analogues and simultaneously minimize the resulting supermolecule with each molecule invisible to the others (Fig. 2). By appropriate weighting of the spring constants, the molecules can be made to as-

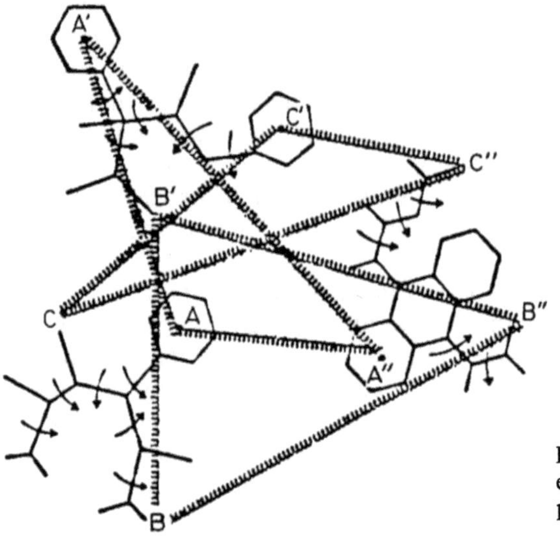

Fig. 2. Constrained minimization to examine existence of pharmacophoric pattern

sume similar three-dimensional arrangements of the three groups (Duchamps 1979). Unfortunately, there are two major deficiencies in such an approach. First, the results are dependent on the starting positions, as only the nearest local minimum in the total energy function is found. Second, no information regarding the global minima or the uniqueness of the solution found is available. It is obviously important to have an estimate of the number of possible pharmacophore hypotheses consistent with the set of assumptions as well as the existence of a possible solution.

Because the constraints on a molecule to induce the appropriate biological response are more stringent than simply high affinity for the active site, which could lead to inhibition only, there is a higher probability of success with the pharmacophore assumption with agonists than with antagonists. One approach to the question of whether agonists and antagonists bind to the same site in the same state would be to analyze antagonist and agonist data separately and compare the resulting models to see whether a consistent view arises. Klunk et al. (1983) have recently made independent analyses for a set of picrotoxinin and a set of gamma butyrolactone convulsants. Their data are consistent with a common binding mode at a common receptor, with the lactone rings in the two sets of compounds interacting in a similar fashion. Recent radioligand studies indicate displacement of the same ligand by both picrotoxinin and gamma butyrolactones from brain membranes (Levine et al. 1985).

3 Orientation Space

In order to search efficiently for common patterns available to a set of drugs interacting with the same receptor, a methodology (Motoc et al. 1985) independent of the molecular framework and rotation of the compounds is desirable. By trans-

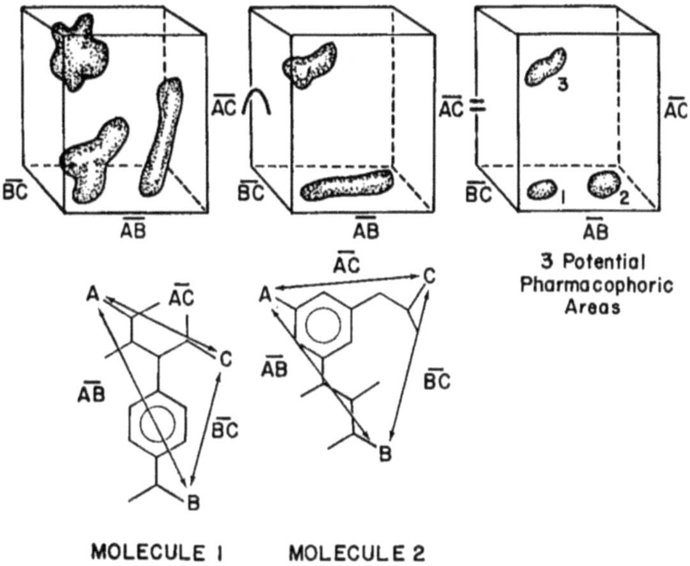

Fig. 3. Three-dimensional orientation space maps with each axis representing the distance between two of three pharmacophoric groups. Intersection of maps identifies common three-dimensional patterns

forming each conformation (which could be expressed either in terms of internal degrees of freedom, i.e., torsional rotations, or by absolute coordinates) into a relative distance space in which the distances between pharmacophoric groups become the metric, compounds of different congeneric series can be compared independently of their absolute orientations. This relative distance space focuses on the *orientation* of important groups relative to each other, i.e., potential pharmacophoric patterns; hence the name, orientation space. A three-group pharmacophore can be considered as a triangle, which can be represented by a single point in an orientation space with a dimensionality of three. By intersecting the orientation space maps for a set of active analogues, one can determine whether a common pharmacophoric pattern or patterns can be assumed by all the analogues (Fig. 3). In other words, for each sterically allowed conformation available to an analogue, a point in orientation space is generated. This represents the three-dimensional arrangement of the groups designated by the chemist to be responsible for activity for that particular conformer. The set of such points represents all the possible arrangements available to the analogue. Since our hypothesis of a pharmacophore implies a common pattern among the set of active analogues, the corresponding point in orientation space must be occupied in each orientation space map generated for each analogue. The common set of points represents the set of pharmacophore patterns consistent with the assignments of pharmacophoric groups and the set of analogues examined.

4 Receptor Mapping

Besides the ability to present an appropriate message, the pharmacophore, other criteria are necessary for activity. Sufficient affinity must be present to distinguish the activity over background noise attributable to nonspecific interactions, and this affinity can be severely compromised by a negative steric interaction with the receptor. In other words, the correct pattern may be present on the key, but the key blank may not fit the lock. Comparison of the set of key blanks which work will outline some of the space available for successful key blanks when aligned with the common pattern (Fig. 1). The assumption is made, therefore, that the common pharmacophoric pattern represents a common binding mode and can be used to align the set of analogues in a common frame of reference. The union of the volume of the parts of each analogue which are fixed during presentation of the pharmacophore defines a minimum volume available at the receptor.

According to the above arguments, one reason for inactivity could be the competition between the receptor and the analogue for common space when the analogue has assumed the appropriate conformation to present the pharmacophore. This becomes another basis for a check of consistency as well as an indication of the receptor orientation relative to the pharmacophore. If an inactive analogue requires no novel volume while presenting the pharmacophore besides that defined by the union of actives, then something is wrong somewhere. The assumption of a common mode of action, the trial pharmacophore hypothesis, assignment of correspondence between functional groups, and/or measurement of activity all become suspect. In general, an alternative pharmacophore hypothesis is explored for consistency. If there are good pharmacological data suggesting a common site of action, i.e., competitive binding assays, and either a null set occurs for the orientation map analysis or an inconsistency cannot be avoided in receptor mapping, then a more complicated interpretation, e.g., multiple binding modes, must be explored.

5 Beyond the Pharmacophore

The strict pharmacophore hypothesis is clearly an oversimplification of what our experience suggests to be the general case. Receptor sites are multipotential with respect to modes of binding of conformers of a drug. The next level of assumption is to assume that the receptor site is relatively static, and to explore how one can derive site models consistent with the available data. The approach developed by Crippen allows user specification of site points (Crippen 1981), which could be computer-assisted. One can extend the methodology of the active analogue approach by systematically searching for coincidence of sites capable of interacting with functional groups rather than for overlapping of those functional groups. To give an example, detailed consideration of the opioid mu receptor by Fries and Portoghese (1976) has led to a proposal of multiple binding modes for substituted piperidine opioids. Humblet and Marshall (1981) were led to a similar conclusion by extending the lone pair on the nitrogen to a distance capable of hydrogen bonding to an oxygen atom and searching for overlap of the postulated receptor

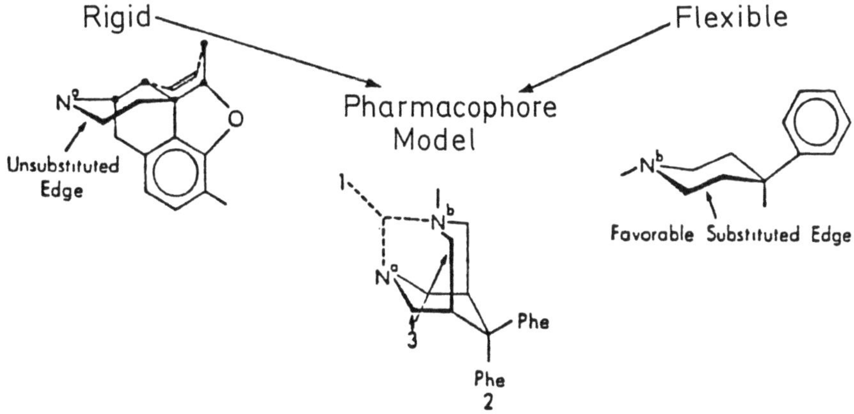

Fig. 4. Proposed model for binding to opioid mu-receptor

site oxygen. This, plus an additional phenyl-binding site which was clearly indicated by structure-activity data, forms the current basis of their model of the mu receptor (Fig. 4). Such an extension is clearly justified in the case of angiotensin-converting enzyme inhibitors by extending the sulfhydryl function of captopril and the carboxylate functionality of enalopril to include the zinc atom, Z; the C-terminal carboxylate to include the positively charged site point, X; and the carboxyl group to include the hydrogen bond donor, Y (Fig. 5). Studies of a set of angiotensin-converting enzyme (ACE) inhibitors (Mayer et al. 1986) led to a unique arrangement for groups X, Y, and Z. Confidence in this potential geometry for the active site of ACE arises from the fact that this site can bind thiorphan, an inhibitor of both ACE and enkephalinase, but not retrothiorphan, a specific inhibitor of enkephalinase (Roques et al. 1983).

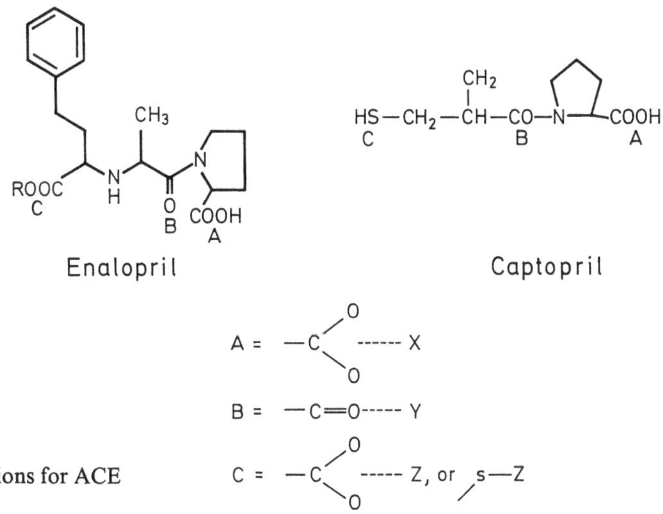

Fig. 5. Site model extensions for ACE inhibitors

Why not include such elaborations in the initial analysis? The number of assumptions is clearly greater. The number of degrees of freedom for systematic search has to be increased which can be computationally crippling. But more importantly, the accumulated structure-activity data often are not sufficient to rule out a much simpler hypothesis. What one is attempting is the use of analogues to probe the receptor site in an effort to deduce as much as possible about its properties. Based on the parlor game of Twenty Questions, one can clearly derive a great deal of information by careful selection of questions and pruning of the combinatorial tree of possibilities depending on the answers. There are many systems, such as the opioid or dopamine receptor, where the medicinal chemist has synthesized and had the activity measured on thousands of compounds. Clearly, we are novices at this version of Twenty Questions, but there are glimmers of a successful strategy.

6 Caveats

Several implicit assumptions underlie the static pharmacophore approach outlined above, which can be seriously challenged. The assumption of a common binding mode is clearly oversimplified. Receptor sites are multifaceted and capable of generating comparable binding affinities by interaction with combinations of subsites. One is forced, however, by Occam's razor (Russel 1945) to assume the simplest site until the accumulated data force a more complicated interpretation. One advantage which arises from this approach is the lack of emphasis on accurate energy calculations. Difficulties arise when one is attempting to determine the details of molecular energetics attributable to limitations in force field parameters, inappropriate treatment of the dielectric constant (Greenberg et al. 1978), and lack of consideration of solvation and entropic effects.

7 Conclusions

A molecular understanding of drug-receptor interactions is clearly desirable as a basis for drug design. Lack of correlation between experimental and theoretical studies and observed activities can be seen to be due to oversimplified assumptions, technical limitations such as the local minima problem, and lack of detailed information about the receptor itself. The use of a systematic search strategy and the assumption of a pharmacophore provides a rational basis on which to examine simple hypotheses regarding features responsible for a given activity. Consistency and predictability are the primary criteria by which one can judge such simplified ideas. While the scientific method requires the use of such a simple-minded approach, one must keep in mind that evolution has had multiple opportunities to develop complicated mechanisms. In other words, Mother Nature never shaved with Occam's razor; and we must view our simplified hypotheses simply as a means of gaining more insight into the more complicated mechanisms which underlie both molecular recognition and pharmacological activity.

Acknowledgements. The concepts, developments, and results represented are the results of the efforts and contributions of a multidisciplinary group at Washington University whose names appear in the references. Without them and the support of the National Institutes of Health (GM 24483), our understanding of molecular recognition would be even more limited.

References

Bierzynsk A, Kim PS, Ballwin RL (1982) A salt bridge stabilizes the helix formed by isolated C-peptide of RNase A. Proc Natl Acad Sci USA 79:2470–2474

Crippen GM (1981) Distance geometry and conformational calculations. In: Bawden D (ed) Chemometrics research studies series, vol 1. Wiley, Chichester

Duchamp DJ (1979) Molecular mechanics and crystal structure analysis in drug design. In: Olson EC, Christoffersen RE (eds) Computer-assisted drug design. ACS symposium series 112. American Chemical Society, Washington, DC, pp 79–102

Fries DS, Portoghese PS (1976) Stereochemical studies on medicinal compounds. 20. Absolute configuration and analgetic potency of alpha-promedol enantiomers. The role of the C-4 chiral center in conferring stereoselectivity in axial- and equitorial-phenyl prodine congeners. J Med Chem 19:1155–1158

Greenberg DA, Barry CD, Marshall GR (1978) Investigation and parameterization of a molecular dielectric function. J Am Chem Soc 100:4020–4026

Gund P (1979) Pharmacophore pattern searching and receptor mapping. Ann Rep Med Chem 14:299–308

Hansch C (1969) A quantitative approach to biochemical structure-activity relationships. Acc Chem Res 2:232–239

Humblet C, Marshall GR (1981) Three-dimensional computer modeling as an aid to drug design. Drug Dev Res 1:409–434

Klunk WE, Kalman BL, Ferrendelli JA, Covey DF (1983) Computer-assisted modeling of the picrotoxinin and gamma-butyrolactone receptor site. Mol Pharmacol 23:511–518

Levine JA, Ferrendelli JA, Covey DF (1985) Convulsant and anti-convulsant gammabutyrolactones bind to the picrotoxinin/t-butylbicyclophosphorothionate (TBPS) receptor. Biochem Pharmacol 34:4187–4190

Marshall GR, Barry CD, Bosshard HE, Dammkoehler RA, Dunn DA (1979) The conformational parameter in drug design: the active analog approach. In: Olsen EC, Christoffersen RE (eds) Computer-assisted drug design. ACS symposium series 112. American Chemical Society, Washington, DC, pp 205–226

Mathews DA, Bolin JT, Burridge JM, Filman DJ, Volz KW, Kaufman BT, Beddell CR, Champness JN, Stammers DK, Kraut J (1985) Refined crystal structures of *Escherichia coli* and chicken liver dihydrofolate reductase containing bound trimethoprim. J Biol Chem 260:381–391

Mayer D, Motoc I, Marshall GR (1986) Determination of an active site model of angiotensin converting enzyme. J Med Chem (in press)

Motoc I, Dammkoehler RA, Marshall GR (1985) Three-dimensional structure-activity relationships and biological receptor mapping. In: Trinajstic N (ed) Application of mathematical concepts to chemistry. Ellis Horwood, Chichester (in press)

Parthasarathy R, Fridey SM (1984) Conformational variability of NAD+ in the free and bound states: a nicotinamide sandwich in NAD+ crystals. Science 226:969–971

Roques BP, Lucas-Soroca E, Chaillet P, Costentin J, Fournie-Zaluski J (1983) Complete differentiation between enkephalinase and angiotensin-converting enzyme inhibition by *retro*-thiorphan. Proc Natl Acad Sci USA 80:3178–3182

Russell B (1945) A history of western philosophy. Simon and Schuster, New York, p 472

Synthesis of New Peptides Based on Models of Receptor-Bound Conformation

R. M. FREIDINGER [1], S. F. BRADY [1], W. J. PALEVEDA [1], D. S. PERLOW [1], C. D. COLTON [1], W. L. WHITTER [1], R. SAPERSTEIN [2], E. J. BRADY [2], M. A. CASCIERI [2], and D. F. VEBER [1]

1 Introduction

About three dozen small peptides (mostly 2–40 residues) have been identified in the nervous system (Iversen 1983, 1984; Krieger 1983). The neuropeptides mediate a wide range of endocrine, motor, and behavioral responses (Snyder 1980; Krieger 1983). These substances control such diverse functions as growth, reproduction, digestion, metabolism, and the dynamics of the cardiovascular system. Immunostaining techniques have been used to visualize and map the distribution of peptides, in particular neuronal pathways. Many of these substances have also been shown to occur in peripheral regions, such as the gastrointestinal tract. The role of many of these agents is largely unknown, but their potential utility in therapy is great.

There are a number of shortcomings, however, which limit the application of native peptides as drugs. These limitations include rapid degradation by proteases, lack of specificity, poor transport from gastrointestinal tract to blood and from blood to brain, and rapid excretion by liver and kidneys. The challenge is to learn how to overcome these problems and develop useful agents based on these peptide leads.

One approach to potentially solving all of these problems is random screening for a substance (probably nonpeptide) which is an agonist or antagonist of the particular peptide of interest. The opiate alkaloid analgesics which mimic the endogenous enkephalins are one such example. A second approach, which will be the focus of the present discussion, is rational drug design based on a knowledge of the peptide structure. The focus of this conformation-activity approach is the receptor-bound or bioactive conformation of the peptide (conformation at a given receptor at the instant that a given response is elicited). From information about the bioactive conformation, properties of the biological receptor itself can be inferred.

The initial attack on a particular problem requires the generation of a data base of new peptide analogues by chemical synthesis, followed by conformational and biological evaluation of these compounds. The results can lead to a first working hypothesis for the bioactive conformation. The hypothesis can then be tested by synthesis of conformationally constrained analogues and revised as appropriate. Besides giving information about the bioactive conformation, con-

Merck Sharp & Dohme Research Laboratories, [1] West Point, PA 19486 and [2] Rahway, NJ 07065, USA.

Clinical Pharmacology in Psychiatry
Editors: Dahl, Gram, Paul, Potter
(Psychopharmacology Series 3)

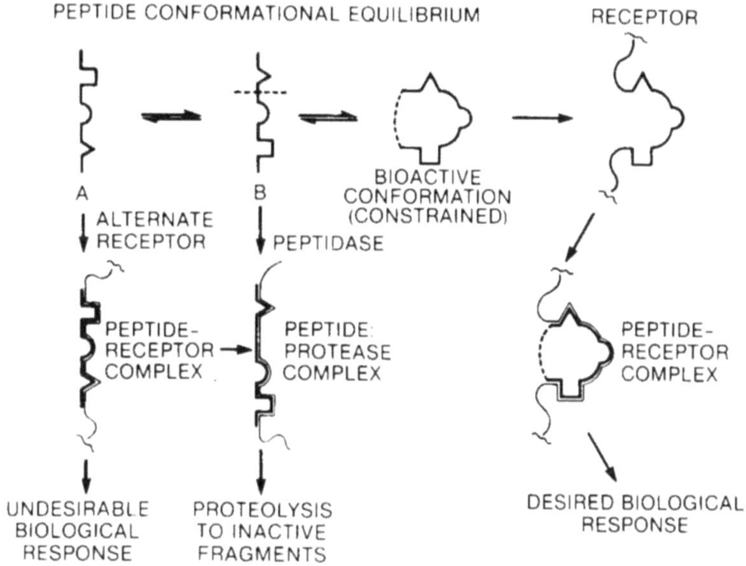

Fig. 1. Conformational constraint stabilizing the bioactive conformation over alternative conformations. [From Veber and Freidinger (1985) with permission. Copyright 1985 by Elsevier Science Publishers, B.V., Amsterdam]

formational constraints can also help to overcome some of the problems discussed above. Stability to proteases may be increased by destabilizing a metabolized conformer. Similarly, selectivity may be improved by destabilizing a conformer that interacts with a receptor which produces an unwanted response. Potency may be raised by increasing the proportion of molecules with the bioactive conformation available to interact with the receptor of interest. Often structural simplification is possible by removing amino acids whose main role (conformational) is now performed by the constraint (see Fig. 1). The application of this approach to three different peptide systems will be described.

2 Somatostatin

This macrocyclic 14-peptide inhibits the release of numerous substances, including insulin, glucagon, and growth hormone (Veber and Saperstein 1979). It is also found in the central nervous system (CNS) and is attracting interest as a neuropeptide (Srikant and Patel 1981). It is rapidly degraded in vivo and is only useful clinically when given by infusion. Structure modification studies have been quite successful in attaining simplified and metabolically stable analogues culminating in cyclic hexapeptides of greater potency than somatostatin (Veber et al. 1981; Fig. 2).

Using biological results from numerous analogues, nuclear magnetic resonance (NMR), and computer modeling techniques, a working model for the bioactive conformation of the latter compounds has been developed. This model

H-Ala-Gly-Cys-Lys-Asn-Phe-Phe-Trp
HO-Cys-Ser-Thr-Phe-Thr-Lys

Somatostatin

⇓

X-Phe-D-Trp
Phe-Thr-Lys

X = Pro
X = N^{α}-Me-Ala

Fig. 2. Somatostatin and simplified analogs

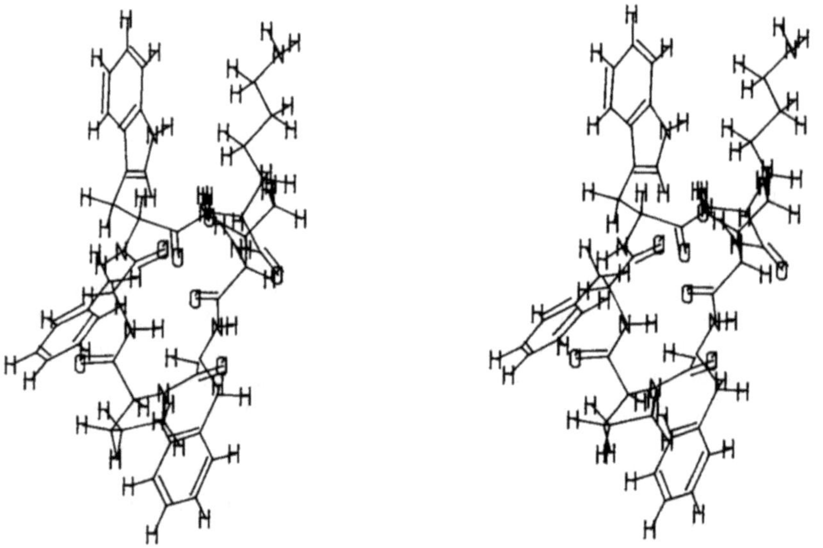

Fig. 3. Stereo view of bioactive conformational model of cyclo-(Phe-D-Trp-Ly-Thr-Phe-Pro). [From Freidinger et al. (1984), with permission. Copyright 1983 by Munksgaard International Publishers Ltd., Copenhagen, Denmark]

is characterized by two reverse turns (beta turns) and certain side chain proximities (see Fig. 3). It was of interest to test the validity of this model with conformational modifications to sharpen the view of the somatostatin receptor's requirements for a potent ligand.

2.1 Bicyclic Analogues

Certain side chains in the model are relatively close in space. Locking these proximities with a covalent bridge tests the validity of this aspect of conformation. The beta carbons of Phe-11 and Pro-6 (somatostatin numbering) are 4.7 Å apart in the model, and computer superposition shows they are properly positioned for

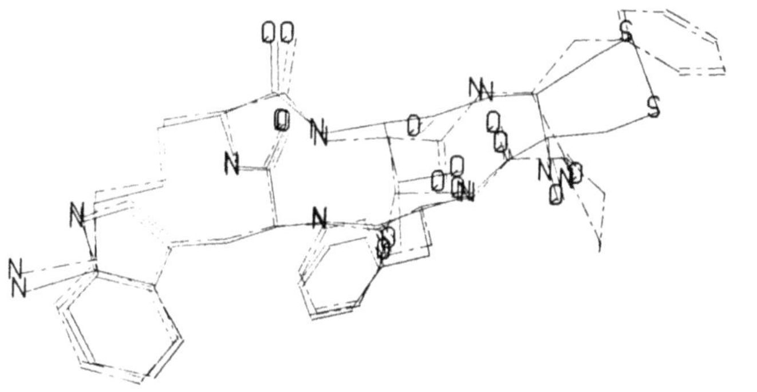

Fig. 4. Comparison of cyclo-(Phe-D-Trp-Lys-Thr-Phe-Pro) (dashed) with bicyclic analog cyclo-(Phe-D-Trp-Lys-Thr-Cys-Cys) (solid)

connection by a disulfide linkage. Such a bridge would result from incorporation of cystine in place of these two amino acids. Furthermore, the disulfide group would fall into the same region and occupy about the same amount of space as the essential phenyl side chain of Phe. This conformational modification then tests one of the beta turns and the position of the side chain in the model (see Fig. 4).

This new analogue cyclo-(Cys-Cys-Phe-D-Trp-Lys-Thr) was synthesized, and its biological activity for inhibition of release of insulin, glucagon, and growth hormone was found to parallel the parent structure. These results lend additional credence to the hypothesized bioactive conformation.

2.2 Retrocycloisomeric Analogues

It was of interest to test whether the backbone of the cyclic hexapeptide has a role in binding to the receptor or simply serves to position the key side chain binding elements properly. This question was addressed through design of analogues based on the retroenantiomer hypothesis (Goodman and Chorev 1979). In simplest terms, this concept involves reversing the direction of the peptide backbone and inverting the configuration of each amino acid in the hope that the side chains of the resultant peptide will occupy the same positions as in the starting structure. This approach was originally explored as a way of stabilizing peptides to proteases with D-amino acids while retaining biological activity. Although the side chain conformations of a peptide and its retroenantiomer cannot in fact be the same (Freidinger and Veber 1979), they may be similar, and it might be possible to retain the biological activity of the parent compound through application of the hypothesis based on conformational considerations.

To examine this possibility, retrocycloisomers of the potent analog cyclo-(*N*-Me-Ala-Phe-D-Trp-Lys-Thr-Phe) were prepared (see Fig. 5). The first analogue, cyclo-(D-Phe-D-Thr-D-Lys-L-Trp-D-Phe-*N*-Me-D-Ala), resulting from strict application of the hypothesis, was only about 0.1% as potent as the parent. This outcome was expected, since the working conformational model contains a *cis*-peptide linkage between *N*-Me-Ala and Phe, and misplacement of the *N*-methyl

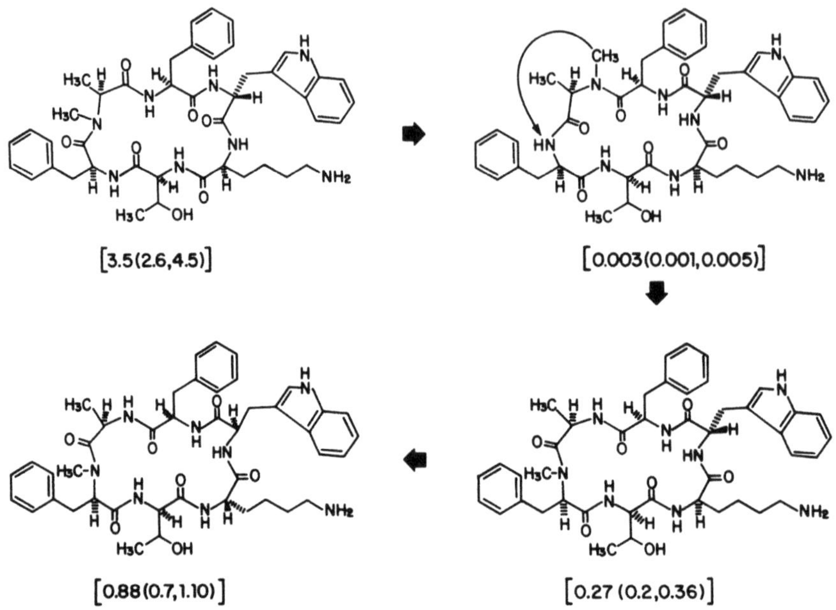

Fig. 5. Design of retro cycloisomeric hexapeptide analogues of somatostatin. Potency for inhibition of release of growth hormone in an in vitro pituitary cell system (somatostatin = 1) is in brackets

group from the middle of the beta turn in the new analogue would result in a probable *trans*-amide and a substantial change in the shape of the molecule. Examination of molecular models revealed that the desired two beta turn conformation might be restored by moving the *N*-methyl group from D-Ala-6 to D-Phe-11 in this compound. This change would permit the key *cis*-peptide bond to form in the proper location in the backbone, which should result in the achievement of better overall side chain correspondence with the parent compound. The resultant structure, cyclo-(*N*-Me-D-Phe-D-Thr-D-Lys-L-Trp-D-Phe-D-Ala), was synthesized and in fact displayed a full biological response and had about 10% of the potency of the parent peptide and 25% of that of somatostatin for inhibition of growth hormone, glucagon, and insulin release. A final adjustment in the backbone was inversion of the Lys and Trp residues to produce cyclo-(*N*-Me-D-Phe-D-Thr-L-Lys-D-Trp-D-Phe-D-Ala), which is now stable to the action of proteases and comparable in potency to somatostatin itself. NMR studies have shown that this peptide also assumes the predicted conformation in solution.

The correspondence in side chain topography for the bioactive conformations of this compound and the parent cyclic hexapeptide must be quite good, because these relative potencies reflect a difference of less than 1 kcal/mol of receptor-binding energy. This is remarkable since the former analogue retains only five of the original amino acids of somatostatin and all but one has the D-configuration. The results indicate that the peptide backbone contributes only minimally to receptor binding by somatostatin and its analogues. The main role of the backbone must be the proper positioning of the key side chains for interaction with the receptor, thus raising the possibility that a nonpeptide "backbone" could be designed to perform the same function. Such an accomplishment could provide a further advance to a useful therapeutic agent, but this possibility remains to be tested.

3 Luteinizing Hormone-Releasing Hormone

Luteinizing Hormone-Releasing Hormone (LH-RH) or Glp-His-Trp-Ser-Tyr-Gly-Leu-Arg-Pro-Gly-NH_2, has been the subject of intensive studies as a novel approach to fertility control. Despite the synthesis of hundreds of agonist and antagonist analogues, it has not proven possible to reduce the size of the peptide significantly while retaining activity. Several of the existing analogues have suggested the presence of a Tyr-Gly-Leu-Arg type II′ beta turn in the bioactive conformation of agonist and/or antagonist analogues (Freidinger et al. 1980). This turn is the same type as for Phe-D-Trp-Lys-Thr in the working model of somatostatin analogues discussed above. It therefore appeared possible to stabilize this turn in a cyclic hexapeptide, and the structure selected and synthesized to test this possibility was cyclo-(Tyr-D-Trp-Leu-Arg-Trp-Pro). The Trp-Pro sequence was chosen to complete the ring for two reasons: Pro in this position should permit a *cis*-peptide bond and the same backbone conformation as in the somatostatin analogues, and the Trp may provide a hydrophobic binding element to replace the first three residues of LH-RH, which have been deleted. In addition, D-Trp in place of Gly is a known potency-enhancing element.

The new peptide was expected to be an antagonist, since deletion of His-2 generally furnishes antagonists. In fact, this was shown to be the case in an in vitro pituitary cell culture system, and no agonist activity was observed even at high doses. A dose of this analogue 400 times that of LH-RH is required to reduce LH-RH-mediated secretory rates by 50%. This compound is a weak antagonist by present-day standards, but it is the smallest analogue to have demonstrated antagonism to LH release by LH-RH in an in vitro assay. This result further emphasizes the importance of the positions 5–8 beta turn in LH-RH, and suggests it should be a focus of further design studies toward orally effective antagonists. This result also demonstrates that the conformation/activity approach to analogue design used successfully in the somatostatin work can be extended to other peptide/receptor systems, particularly including noncyclic peptides.

4 Tachykinins

These peptides are a family, which shares the carboxyl terminal sequence Phe-X-Gly-Leu-Met-NH_2 and which causes contraction of various smooth muscle systems. Substance P, H-Arg-Pro-Lys-Pro-Gln-Gln-Phe-Phe-Gly-Leu-Met-NH_2, is a mammalian peptide which has been shown to be widely located in synaptic vesicles in both the central and peripheral nervous systems. It is likely that it functions as a neurotransmitter or modulator in the CNS. Eledoisin is a tachykinin of amphibian origin with the sequence Glp-Pro-Ser-Lys-Asp-Ala-Phe-Ile-Gly-

Leu-Met-NH_2. The minimum fully potent sequence for tachykinins is known to be the carboxy terminal hexapeptide.

It has been proposed that there may be two subtypes of tachykinin receptors (Lee et al. 1983). In "P" type tissues, substance P and eledoisin are nearly equipotent, while in "E" type tissues, eledoisin is 10–100 times more potent than substance P. It has been shown that ^{125}I-Bolton Hunter-conjugated substance P (^{125}I-BH-SP) and ^{125}I-Bolton Hunter-conjugated eledoisin (^{125}I-BH-eledoisin) bind to pharmacologically distinct sites in rat brain cortex membranes (Cascieri and Liang 1984; Cascieri et al. 1985). Thus, there are at least two distinct tachykinin receptors in the mammalian CNS.

The conformational requirements of these receptors were examined with constrained analogues. Since the presence of a Gly residue may favor a turn in the peptide backbone, several conformationally restricted analogues of substance P hexapeptide designed to test this possibility for the bioactive conformation were prepared. The two isomeric compounds containing a lactam bridge between the nitrogen of Leu and the alpha carbon of Gly were especially interesting (Fig. 6, Table 1). The RS diastereomer is a potent ^{125}I-BH-eledoisin receptor selective agonist. The SS diastereomer has little activity in either substance P or eledoisin assays. Lactams have previously shown utility in stabilizing turn conformations (Freidinger 1981). These results indicate that the conformational requirements for the ^{125}I-BH substance P and ^{125}I-BH eledoisin receptors are different, and provide additional support for the observation of multiple tachykinin receptors. A turn conformation probably involving X-Gly-Leu-Met is favored by the latter receptor, and evidence for such a turn in solution has been obtained using NMR spectroscopy. For the substance P receptor, a different conformation from the two turn structures examined here must apply. The RS isomer is a useful receptor

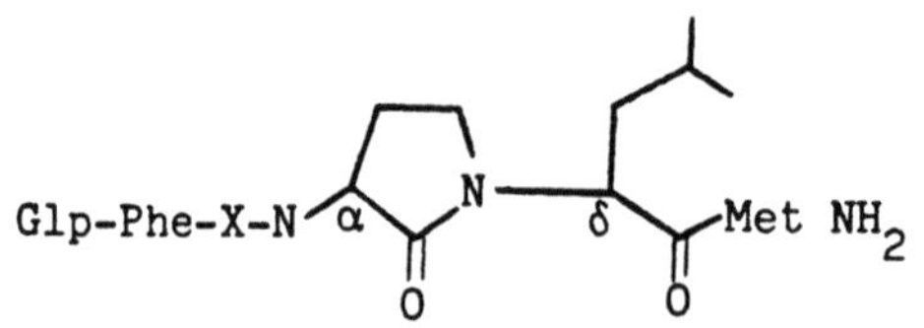

Fig. 6. General structure formula for lactam-containing tachykinin hexapeptides

Table 1. Receptor affinities and biological potencies of lactam-containing tachykinin hexapeptides

X	α	δ	IC_{50} (*M*) Mean ± SD (*n*) ^{125}I-BH-SP	^{125}I-BH-Eledoisin	ED_{50} Guinea pig ileum (n*M*)	Salivation (nmol/rat)
Phe	R	S	$1.6 \pm 0.5 \times 10^{-5}$	$3.2 \pm 2.1 \times 10^{-8}$ (11)	1.2	>100
Phe	S	S	$>6 \times 10^{-5}$ (3)	$3.0 \pm 0.4 \times 10^{-5}$ (2)	≧1000	> 65
Substance P			$1.0 \pm 0.5 \times 10^{-8}$ (7)	$2.1 \pm 1.6 \times 10^{-7}$ (4)	0.44	0.2
Eledoisin			$3.6 \pm 0.5 \times 10^{-7}$ (3)	$3.1 \pm 2 \times 10^{-8}$ (4)	1.6	0.4

probe and should facilitate determination of the physiological roles of these receptor subtypes.

Conclusions

It has been shown in three different peptide systems that a constrained analogue approach can provide useful information about the bioactive conformation of a peptide, while concomitantly leading to analogues with improved properties. In the case of somatostatin, a highly potent analogue developed in this way is now undergoing clinical evaluation (Veber et al. 1984). From the conformational information developed using this approach, characteristics of the biological receptors for these ligands can be inferred.

References

Cascieri MA, Liang T (1984) Binding of [^{125}I]Bolton Hunter conjugated eledoisin to rat brain cortex membranes – evidence for two classes of tachykinin receptors in the mammalian central nervous system. Life Sci 35:179–184

Cascieri MA, Chicchi GG, Liang T (1985) Demonstration of two distinct tachykinin receptors in rat brain cortex. J Biol Chem 260:1501–1507

Freidinger RM (1981) Computer graphics and chemical synthesis in the study of conformation of biologically active peptides. In: Rich DH, Gross E (eds) Peptides: synthesis-structure-function. Pierce Chemical Company, Rockford, pp 673–683

Freidinger RM, Veber DF (1979) Peptides and their retro enantiomers are topologically non-identical. J Am Chem Soc 101:6129–6131

Freidinger RM, Veber DF, Perlow DS, Brooks JR, Saperstein R (1980) Bioactive conformation of luteinizing hormone releasing hormone: evidence from a conformationally constrained analog. Science 210:656–658 and references cited therein

Freidinger RM, Perlow DS, Randall WL, Saperstein R, Arison BH, Veber DF (1984) Conformational modifications of cyclic hexapeptide somatostatin analogs. Int J Pept Protein Res 23:142–150

Goodman M, Chorev M (1979) On the concept of linear modified retro-peptide structures. Accounts of Chemical Research 12:1–7

Iversen LL (1983) Nonopiod neuropeptides in mammalian CNS. Annu Rev Pharmacol Toxicol 23:1–27

Iversen LL (1984) Amino acids and peptides: fast and slow chemical signals in the nervous system? Proc R Soc London [Biol] 221:245–260

Krieger DT (1983) Brain peptides: what, where, and why? Science 222:975–985

Lee CM, Iversen LL, Hanley MR, Sandberg BEB (1983) The possible existence of multiple receptors for substance P. Naunyn-Schmiedebergs Arch Pharmacol 318:281–287

Snyder SH (1980) Brain peptides as neurotransmitters. Science 209:976–983

Srikant CB, Patel YC (1981) Somatostatin receptors: identification and characterization in rat brain membranes. Proc Natl Acad Sci USA 78:3930–3934

Veber DF, Freidinger RM (1985) The design of metabolically stable peptide analogs. Trends Neurosci 8:392–396

Veber D, Saperstein R (1979) Somatostatin. Annu Rep Med Chem 14:209–219

Veber DF, Freidinger RM, Perlow DS, Paleveda WJ, Holly FW, Strachan RG, Nutt RF, Arison BH, Homnick C, Randall WC, Glitzer MS, Saperstein R, Hirschmann R (1981) A potent cyclic hexapeptide analogue of somatostatin. Nature 292:55–58

Veber DF, Saperstein R, Nutt RF, Freidinger RM, Brady SF, Curley P, Perlow DS, Paleveda WJ, Colton CD, Zacchei AG, Tocco DJ, Hoff DR, Vandlen RL, Gerich JE, Hall L, Mandarino L, Cordes EH, Anderson PS, Hirschmann R (1984) A super active cyclic hexapeptide analog of somatostatin. Life Sci 34:1371–1378

Molecular Approach to the Mechanism of Action of Antidepressant Drugs

A. WÄGNER[1,2] and P. Fork[1]

1 Drug-Receptor Interactions and Molecular Structures

In any attempt to explain the action of psychoactive drugs and neurotransmitters at the molecular level, in particular the binding and interaction with the receptor sites, it is of primary importance to elucidate the characteristic structural and conformational features of these compounds. This can be accomplished by analysis of SAR data (structure-activity relationship) for different types of drugs and related compounds.

It is generally thought that these drugs and transmitters act in a "preferred" or "favored" conformation in order to achieve optimal interaction with the specific receptors. Furthermore, if the receptors can be assumed to be in some way complementary to the acting compounds – and this is generally thought to be the case – information about the topography of the receptor sites can be gained from the knowledge of these preferred conformations.

The exact topography of the receptors can probably not be known until the receptors have been isolated, and preferably also the drug-receptor complexes. X-ray structure analysis of these macromolecules would then provide the desired information.

However, the use of X-ray crystallographic techniques, energy calculations and molecular graphic techniques on psychoactive drugs and related compounds can yield the following information in the context of drug-receptor interaction (Wägner 1980a):

1. One possible conformation, viz. the one observed in the crystal, usually energetically favorable, is established with high accuracy (see Fig. 1).
2. With this conformation as a starting point, energy calculations can be performed and the behavior of the molecule in solution can be performed (see Fig. 2).
3. No precise knowledge is available about the conformation of a drug in the physiological environment of the receptor, but it is reasonable to assume that complex hydrogen bonding systems arising in the crystal structure mimic those probably existing in solution (see Fig. 3).
4. If the studied molecules are rigid, or semirigid, the structure results obtained can be extended to the conformation in solution and the conformation engaging the receptor.

[1] Department of Structural Chemistry, Arrhenius Laboratory, University of Stockholm, S-106 91 Stockholm, Sweden.
[2] Department of Psychiatry and Psychology, Karolinska Institute, Karolinska Hospital, S-104 01 Stockholm, Sweden.

Clinical Pharmacology in Psychiatry
Editors: Dahl, Gram, Paul, Potter
(Psychopharmacology Series 3)

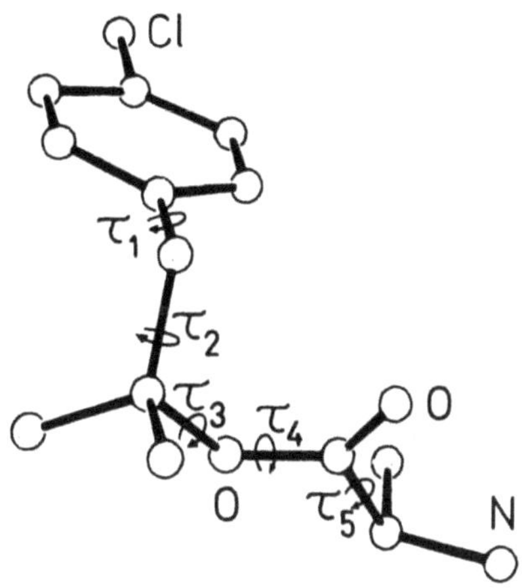

Fig. 1. Solid state conformation of alaproclate obtained from crystal data. *Arrows* indicate where free rotation around a bond is possible. (Wägner 1980 b)

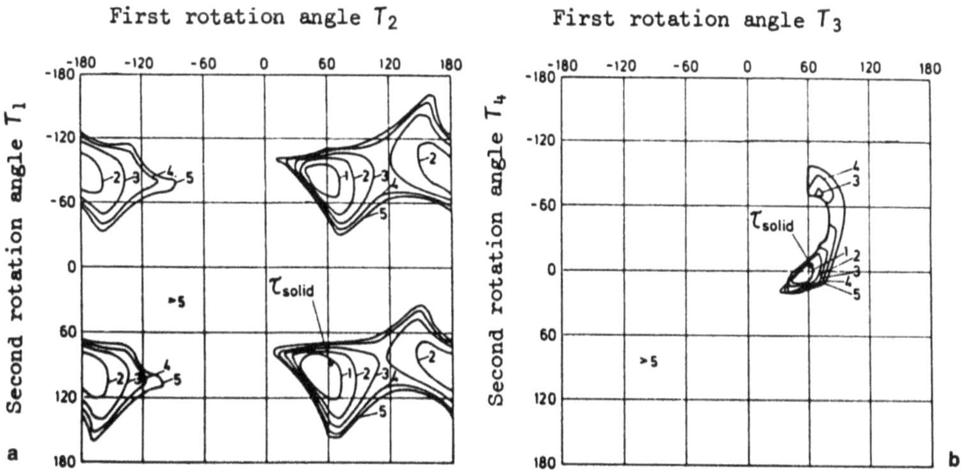

Fig. 2 a, b. Potential energy maps for alaproclate. Only energy regions below 5 kcal are plotted. **a** Rotation around T_1 and T_2 gives a symmetrical map indicating two energy minima. **b** Rotation around the T_3 and T_4 bonds results in a very narrow low-energy region, implying that rotation around these bonds is restricted. (Wägner 1980 b)

5. By studying series of pharmacologically active substances and related compounds acting at a common receptor, geometrical parameters intended to describe the molecular conformation and configuration of the relevant pharmacophore groups can be calculated for the compounds studied (see discussion below and Fig. 6).
6. As a consequence, the spatial arrangement of the reactive groups on the receptor surface may be estimated.
7. The results of the crystal structure determinations can also serve as input to charge distribution calculations which yield the internal electronic configuration of the compounds, and this may extend our knowledge about the interac-

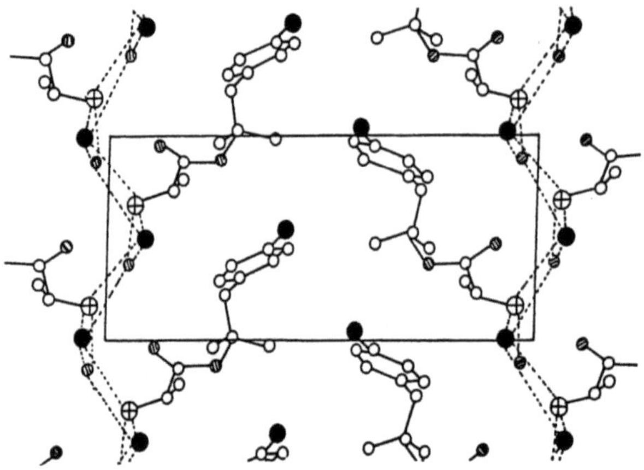

Fig. 3. Hydrogen bond system of alaproclate in the crystal structure. Hydrogen bonds are formed between the amino group (○), the Cl ion (●), and the water molecules (○). (Wägner 1980a)

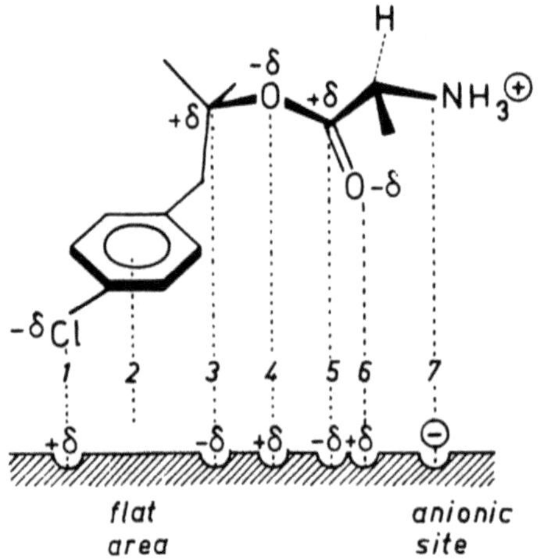

1. electrostatic forces?
2. van der Waals interactions?
   π-π interactions?
   charge transfer?
3. dipole-dipole/dipole-ionic interactions?
4. dipole-dipole/dipole-ionic interactions?
5. dipole-dipole/dipole-ionic interactions?
6. dipole-dipole/dipole-ionic interactions?
   charge transfer?
7. ionic binding?

alaproclate

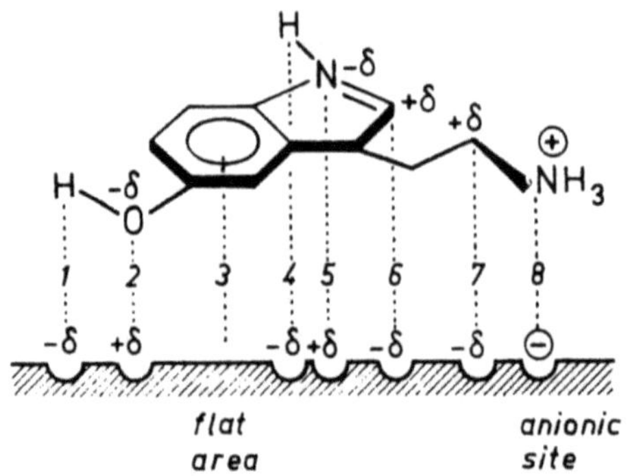

1. hydrogen bonding?
2. electrostatic forces?
3. van der Waals interactions?
   π-π interactions?
   charge transfer?
4. hydrogen bonding?
5. electrostatic forces?
6. charge transfer?
7. dipole-dipole/dipole-ionic interactions?
8. ionic binding?

5-hydroxytryptamine

Fig. 4. Electronic properties of alaproclate and 5-HT, implying different binding possibilities to the receptor surface. Charge distributions are taken from calculated data published elsewhere (Wägner 1980a). Possible binding and energy forces are indicated

tion and binding possibilities of the studied compounds at the receptor level (see Fig. 4).
8. When the conformational and electronic characteristics of a compound or a series of compounds have been ascertained with reasonable certainty, hypotheses about the complementary characteristics of the receptor, in terms of geometrical and electronic properties, can be formulated.

2 Selective Inhibitors of 5-HT

Molecular graphic techniques (e.g., Chemgraph[1]) can facilitate the handling and analysis of structure information. As an example, we present some preliminary results concerning molecular differences between 5-HT (5-hydroxytryptamine) and selective 5-HT uptake blockers (with established clinical antidepressant effect).

Assuming that 5-HT and the uptake blockers compete for the same site, i.e., for the presynaptic membrane-bound 5-HT uptake carrier, there should be some structural similarities between 5-HT and these drugs, but also some differences that could account for the antagonist action. From SAR data it is known that in the case of alaproclate, an aromatic ring system with an electronegative substituent and a primary amino group are important for pharmacological activity (Lindberg et al. 1978). We assume that these two groups are of importance for the binding properties. Figure 5 shows how three selective 5-HT uptake blockers (alaproclate, zimelidine, fluoxetine) can be superimposed on the 5-HT molecule with the two important reactive groups in a common position. This fit is achieved by allowing the molecules to rotate within 5 kcal from their calculated minimum energy conformations. The van der Waals' volumes of these compounds have

[1] Created by Davis EK working in the Chemical Crystallography Laboratory, Oxford England; developed and distributed by Chemical Design Ltd in the July 1985 version.

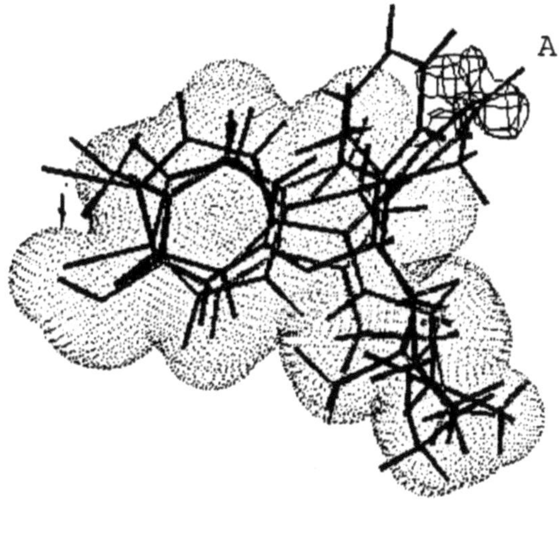

Fig. 5. Superimposition of alaproclate, zimelidine, and fluoxetine on the 5-HT molecule. The volume element *A* represents the common van der Waals' volume present in these drugs but not in 5-HT

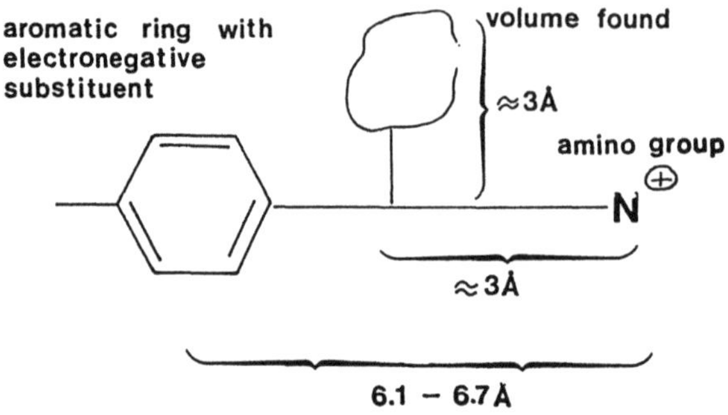

Fig. 6. Postulated pharmacophore responsible for the 5-HT uptake antagonism in the central nervous system

been calculated and the volume element A in Fig. 5 represents the volume that the three drugs have in common but is not present in the 5-HT molecule.

We postulate that this volume provides a third interaction and that this part of the molecule is responsible for the antagonism of the 5-HT uptake. The pharmacophore would then contain (a) an aromatic nucleus with an electronegative substituent; (b) a positively charged amino group; and (c) a geometrically well-defined locus which probably interacts sterically with the 5-HT uptake site, since no immediate common electronic properties can be discerned at this locus in the three drugs (see Fig. 6).

However, further studies with more compounds with different degrees of selectivity in the action on the 5-HT and noradrenaline uptake, such as the classical tricyclic antidepressants, are needed before any definite conclusions can be drawn. Such studies are in progress.

3 Comments and Conclusions

Geometrical parameters are important for the activity of drugs, e.g., in the case of optical and geometrical isomers. In the case of *cis/trans* isomerism the difference in activity might be explained by differences in distances between important reactive groups in the pharmacophore. One possible advantage of the *cis* conformation could be that the reactive groups are simultaneously available for binding to the receptor without chemical groups intervening as would be the case in the *trans* form. For instance, zimelidine in the *cis* form is more potent in blocking the 5-HT uptake than its *trans* form (Ross and Renyi 1977). The *cis* forms of 10-hydroxyamitriptyline, 10-hydroxynortriptyline, and zimelidine are more potent in blocking ^{3}H-imipramine binding than the corresponding *trans* forms (Langer et al. 1980). The same reasoning would also be true for different enantiomers (R and S configurations).

Although structural and geometrical parameters are of primary importance, other factors must be taken into consideration in the analysis of drug-receptor interaction.

Compounds with rather similar conformations may show different activities or even different pharmacological profiles, which suggests the importance of electronic properties for the interaction with the receptor sites. Introduction of a Cl atom in the tricyclic framework of rigid spiro amines completely alters the pharmacological profile from antidepressant to neuroleptic (Carnmalm et al. 1976), but this has only a minor influence on the overall conformation (Wägner 1980c). Although the metabolite 10-hydroxynortriptyline retains the noradrenaline and 5-HT uptake blocking capability of nortriptyline, the presence of the hydroxyl group in the metabolite drastically changes the affinity for the muscarinic receptor (Wägner et al. 1984). Horn et al. (1975) reported a distance of 6 Å between the nitrogen atom and the benzene ring in a series of tricyclic compounds belonging to the neuroleptic class, in both active and inactive compounds.

Consequently, geometrical parameters are not sufficient for the characterization of pharmacological profiles or pharmacophores. It would thus be interesting to achieve some form of characterization of the electronic profiles of compounds, together with information on how binding and interaction possibilities are coupled to local electron density properties. Charge distribution calculations combined with structural results can be seen as a first step in this direction.

It must also be pointed out that the optimal conformation for activity of the pharmacophore is not necessarily a low-energy or minimum-energy conformation; another conformation with higher energy might be favored. Energy calculations can be used to estimate energy differences involved when flexible molecules with several possible conformations (in solution under physiological conditions) are studied. This problem can be overcome by studying rigid analogues with a side chain locked in a specific position, for example (e.g., comparison between dopamine and apomorphine in Wägner 1980a).

Thermodynamic binding studies can help in the further estimation of energy conditions. For instance, Reith et al. (1984) have shown that the energies involved in the binding of selective 5-HT uptake blockers and tricyclic antidepressants to the ^{3}H-imipramine binding sites are quite different, suggesting different types of binding interactions.

References

Carnmalm B, Johansson L, Rämsby S, Stjernström NE, Ross SB, Ögren SO (1976) Stereoselective effects of the potentially neuroleptic rigid spiro amines. Nature 263:519–520

Horn AS, Post ML, Kennard O (1975) Dopamine receptor blockade of the neuroleptics, a crystallographic study. J Pharm Pharmacol 27:553–563

Langer SZ, Raisman R, Briley MS (1980) Stereoselective inhibition of ^{3}H-imipramine binding by antidepressant drugs and their derivatives. Eur J Pharmacol 64:89–90

Lindberg UH, Thorberg SO, Bengtsson S, Renyi AL, Ross SB, Ögren SO (1978) Inhibitors of neuronal monoamine uptake. 2 Selective inhibition of 5-hydroxytryptamine uptake by α-aminoacid esters of phenethyl alcohols. J Med Chem 21:448–456

Reith MEA, Sershen H, Lajtha A (1984) Thermodynamics of the interactions of tricyclic drugs with the binding sites for ^{3}H-imipramine binding in mouse cerebral cortex. Biochem Pharmacol 33:4101–4104

Ross SB, Renyi AL (1977) Inhibition of the neuronal uptake of 5-hydroxy-tryptamine and noradrenaline in rat brain by (Z)- and (E)-3-(4-bromophenyl)-N,N-dimethyl-3(3-pyridyl)-allylamines and their secondary analogues. Neuropharmacology 16:57–63

Wägner A (1980a) On the molecular structure of some psychoactive drugs. Studies of the antidepressant alaproclate and two potentially neuroleptic rigid spiro amines. Thesis. Chem Commun 5:1–61

Wägner A (1980 b) Structure and absolute configuration of (R)-alaproclate[2-(4-chlorophenyl)-1,1-dimethyl-2-amino propanoate] hydrochloride, a selective inhibitor of neuronal 5-hydroxytryptamine uptake. Acta Cryst B36:77–81
Wägner A (1980 c) Crystal structure and absolute configuration of the hydrochloride of a dopamine receptor blocking rigid spiro amine: (1S,4R)-3′-chloro-N,N-dimethyl spiro [2-cyclohexene-1,5′-[5H]dibenzo(a,d)cyclohepten]4-amine. Acta Crystallogr Sect B:1113–1117
Wägner A, Ekqvist B, Bertilsson L, Sjöqvist F (1984) Weak binding of 10-hydroxymetabolites of nortriptyline to rat brain muscarinic receptors. Life Sci 35:1379–1383

Anxiolytics

Modulation of the Benzodiazepine-GABA Receptor Chloride Ionophore Complex by Multiple Allosteric Sites: Evidence for a Barbiturate "Receptor"

P. Skolnick[1], H. Havoundjian[1], and S. M. Paul[2]

1 Introduction

The discovery of specific recognition sites (receptors) for benzodiazepines in the central nervous system has resulted in a better understanding of the molecular pharmacology of benzodiazepines, barbiturates, and related compounds. Within the past 5 years it has become apparent that the benzodiazepine receptor is one component of a "supramolecular complex" consisting of multiple allosteric recognition sites which play a critical role in the regulation of transmembrane potential. Both neurochemical and electrophysiological studies support the notion that occupation of either the benzodiazepine-GABA receptor complex or distinct, allosteric sites for compounds such as barbiturates and cage convulsants (which are probably located on or near the chloride ionophore) can regulate the properties of this chloride channel. This chapter will review neurochemical evidence that demonstrates a functional coupling of the recognition components of the benzodiazepine-GABA receptor chloride ionophore complex (supramolecular complex) and summarize recent findings from our laboratory demonstrating that the "effector" component of this complex, the chloride ionophore, is rapidly altered by stress.

2 The Benzodiazepine-GABA Receptor Chloride Ionophore Complex: Evidence for Multiple Allosteric Regulatory Sites

In 1978, Tallman et al. demonstrated that GABA and the GABAmimetic muscimol increased the apparent affinity of [^{3}H]diazepam for benzodiazepine receptors in tissue that had been washed free of endogenous GABA. This study provided the first neurochemical evidence of a functional link between benzodiazepine and GABA receptors and supported earlier electrophysiological findings (cf. Haefely and Polc 1983, for review) that benzodiazepines can augment the actions of GABA. Subsequent studies have demonstrated that benzodiazepines can increase either the apparent affinity or the number (dependent upon both the assay conditions and tissue preparation) of low-affinity GABA receptors (Skerritt and

[1] Laboratory of Bioorganic Chemistry, NIADDK and
[2] Clinical Neuroscience Branch, NIMH, National Institutes of Health, Bethesda, MD 20205, USA.

Clinical Pharmacology in Psychiatry
Editors: Dahl, Gram, Paul, Potter
(Psychopharmacology Series 3)

Johnston 1983; Biggio 1983; Guidotti et al. 1983). The latter findings may more precisely reflect electrophysiological observations, and further demonstrate that occupation of either the benzodiazepine or GABA recognition site can alter the kinetic characteristics of the other. Biochemical investigations have unequivocally shown that recognition sites for benzodiazepines and GABA reside on the same protein with a molecular weight of ~50–60 kd (Gavish and Snyder 1981; Mohler et al. 1984; Schoch et al. 1984).

In 1979, Costa et al. demonstrated that halides such as bromide, iodide, and chloride increase the apparent affinity of [^{3}H]diazepam. Similar increases were not observed with ions that have a low permeability for chloride channels, such as acetate, citrate, and maleate, thus providing a neurochemical link between chloride channels and benzodiazepine receptors. This link was further supported by the observation that barbiturates (such as pentobarbital) can also increase the apparent affinity of [^{3}H]benzodiazepines for their receptors (Skolnick et al. 1980, 1981; Leeb-Lundberg et al. 1980) and that this effect was dependent on the presence of chloride ions. Furthermore, concentrations of pentobarbital lower than those required to directly enhance [^{3}H]benzodiazepine binding were found to potentiate the stimulatory effect of GABA on [^{3}H]benzodiazepine binding (Skolnick et al. 1980, 1981; Skerritt et al. 1983). Barbiturates have also been shown to increase [^{3}H]GABA binding in a chloride-dependent fashion (Asano and Ogasawara 1981; Olsen and Snowman 1982). Other compounds, such as the pyrazolopyridines SQ 65,396 and SQ 20,009, which share common pharmacologic actions with barbiturates and benzodiazepines, were also found to enhance [^{3}H]benzodiazepine and [^{3}H]GABA binding in a chloride-dependent fashion (Supavilai and Karobath 1979, 1980; Meiners and Salama 1982; Placheta and Karobath 1980). These findings, together with studies of highly purified receptor preparations, have provided evidence that recognition sites for benzodiazepines and GABA are present on the same molecule and functionally linked to a chloride ionophore (containing multiple allosteric recognition sites for barbiturates, cage convulsants, pyrazolopyridines, and perhaps ethanol).

During the past year, the functional relationships between the benzodiazepine-GABA receptor and the associated chloride ionophore have been studied in a cell-free (synaptoneurosome) preparation by Schwartz et al. (1985 a, b). These investigators have reported that GABAmimetics and barbiturates increase both the efflux and the uptake of ^{36}Cl in this preparation (Schwartz et al. 1985 a,b). A statistically significant correlation was found between the potencies of a series of barbiturates to enhance ^{36}Cl flux in synaptoneurosomes and their potencies in enhancing [^{3}H]diazepam binding in membranes. Further, there was a significant correlation between the potencies of these barbiturates to enhance $^{36}Cl^-$ flux and their anesthetic potencies in mice (Schwartz et al. 1985 a, b). This technique has considerable potential, since it provides a ready means of biochemically measuring the functional relationship between components of this supramolecular complex.

At the present time, it is not possible to measure recognition sites for barbiturates *directly*, probably due to the relatively low affinities of these compounds. Nonetheless, both neurochemical and electrophysiological evidence supports the contention that there are stereoselective recognition sites for barbiturates that are coupled to benzodiazepine and GABA receptors and an associated chloride ionophore. Ticku et al. (1978 a, b) demonstrated that a reduced form of the cage convulsant picrotoxinin (α-dihydropicrotoxinin) labeled a set of sites that could be stereospecifically affected by barbiturates (Ticku 1981). Electrophysiological evidence strongly suggests that picrotoxinin does not act directly at GABA receptors, but at a discrete locus on or near the chloride ionophore (Nicoll and Wojtowicz 1980; Akaike et al. 1985). Unfortunately, the relatively low affinity of [^{3}H]α-dihydropicrotoxinin, coupled with the unfavorable "signal to noise" of this radioligand, severely limited investigation of this site. In 1983, Squires et al. reported that a related cage convulsant, [^{35}S]*t*-butylbicyclophosporothionate (TBPS), labeled a population of sites with characteristics similar to those identified with α-

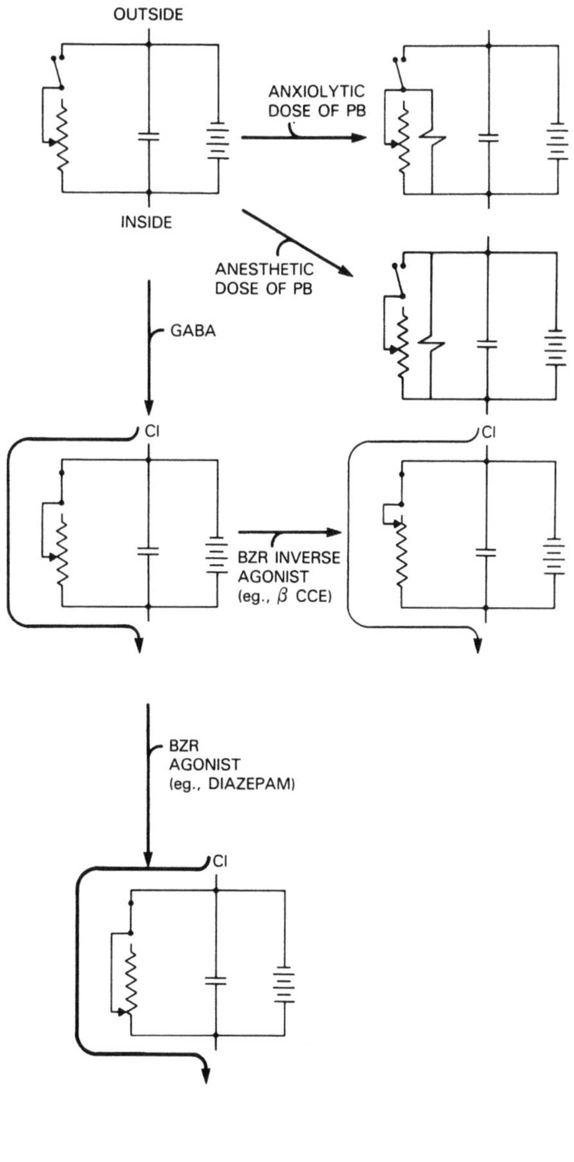

Fig. 1. Representation of the benzodiazepine-GABA receptor chloride ionophore complex as a "wiring diagram." See text for details

dihydropicrotoxinin, but with a much higher affinity ($K_d \sim 40$ n*M*) and a more favorable signal to noise than the latter radioligand. [^{35}S]TBPS binding is competitively inhibited by picrotoxinin with a Hill coefficient close to unity, suggesting that TBPS and picrotoxinin bind to the same population of sites. [^{35}S]TBPS binding is dependent upon the presence of halide ions (Squires et al. 1983) and is inhibited by a number of compounds, including barbiturates and pyrazolopyridines. Although barbiturates and pyrazolopyridines inhibit [^{35}S]TBPS binding, this probably occurs through an allosteric site, since this inhibition does not follow the law of mass action (Ramajaneyulu and Ticku 1984; Trifiletti et al. 1984). Thus, [^{35}S]TBPS binding appears to be a useful probe for monitoring changes in the chloride ionophore, which possesses specific recognition sites for barbiturates, the so-called barbiturate receptors.

Many models of the benzodiazepine-GABA receptor chloride ionophore complex have been proposed. We have chosen to illustrate this supramolecular complex as a "wiring diagram" (Fig. 1) rather than in molecular terms (e.g., Olsen 1981; Skolnick and Paul 1983; Guidotti et al. 1983). In our current model, the membrane is represented by a capacitor and the overall electrochemical gradient for chloride by a battery. The GABA receptor may be envisioned as a "switch," completing a circuit that permits chloride ions into the cell when this site is occupied by GABA or a GABAmimetic. The benzodiazepine receptor may best be illustrated as a rheostat. Thus, when the benzodiazepine receptor is occupied by an "agonist" (i.e., a benzodiazepine-like compound), and the switch is on (i.e., there is GABAergic tone), the resistance through its circuit is decreased, resulting in an increased chloride influx and hyperpolarization. In contrast, when the benzodiazepine receptor is occupied by an "active antagonist" ("inverse agonist") such as 3-carbomethoxy-β-carboline, the chloride flux will be reduced under the same GABAergic tone (Fig. 1). Barbiturates at low (e.g., anxiolytic) concentrations will also increase conductance by augmenting GABAergic transmission in a way analogous to a shunt, while at higher (hypnotic-anesthetic) concentrations they will "short-circuit" the benzodiazepine-GABA receptor to directly increasing conductance.

3 Is the "Supramolecular Complex" Involved in the Physiological Control of Anxiety?

Many studies have attempted to demonstrate an alteration in the benzodiazepine receptor after stressful or anxiety-provoking situations. Alterations in benzodiazepine receptors might intuitively be expected if these receptors were involved in the physiologic control of anxiety. However, the changes in radioligand binding to benzodiazepine receptors observed after stress have for the most part been modest and bidirectional. If benzodiazepine receptors were involved in the control or generation of anxiety, it could be argued that the *effector* component of the receptor would be altered, rather than the recognition site itself. Since the chloride ionophore may be viewed as the effector component of the supramolecular complex, we recently embarked on studies designed to test this hypothesis.

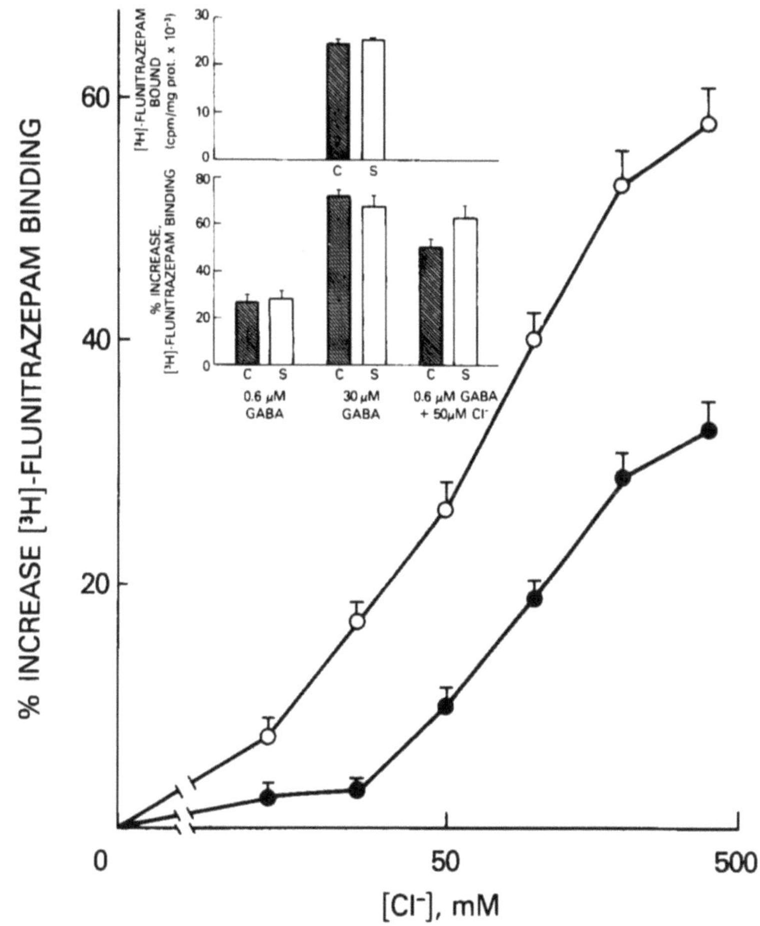

Fig. 2. Effects of stress on chloride-mediated enhancement of [^{3}H]flunitrazepam binding to cerebral cortical membranes: Rats were subjected to a 10-min swim stress (25 °C), and cerebral cortical membranes prepared from these rats and naive animals were washed five times. [^{3}H]Flunitrazepam binding (0.7 n*M*) was assayed in the presence of various concentrations of chloride ions. *Closed circles*, naive rats; *open circles*, stressed rats. Both the maximum enhancement of [^{3}H]flunitrazepam binding by chloride ions and the potency of chloride ions to enhance [^{3}H]flunitrazepam binding were significantly increased ($P<0.001$) by swim stress. These values are means ±SEM for 6–12 rats. *Inset: Upper panel*, [^{3}H]flunitrazepam binding in cortical membranes from naive (*C*) and swim-stressed (*S*) rats. This tissue was assayed in the absence of chloride ions. *Lower panel*, effects of stress on GABA-enhanced [^{3}H]flunitrazepam binding. No significant differences in [^{3}H]flunitrazepam binding were observed in the presence of suboptimal or optimal concentrations of GABA between the naive (*C*) and swim-stressed (*S*) rats. Addition of 50 m*M* NaCl to the incubation medium revealed a slightly more pronounced effect of GABA in the stressed group. This effect is due to the ability of chloride ions to potentiate GABA-enhanced [^{3}H]flunitrazepam binding. Values are means ±SEM for 6–7 animals. The tissue was assayed in the presence of 0.7 n*M* flunitrazepam. (From Havoundjian et al. 1985a, b)

In these studies, rats were subjected to a brief, ambient temperature (25 °C) swim as a model stressor. As had previously been reported with a number of other stressors, no statistically significant changes in the basal binding of [^{3}H]flunitrazepam were observed in cerebral cortical membranes of the swim-stressed rats compared with naive animals (Fig. 2, inset). Furthermore, GABA-enhanced [^{3}H]flunitrazepam binding (measured in the absence of chloride ions) was also unchanged (Fig. 2, inset), suggesting that the population of GABA receptors linked to benzodiazepine receptors (cf. Gallager et al. 1984) was also unaffected by stress. In contrast, the potency and efficacy of chloride ions in enhancing [^{3}H]flunitrazepam binding were markedly increased in the swim-stressed animals (Fig. 2). Scatchard analyses of chloride-enhanced [^{3}H]flunitrazepam binding demonstrated significantly greater increases in the apparent affinity of [^{3}H]flunitrazepam in cortical tissue from stressed compared with naive animals (Havoundjian et al. 1985 a). A similar phenomenon was also observed with other Eccles permeable ions (e.g. Br^-, I^-), but not with anions such as acetate, which do not penetrate chloride channels well (Havoundjian et al. 1985 b).

These findings suggested that acute stress produces a rapid and robust change in either the coupling between chloride channels and benzodiazepine receptors or the chloride channel itself. Since [^{35}S]TBPS binding is thought to measure sites associated with benzodiazepine-GABA receptor-coupled chloride channels, we then examined [^{35}S]TBPS binding in cerebral cortical membranes from swim-stressed and naive rats. A statistically significant increase in both the maximum number of [^{35}S]TBPS-binding sites (~40%) and the apparent affinity of [^{35}S]TBPS (~25%) was observed (Table 1) (Havoundjian et al. 1985 b), which strongly suggests the chloride ionophore is altered by stress.

These studies support the concept that the supramolecular complex is involved in the physiological response to stress. However, at the present time it is not known whether these changes are consequential or compensatory. Furthermore, it is not known whether benzodiazepine or GABA receptors must be occupied to effect these stress-induced changes in the chloride ionophore. However, kinetic studies from our laboratory have revealed a striking similarity between tis-

Table 1. Effects of swim stress on the kinetics of [^{3}H]flunitrazepam and [^{35}S]TBPS binding

	Naive		Swim-stress	
	K_D (nM)	B_{max} (pmol/mg prot.)	K_D (nM)	B_{max} (pmol/mg prot.)
[^{3}H]Flu	2.16±0.13	2.93±0.29 (5)	1.88±0.05*	3.11±0.18 (6)
[^{35}]TBPS	37.2±3.0	2.03±0.06 (4)	28.6±1.6*	2.72±0.06 (4)**

Animals were subjected to a 10-min swim stress (25 °C) as described elsewhere (Havoundjian et al. 1985a, b). [^{3}H]Flunitrazepam binding to cortical membranes was performed in the presence of 100 mM NaCl using 0.3–9.2 nM radioligand. [^{35}S]TBPS binding was performed in the presence of 200 mM NaCl using 5–165 nM radioligand. Detailed methods have been described by Havoundjian et al. (1985a, b). Values are means ±SEM, with the number of animals in parentheses.
* $P<0.05$; ** $P<0.001$ compared with naive animals (Student's t-test).

sue from stressed animals and tissue from naive animals incubated with pentobarbital (Havoundjian et al. 1985 b). This similarity may be interpreted as the stressor promoting a compensatory (directed at dampening the effects of stress) increase in the conductance of chloride channels, which is observed (electrophysiologically) with barbiturates such as pentobarbital. These findings suggest that inappropriate responses to stress that are (eventually) manifest as pathologic anxiety may well involve a molecular defect in one or more components of the supramolecular complex.

Acknowledgments. H. H. was a Morehead Fellow in Medicine and a Howard Hughes Medical Scholar during these investigations.

References

Akaike N, Hattori Y, Oomura Y, Carpenter D (1985) Bicuculline and picrotoxin block γ-aminobutyric acid and gated Cl^- conductance by different mechanisms. Experientia 41:70–71

Asano T, Ogasawara N (1981) Chloride-dependent stimulation of GABA and benzodiazepine receptor binding by pentobarbital. Brain Res 225:212–216

Biggio G (1983) The actions of stress, β-carbolines, diazepam, and Ro 15-1788 on GABA receptors in the rat brain. In: Biggio G, Costa E (eds) Benzodiazepine recognition site ligands: biochemistry and pharmacology. Raven, New York, pp 105–120

Costa T, Rodbard D, Pert C (1979) Is the benzodiazepine receptor coupled to a chloride ion channel? Nature 277:315–317

Gallager D, Lakoski J, Gonsalves S, Rauch S (1984) Chronic benzodiazepine treatment decreases postsynaptic GABA sensitivity. Nature 398:74–77

Gavish M, Snyder SH (1981) Gamma-aminobutyric acid and benzodiazepine receptors: Copurification and characterization. Proc Natl Acad Sci USA 78:1939–1942

Guidotti A, Corda M, Wise B, Vaccarino F, Costa E (1983) GABAergic synapses: supramolecular organization and biochemical regulation. Neuropharmacology 22:1471–1479

Haefely W, Polc P (1983) Electrophysiological studies on the interaction of anxiolytic drugs with GABAergic mechanisms. In: Malick J, Enna S, Yamamura H (eds) Anxiolytics: neurochemical, behavioral and clinical perspectives. Raven, New York, pp 113–145

Havoundjian H, Paul SM, Skolnick P (1985 a) Rapid, stress induced modulation of the benzodiazepine receptor coupled chloride ionophore. Brain Res 375:401–406

Havoundjian H, Paul SM, Skolnick P (1985 b) Acute, stress-induced changes in the benzodiazepine-GABA receptor complex are confined to the chloride ionophore. J Pharmacol Exp Ther 237:787–793

Leeb-Lundberg F, Snowman A, Olsen R (1980) Barbiturate receptor sites are coupled to benzodiazepine receptors. Proc Natl Acad Sci USA 77:7468–7472

Meiners B, Salama A (1982) Enhancement of benzodiazepine and GABA binding by the novel anxiolytic, tracazolate. Eur J Pharmacol 78:315

Mohler H, Schoch P, Haring P, Takacs B, Stahli C (1984) A purified GABA/benzodiazepine receptor: biochemical, pharmacological and immunological characterization. Clin Neuropharmacol 7 [Suppl 1]:S-307

Nicholl R, Wojtowicz J (1980) The effects of pentobarbital and related compounds on frog motorneurons. Brain Res 191:225–237

Olsen RW (1981) GABA-benzodiazepine-barbiturate receptor interactions. J Neurochem 37:1–13

Olsen R, Snowman A (1982) Chloride-dependent enhancement by barbiturates of gamma-aminobutyric acid receptor binding. J Neurosci 2:1812–1823

Placheta P, Karobath M (1980) In vitro modulation of SQ 20,009 and SQ 65,390 GABA receptor binding in rat CNS membranes. Eur J Pharmacol 62:225–228

Ramanjaneyulu R, Ticku M (1984) Binding characteristics and interactions of depressant drugs with [^{35}S]*t*-butylbicyclophosphorothionate, a ligand that binds to the picrotoxinin site. J Neurochem 42:221–229

Schoch P, Haring P, Takacs B, Stahli C, Mohler H (1984) A GABA/benzodiazepine receptor complex from bovine brain: purification, reconstitution and immunological characterization. J Recept Res 4:189–200

Schwartz R, Jackson J, Weigart D, Skolnick P, Paul SM (1985a) Characterization of barbiturate-stimulated chloride efflux from rat brain synaptoneurosomes. J Neurosci (in press)

Schwartz R, Skolnick P, Seale T, Paul SM (1985b) Demonstration of GABA/barbiturate-receptor-mediated chloride transport in rat brain synaptoneurosomes: a functional assay of GABA receptor-effector coupling. In: Biggio G, Costa E (eds) Advances in biochemical psychopharmacology. GABAergic transmission and anxiety. Raven, New York (in press)

Skerritt J, Johnston G (1983) Enhancement of GABA binding by benzodiazepines and related anxiolytics. Eur J Pharmacol 89:193–198

Skerritt J, Johnston G, Katsikas T, Tabar J, Nicholson G, Andrews P (1983) Actions of pentobarbitone and derivatives modified 5-butyl substituents on GABA and diazepam binding to rat brain synaptosomal membranes. Neurochem Res 8:1337–1350

Skolnick P, Paul S (1983) New concepts in the neurobiology of anxiety. J Clin Psychiatry 44:12–19

Skolnick P, Paul S, Barker J (1980) Pentobarbital potentiates GABA-enhanced [^{3}H]diazepam binding to benzodiazepine receptors. Eur J Pharmacol 65:125–127

Skolnick P, Moncada V, Barker J, Paul S (1981) Pentobarbital has dual actions to increase brain benzodiazepine receptor affinity. Science 211:1448–1450

Squires RF, Casida JE, Richardson M, Saederup E (1983) ^{35}S t-Butylbicyclophosphorothionate binds with high affinity to brain specific sites couples to gamma-aminobutyric acid-A and ion recognition sites. Mol Pharmacol 23:326–336

Supavilai P, Karobath M (1979) Stimulation of benzodiazepine receptor binding by SQ 20,0009 is chloride dependent and picrotoxin-sensitive. Eur J Pharmacol 60:111–113

Supavilai P, Karobath M (1980) Interaction of SQ 20,009 and GABA-like drugs as modulators of benzodiazepine receptor binding. Eur J Pharmacol 62:229–233

Tallman J; Thomas J, Gallager D (1978) GABAergic modulation of benzodiazepine binding site sensitivity. Nature 274:383–385

Ticku M (1981) Interaction of stereosiomers of barbiturates with [^{3}H]dihydropicrotoxinin binding sites. Brain Res 211:127–133

Ticku MK, Ban M, Olsen RW (1978a) Binding of [^{3}H]α-dihydropicrotoxinin, a gamma-aminobutyric acid synaptic antagonist, to rat brain membranes. Mol Pharmacol 14:391–402

Ticku MK, Van Ness FC, Haycock JW, Levy WB, Olsen RW (1978b) Dihydropicrotoxinin binding sites in rat brain: comparison to GABA receptors. Brain Res 150:642–647

Trifiletti R, Snowman A, Snyder S (1984) Barbiturate recognition sites on the GABA/benzodiazepine receptor complex is distinct from the picrotoxinin/TBPS recognition site. Eur J Pharmacol 106:441–447

β-Carbolines: New Insights into the Clinical Pharmacology of Benzodiazepine Receptor Ligands

R. Dorow, T. Duka, N. Sauerbrey, and L. Höller

1 Introduction

With the discovery of benzodiazepine receptors it became evident that benzodiazepines produce their various pharmacological effects through interactions with these binding sites. This major finding was followed by numerous biochemical, histological, and electrophysiological studies, which then showed that the benzodiazepine receptor is an allosteric modulatory site that is functionally coupled to, and located on, a subgroup of GABA receptors that gate a chloride channel. The benzodiazepines' primary target is thus located on neurons that are modulated by the GABAergic neurons containing the GABA-benzodiazepine receptor-chloride channel (GBC) complex. (For review see P. Skolnick et al., this volume.)

A further step towards a better understanding of these receptor systems and their physiological function was the discovery of specific benzodiazepine receptor antagonists such as the imidazobenzodiazepinone Ro 15–1788, which has become an important tool in experimental pharmacology (Hunkeler et al. 1981). In addition, the recent development of monoclonal antibodies directed at proteins of the benzodiazepine-receptor complex has provided scientists with a deeper insight into the molecular structure and localization of benzodiazepine receptors in the CNS (Schoch et al. 1985). Moreover, the significance of the GBC complex was further unerlined after the characterization of an endogenous peptide binding to the benzodiazepine receptor, which was found to be widely distributed in the CNS of rats and had pharmacological effects in this species (Ferrero et al. 1984). Finally, the discovery of the β-carbolines and their subsequent characterization in biochemical and pharmacological studies were of major relevance.

2 Benzodiazepine Receptors: Studies of FG 7142 in Human Volunteers

In the search for endogenous ligands, Braestrup et al. (1980) isolated a β-carboline (β-CCE) from human urine, which although it was an artifact formed during the purification procedure had high affinity for the benzodiazepine receptors.

Research Laboratories of Schering AG, Berlin (West)/Bergkamen, Federal Republic of Germany.

Clinical Pharmacology in Psychiatry
Editors: Dahl, Gram, Paul, Potter
(Psychopharmacology Series 3)

When tested in animal experiments, β-CCE turned out to possess none of the pharmacological properties known of benzodiazepines, such as anticonvulsant, anticonflict, and ataxiogenic properties. On the contrary, this compound antagonized the effects of diazepam and seemed to have a pharmacological activity of its own (Oakley and Jones 1980; Tenen and Hirsch 1980; Cowen et al. 1981; Cepeda et al. 1981). A problem encountered when using β-CCE for experiments in rodents is its short half-life and low bioavailability after oral administration. In the search for longer acting and metabolically more stable congeners, *N*-methyl-β-carboline carboxamide (FG 7142) was synthesized. When first tested in animals, FG 7142 was shown to have a pharmacological profile comparable with that of β-CCE, inasmuch as it antagonized effects induced by benzodiazepines and increased motor activity in rats (Petersen et al. 1982).

FG 7142 was first tested in humans in early 1981, when it was still thought to bear some resemblance to a potential endogenous ligand. Surprisingly, when the first compound from the new series of β-carboline benzodiazepine receptor ligands was studied, it turned out to exhibit an activity opposite to that known for benzodiazepines. It induced anxiety attacks, which correlated with the occurrence of high plasma levels of the compound. Symptoms described by two volunteers were similar to those experienced in panic attacks or severe generalized anxiety disorders (see Table 1). The effects of this compound could be reversed instantaneously by an i.v. dose of lormetazepam, a potent benzodiazepine hypnotic, indicating that these effects were mediated by benzodiazepine receptors (Dorow et al. 1983). This observation and subsequent animal studies indicated the existence of benzodiazepine receptor ligands that mediate the opposite effects to those known for benzodiazepines, i.e., anxiety and convulsions, via the same receptor. Although the limited experiments with FG 7142 warrant caution in interpretation of the results, it can be said that the effects were quite dramatic, and for this reason all ongoing investigations in humans were stopped.

Major difficulties met with the use of FG 7142 as a test drug for induction of anxiety were its unpredictable biovailability after oral administration and its poor solubility even in strong lipophilic solvents, such as propylene glycol. A maximum i.v. dose of 5 mg FG 7142 (limited by the local tolerance of propylene glycol solutions) resulted in plasma levels that were clearly below those observed in the two cases in which anxiety occurred after oral ingestion. No marked effects were observed when this i.v. dose of FG 7142 was administered to volunteers. In fact, this

Table 1. Common symptoms experienced after ingestion of FG 7142 in two volunteers and by patients suffering from anxiety disorders according to DSM III

Central effects	Autonomic hyperactivity	Vigilance and scanning
Fear of impending doom	Sweating	Difficulty in concentrating
Inner tension	Palpitations	Irritability
Strained face	Chest pain	Impatience
Restlessness	Choking sensations	
Excitation	Paresthesias	
Dizziness	Hot and cold flashes	
	Trembling or shaking	

dose could not reverse the sedative and muscle-relaxant effects of 1 mg lormetazepam i.v. (Dorow et al. 1984). Compounds such as β-CCE and FG 7142 have been termed "inverse" agonists or "active" antagonists in attempts to explain their activity, which is inverse or opposite to that of benzodiazepines though mediated by the same receptors (Polc et al. 1982; Braestrup et al. 1982). These findings and the observation that the benzodiazepine antagonist Ro 15-1788 could antagonize both agonist and inverse agonist effects led to the introduction of a new concept of bidirectional activity forwarded at a single receptor.

It should be mentioned at this point that in the early pharmacological and toxicological studies conducted with FG 7142 no anxiety-related effects in animals had been detected. Furthermore, as little is known about the extent to which experimental procedures in animals resemble anxiety in humans, FG 7142 and other inverse agonists have been used to validate animal models thought to be predictive for anxiety (for review see Pellow and File 1984). The finding that anxiety could be induced in humans with FG 7142 shows that clinical pharmacology can indeed lead to profound new insights into the understanding of basic CNS functions, e.g., mechanisms underlying anxiety (Dorow et al. 1983).

As more β-carbolines were synthesized it became evident that a continuum of pharmacological effects (anxiolysis to anxiomimesis, anticonvulsant to convulsant action) could be induced by different representatives of this group (Braestrup et al. 1984; Stephens and Kehr 1985). This led to hopes that pharmacological effects could be singled out from the plethora of benzodiazepine activities. So far the distinction has been made between full and partial agonists, receptor antagonists, and partial and full inverse agonists. A major object of this paper is to show, on the basis of representative compounds from this continuum, that the concept also holds true for human volunteers (see also Table 4).

3 Clinical Pharmacological Studies with Benzodiazepine Receptor Antagonists

A number of specific benzodiazepine receptor antagonists have been described in recent years. The first was the imidazobenzodiazepinone Ro 15-1788 (Hunkeler et al. 1981), a compound that was shown to have pronounced affinity for the benzodiazepine-binding sites in brain homogenates. Ro 15-1788 inhibits the binding of radioligands at benzodiazepine-binding sites, and the distribution of its binding sites in the CNS corresponds to that of benzodiazepine agonists. In animals and humans, Ro 15-1788 has virtually no pharmacological activity when administered in doses that selectively reduce and antagonize the effects of the classic benzodiazepines. For instance, when administered to humans, Ro 15-1788 can reverse the sedative, muscle-relaxant, and amnestic activity of benzodiazepines (Darragh et al. 1981, 1982, 1983; Doenicke et al. 1984; Dorow and Duka 1986; O'Boyle et al. 1983; Scollo-Lavizzari 1982). In the early investigations in humans, Ro 15-1788 was reported to have no effects of its own. However, in a placebo-controlled study, we recently showed that when given i.v. in a dose of 0.1 mg/kg body weight Ro 15-1788 does in fact produce some effect of its own (Dorow and Duka 1986). Some authors have ascribed this to effects produced by the vehicle

(Darragh et al. 1983), but Schöpf et al. (1984) have recently shown that Ro 15-1788 produces some effects in the waking EEG of healthy volunteers, which have been interpreted as an increase of central activation, and Zielger et al. (1985) have reported that the drug reverses slow-wave sleep. There was some evidence in these studies that Ro 15-1788 might have a slight inverse agonist activity. However, preliminary data from the EEG of epileptic patients indicate that Ro 15-1788 might also possess an anticonvulsant effect, which suggest a benzodiazepine-like activity (Scollo-Lavizzari 1984). These data further suggest that depending on the activation/deactivation of the GBC complex, benzodiazepine receptor antagonists might be effective as both agonists and inverse agonists.

Termination of chronic benzodiazepine treatment in patients may lead to symptoms, e.g., sleep disturbances, dysphoria, anxiety, perceptual disturbances, and feelings of depersonalization, which are considered to be withdrawal reactions (Petursson and Lader 1981; Schöpf 1983). Recently, it was shown that withdrawal reactions could be precipitated by Ro 15-1788 in animals that had been given benzodiazepines over a long period (Emmet-Oglesby et al. 1983; Lukas and Griffiths 1982). Since the severity of these effects seems to be related to the duration of treatment and to dose (Lukas and Griffiths 1984; McNicholas and Martin 1982), we studied the effects of Ro 15-1788 after a single high dose of i.v. benzodiazepines in healthy volunteers. At 15 min after benzodiazepines, 0.1 mg/kg Ro 15-1788 i.v. completely reversed all benzodiazepine effects without precipitating withdrawal reactions. When the subjects were rechallenged with the same dose of Ro 15-1788 24 h later the investigators observed reactions reminiscent of mild withdrawal symptoms (Dorow and Duka 1986). These findings indicate that even 24 h after a single high dose of benzodiazepines slight withdrawal reactions might be precipitated with high doses of Ro 15-1788. Several authors have reported that Ro 15-1788 can rapidly antagonize all the effects of benzodiazepines within minutes of the injection. However, owing to the short half-life of the compound (Klotz et al. 1985) the agonistic effects of high i.v. doses of benzodiazepines relapse after 1–2 h (Doenicke et al. 1984; Dorow and Duka 1986). Thus, attention was turned to finding new longer lasting antagonists.

Recently, other nonbenzodiazepine receptor ligands have been shown to be benzodiazepine receptor antagonists. For instance, CGS 8216, a pyrazolochinoline derivative, was also found to antagonize the effects of benzodiazepine agonists in both experimental animals and humans (Czernik et al. 1982; Bieck et al. 1984). Another β-carboline antagonist, ZK 93426 (5-isopropyl-4-methyl-β-carboline-3-carboxylic acid ethyl ester) was shown to be a potent and specific inhibitor of [^{3}H]flunitrazepam binding to brain membranes. In some animal models of epilepsy it was shown to have no proconvulsant activity. In one such test, the highly sensitive audiogenic seizure test in DBA/2 mice, ZK 93426 was similar to Ro 15-1788 in that it exerted a weak anticonvulsant action (Jensen et al. 1983). Yet the compound had no effect in animals tests for ataxia and sedation (Jensen et al. 1984). In a modified four-plate test which is indicative of anti- or propunishment activity, Stephens and Kehr (1985) showed that ZK 93426 has no activity of its own, but can antagonize the effects of benzodiazepines. However, in a conflict test the compound had a proconflict activity, which indicates a slight inverse agonistic effect (Jensen et al. 1984).

A diversity is also reflected in biochemical tests. The final outcome of interactions with the GBC complex is thought to be an increase or decrease in conductance at the chloride channel. 35[S]-*t*-Butylbicyclophosphorothionate (TBPS) was found to label this channel specifically (Squires et al. 1983), and the ratio of TBPS binding in the presence and absence of high concentrations of benzodiazepine receptor ligand is believed to reflect whether the ligand increases conductance (agonist), decreases conductance (inverse antagonist), or has no effect (antagonist) (Supavilai and Karobath 1983). The TBPS ratio of ZK 93426 is slightly below unity, suggesting a moderate reduction of chloride conductance, which in turn indicates that the compound could act as a weak inverse agonist. Interestingly, the GABA ratio, a biochemical measure that is indicative of the kind of interaction between benzodiazepine receptor ligands and the GBC complex, is enhanced. This indicates that ZK 93426 might have additional effects on the GABA binding, and that agonistic features of the compound can also be expected (Stephens et al. 1985).

In placebo-controlled, double-blind study in 30 healthy male subjects from whom written informed consent had been obtained, vehicle (Intralipid solution), 0.01 mg/kg, or 0.04 mg/kg ZK 93426 was administered ($n=10$ per group), after which safety and drug effects were investigated (Duka T, in preparation). Cardiovascular parameters (e.g., blood pressure), ECG, and vital signs (e.g., respiratory rate) were monitored at regular intervals; blood chemistry and urinalysis were done before and after drug treatment. In addition, psychomotor performance and drug effects were evaluated on the basis of standardized question-

Table 2. Symptoms reported by individual subjects ($n=10$/treatment group) 5–20 min after i.v. administration of ZK 93 426 or placebo

	Placebo	ZK 93 426	
		0.01 mg/kg	0.04 mg/kg
Central effects			
Anxiety	–	1	5**
Restlessness	–	–	5**
Dizziness	1	1	5*
Alertness	2	5	1
Tiredness	–	–	3
Total[a]	2	5	10
Other effects			
Tight chest	–	–	3
Cold hands	–	2	6**
Pins and needles	–	3	6**
Muscle tension	1	1	2
Total[a]	1	4	9

* $P=0.07$; ** $P=0.001$ compared with placebo (Fischer's exact probability test).
[a] Number of subjects presenting with symptoms.

naires [modified Treatment Emergent Symptoms Scale-Write-In (TWIS), Dosage Record and Treatment Emergent Symptom scale (DOTES), and visual analog scales] and of subjective ratings by the physicians in charge of the investigations and the volunteers themselves.

ZK 93426 was well tolerated and no side effects were ascertained; it induced no changes in blood chemistry or urinalysis. There was, however, a slight dose-dependent increase in systolic blood pressure. Table 2 lists some of the effects of treatment with placebo and with ZK 93426. Interestingly, ZK 93426 induced some dose-dependent effects in volunteers which could be ascribed to central activation. The increased restlessness and mild anxiety observed by the volunteers is not comparable with the threatening anxiety attacks seen after FG 7142 treatment. The stimulating effects of ZK 93426 were only observed during the first hour after administration. Interestingly, subjects treated with the high dose of the active drug later seemed to experience effects indicative of anxiolytic activity, as evidenced in the visual analog scales (data not shown). However, it remains to be clarified whether this represents a rebound effect or reflects a dual activity of the compound as indicated by the differences in the GABA and TBPS ratios. Preliminary data from another investigation show that ZK 93426 can reverse the sedative properties of a high dose of i.v. lormetazepam (0.03 mg/kg). These results suggest that ZK 93426 does indeed antagonize the effects of benzodiazepines and may itself act as a weak partial inverse agonist, an observation that has also been reported for another benzodiazepine antagonist, Ro 15-3505 (Haefely 1985).

Benzodiazepine receptor antagonists may be useful tools in the reduction of postoperative sedative effects and anterograde amnesia in patients undergoing surgery with anesthetics including benzodiazepines; in the treatment of accidental overdosages in children; and in the treatment of suicidal intoxications in adults, especially when other drugs besides benzodiazepines have been taken and immediate questioning of the patients is vital. However, care should be taken when the patient is receiving chronic or high-dose benzodiazepine treatment. High doses of antagonists are known to precipitate withdrawal reactions in animal experiments and should be avoided as also suggested by our own studies in humans (Dorow and Duka 1986). The reversal of benzodiazepine effects should therefore be carefully graduated by gradually increasing the dose of the antagonist. If endogenous ligands for the benzodiazepine receptor are found to be involved in the causation of hypersomnolent states such as narcolepsy, antagonists may turn out to be valuable drugs.

4 Partial Agonists at Benzodiazepine Receptors

It is well known that, depending on the dose, benzodiazepines as a group can reduce anxiety, antagonize convulsions, sedate, induce ataxia and muscle relaxation, and even provoke anterograde amnesia in patients. Although a number of biochemical and behavioral studies have shown that benzodiazepines act via specific receptors in the CNS, it is still unclear whether the benzodiazepines achieve their different pharmacological effects via subtypes of central benzodiazepine receptors, whether this is due to a difference in their efficacy, i.e., the effect the benzodiazepines might produce at a given receptor occupancy (Stephens et al. 1985), or whether these compounds have different actions at the molecular level.

The putative existence of subtypes of benzodiazepine receptors has given rise to the hope that the "desirable" anxiolytic or anticonvulsant acvtivities might be mediated by one type, and the undesirable ataxic sedative properties by another type of receptor. This hope has been strengthened by several reports on the pharmacological characteristics of compounds called mixed agonists-antagonists or partial agonists. Such benzodiazepine receptor ligands as Ro 16-6028, Ro 17-1812, and CGS 9895, CGS 9896 were shown to possess anticonvulsant and anticonflict activity in rodents, with little effect in tests for muscle-relaxant and ataxic activity (Haefely 1984; Bennett and Petrack 1984). However, the administration of oral doses as high as 1.0 mg of the first two above-mentioned mixed agonists-antagonists induced deep sedation, marked ataxia, impairment of performance, and amnesia in healthy volunteers (Merz 1984). First clinical observations with Ro 17-1812 indicate that it was not possible to separate the anxiolytic and sedative properties of these compounds in patients (Schubert et al. 1984, Kapfhammer 1984).

4.1 Studies with ZK 91 296

A number of β-carbolines with partial agonistic characteristic have recently been synthesized, two of which (ZK 91 296, 5-benzyloxy-4-methoxymethyl β-carboline-3-carboxylic acid ethyl ester, and ZK 95 962, 5-isopropoxy-4-methoxymethyl-β-carboxylic acid ethyl ester) have also been investigated in humans. ZK 91 296 was shown to possess high affinity for benzodiazepine receptors, and the GABA and TBPS ratios were above unity. Potent anticonvulsant activity was observed in several animal models of epilepsy, and anticonflict effects were established in tests that are held to indicate anxiety. Interestingly, ZK 91 296 showed no effect in animal models of sedation and ataxia (for a summary see Petersen et al. 1984) and was free of muscle-relaxant effect (Klockgether et al. 1985). Similar results were obtained for ZK 95962 (L. Jensen, E. Petersen, D. Stephens, et al. 1984, unpublished results).

Oral doses of up to 600 mg and i.v. doses of up to 0.03 mg/kg ZK 91 296 were administered to healthy male subjects who had been informed about the objectives and risks of the trial. No effects were seen in a number of tests thought to be sensitive to the effects of benzodiazepine treatment. These tests included visual analog scales, a complaints list, the multiple sleep latency test (MSLT), effects on power spectra of EEG recordings (especially changes of alpha and beta frequencies), and subjective ratings by volunteers and physicians. After 100 mg administration of ZK 91 296 p.o., neither the physicians nor the volunteers themselves could ascertain whether active substance or placebo had been ingested (R. Dorow 1984, unpublished results). Low and varying biovailability after oral intake of ZK 91 296 was observed (W. Krause, personal communication) and added some uncertainty to the interpretation of these results. However, 0.03 mg/kg i.v., a dose which led to substantial plasma levels, also resulted in no measurable effects. In a total of 20 subjects no treatment-related changes were seen in either vital signs, such as blood pressure, heart rate (including ECG recordings), and respiratory function, or in blood chemistry and urinalysis.

4.2 Studies with ZK 95962

To evaluate the effects and safety of ZK 95962, another partial benzodiazepine agonist, several independent trials (including placebo-controlled studies) were performed, in which 28 subjects were treated with i.v. (0.005–0.04 mg/kg) and 6 of these volunteeers with oral (20–100 mg) doses of ZK 95962. As in the studies of ZK 91296, no treatment-related effects or behavioral changes, and especially none of the typical benzodiazepine effects, could be ascertained after oral doses of ZK 95962. Low bioavailability following oral administration warranted the selection of the i.v. route to document the drug effects reliably.

In a randomized, double-blind and placebo-controlled study, 30 volunteers were randomly allocated to two treatment groups ($n=15$ per group; 0.04 mg/kg ZK 95962 i.v. or Intralipid vehicle). Standard questionnaires (modified TWIS/DOTES), a complaints list, visual analog scales, and standard neurological examinations were administered before and at 30 and 360 min after treatment. Table 3 presents a summary of the results taken from the questionnaires. As can be seen, only dizziness, ataxic gait, and a sensation of weakness in the legs, and no symptoms of sedation or drowsiness, were observed 20–30 min after administration. Figure 1 presents the results from 100 mm bipolar visual analog scales indicating lack of drive. These data suggest some selectivity of ZK 95962 and show that the compound may indeed resemble a partial agonist. Shortly after the injection, subjects were requested to turn their head with the eyes open; this resulted in blurred vision owing to inappropriate eye movements which were not followed by nystagmus. This may be due to muscle-relaxant effects of external occular muscles leading to spatial disorientation produced by false projection of the visual fields. The parameters of vital function and body chemistry remained unchanged after both

Table 3. Symptoms reported by individual subjects ($n=15$/treatment group) before and during placebo or ZK 95 962 (0.04 mg/kg i.v.) treatment as evaluated by standardized rating scales[a]

Symptoms	Placebo		ZK 95 962	
	Before injection	At 20–30 min after injection	Before injection	At 20–30 min after injection
Drowsiness	8	5	7	8
Agitation	–	–	5	1
Ataxic gait	1	3	4	10**
Blurred vision	–	1	–	4
Weakness in the legs	1	–	1	7***
Dizziness	1	–	1	10***
Numbness	3	4	1	8
Feeling pleasant	10	10	7	12*
Feeling indifferent	6	5	3	7
Floating feeling	1	2	–	5
Total number of subjects presenting with symptoms	13	14	14	15

[a] Modified TWIS/DOTES; for details see text.
* $P<0.1$; ** $P<0.05$; *** $P<0.001$ when placebo was compared with ZK 95 962 (χ^2 test for independent samples).

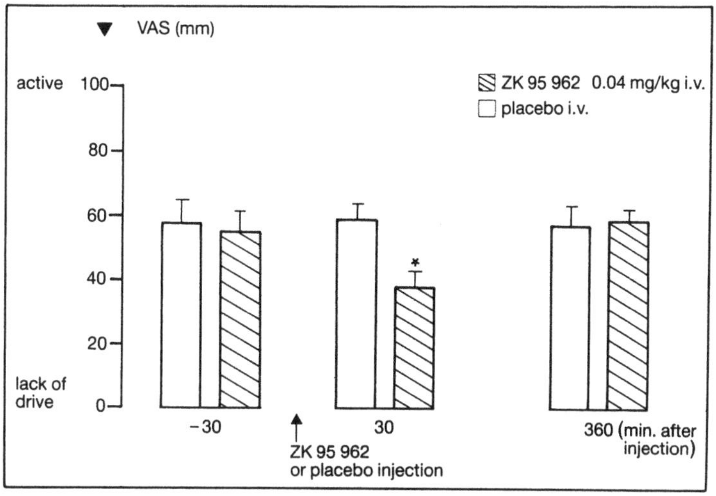

Fig. 1. The effects of ZK 95962 (0.04 mg/kg i.v.) or placebo on a bipolar visual analog scale (active-lack of drive). Changes were only observed 30 min after ZK 95962 administration (* $P<0.05$, Mann-Whitney U test)

oral and i.v. administration, which indicated that the compound was safe and well tolerated. In summary, this study shows that high i.v. doses of ZK 95962 induce slight muscle-relaxant effects without sedation or drowsiness, and thus presents the first evidence that the compound may be a partial agonist; that is to say, it is capable of selectively producing only some of the effects normally observed after benzodiazepine treatment.

In order to test the hypothesis that ZK 95962 at an effective dose lacks major sedative properties, an interaction study was performed with a high dose of lormetazepam administered i.v. Two groups of four volunteers each were treated with 0.03 mg/kg lormetazepam i.v. and 30 min later received either placebo or 0.04 mg/kg ZK 95962 i.v. The above-mentioned psychometric tests and questionnaires were applied and standardized EEG recordings were performed before, during, and after drug administration. The MSLT was performed before and at 2-h intervals after treatment; sleepiness and latencies to stage 1 and 2 sleep were recorded (for a description of methods see Richardson et al. 1978). Figures 2 and 3 exemplify both the vigilosomnograms (staging according to rules of Rechtschaffen and Kales 1968) and the chronospectograms by 20-s power analyses over time, of two subjects treated with either ZK 95962 or placebo. As in this example, three of the four subjects under active treatment, but none under placebo, awoke abruptly from stage 2 or 3 sleep 10–15 min after the second injection. At 60 min after the injection of lormetazepam, all subjects were woken up, examined neurologically, and asked to complete a number of psychometric tests. Marked differences were apparent between the two groups, as judged by both the volunteers and investigators during the trial and after playback of video recordings. While ataxia and muscle relaxation were observed in both groups, behavioral and gesticulatory signs of lormetazepam-induced sedation, e.g., speech, facial expression, and movement, were attenuated only in the group treated with ZK 95962. In the

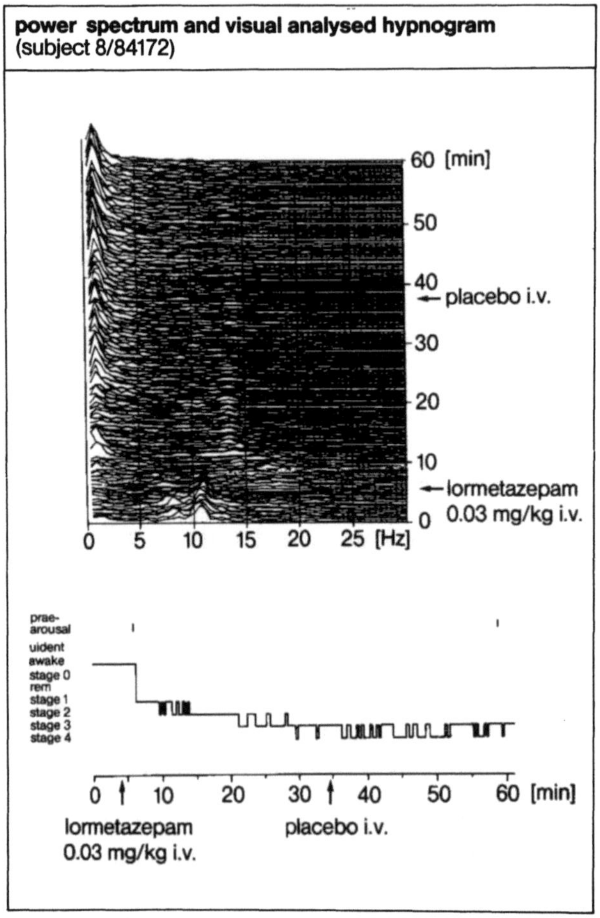

Fig. 2. Time course of lormetazepam effects (0.03 mg/kg i.v.) followed by placebo administration on vigilance, as measured by EEG recordings in a subject. Chronospectrograms of 20-s power spectra and hypnograms evaluated according to Rechtschaffen and Kales (1968)

chronospectograms recorded after lormetazepam, the power of the alpha frequency range was markedly reduced, while the fast beta frequencies were increased, a well-established benzodiazepine effect.

In the course of the experiments, increases in power in the frequency range typical of sleep spindles in stage 2 appeared with a marked increase of delta frequency, indicating slow waves. After the administration of ZK 95962, in the subjects who awoke a normal waking EEG with comparable intensities of alpha power was seen, as shown in Fig. 3. Surprisingly, benzodiazepine-related betafrequencies were not detected. In the MSLTs that were subsequently recorded, a reversal of lormetazepam-induced sleepiness could be seen in the latency to stage 1 (mean values $\pm$SEM 3 h p.a.: placebo = 4.6 $\pm$ 2.3 min; ZK 95962 = 10.5 $\pm$ 3.5 min), which lasted for at least 3 h after ZK 95962, and in the latency to stage 2 (mean values $\pm$SEM 1 h after administration: placebo = 5.8 $\pm$ 2.1 min; ZK 95962 = 10.6 $\pm$ 2.5 min), which lasted for 1 h.

The above findings, although preliminary in character owing to the limited number of volunteers treated, add weight to the hypothesis that ZK 95962 has

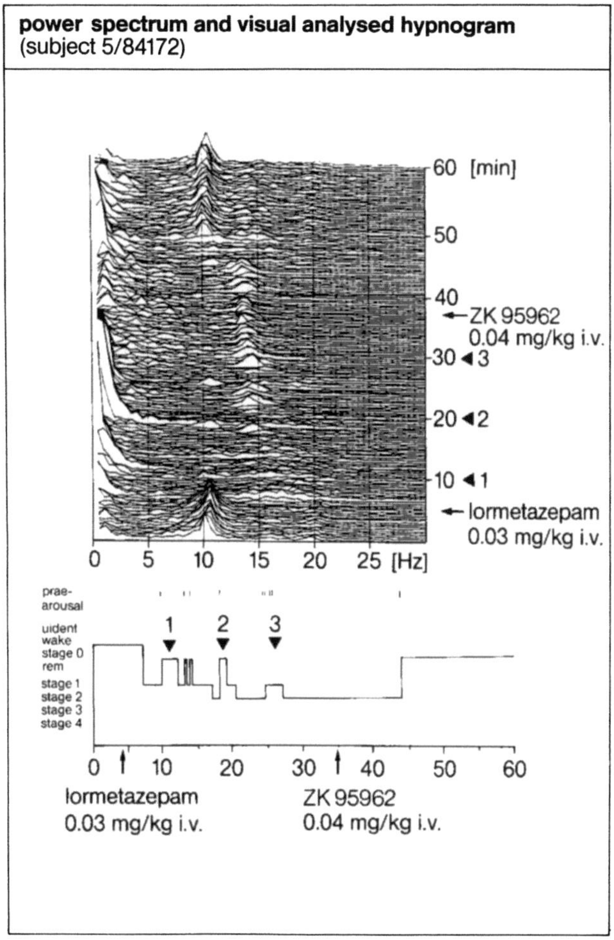

Fig. 3. Time course of lormetazepam effects (0.03 mg/kg i.v.) followed by ZK 95962 (0.04 mg/kg i.v.) administration on vigilance, as measured by EEG recordings in a subject. Chronospectrograms at 20-s power spectra and hypnograms evaluated according to Rechtschaffen and Kales (1968)

the properties of a partial agonist in that it has no sedative properties while exerting muscle relaxation; on the other hand it can even antagonize sedation induced by high i.v. doses of a hypnotic benzodiazepine, while having no effect on lormetazepam's muscle-relaxant activity. Furthermore, subsequent interviews with the volunteers offered some indication that anterograde amnesia induced by lormetazepam was antagonized by ZK 95962.

In the recent literature on the bidirectional effects of β-carbolines in animals, ZK 93423 (6-benzyloxy-4-methoxymethyl-β-carboline-3-carboxylic acid ethyl ester) was shown to be a potent full benzodiazepine agonist (Stephens et al. 1984b; Stephens and Kehr 1985). We have tested a similarly potent compound in volunteers and observed that it produced the full spectrum of benzodiazepine effects; in one case these were readily reversible by ZK 95962, but not to the same extent by Ro 15-1788 as investigated in another subject.

Conclusions

The present studies in healthy volunteers offer additional evidence for the concept of a continuum of bidirectional effects mediated by benzodiazepine receptor ligands (Table 4). Furthermore, clinical pharmacology of individual compounds from the wide range of β-carbolines can promote our understanding of basic CNS mechanisms, e.g., mechanisms underlying anxiety and sleep. When testing benzodiazepine receptor ligands for benzodiazepine-like effects in healthy volunteers, especially partial agonists that are believed to be selective for anticonvulsive and anxiolytic action, the nature of the study determines that only sedative-hypnotic, muscle-relaxant effects and anterograde amnesia (and in some cases anxiolytic activity) can be detected. Anticonvulsant and anxiolytic effects of these compounds cannot be revealed and have to be substantiated in studies with appropriate patients in the clinical setting. However, our findings indicate that compounds like ZK 95962 have a potent activity in reversing some, but not all, effects of lormetazepam, and give rise to hopes that the anxiolytic and anticonvulsant effects observed in animal studies will also be seen in the clinical situation.

A further conclusion of our studies is that partial agonists could have another clinical benefit, i.e., in the control of the sedative component of benzodiazepine-linked anesthesia and intoxications. In such situations, patients would not run the risk of experiencing the precipitation of withdrawal reactions, i.e., anxiety and possibly convulsions.

In summary, our observations in healthy subjects confirm the spectrum of bidirectional effects mediated by benzodiazepine receptor ligands, as represented by the β-carbolines and predicted by numerous animal experiments and biochemical investigations. We think the present studies offer new promise for the clinical application of such compounds, i.e. insight into the mechanism of human anxiety, separation of single effects from the whole benzodiazepine spectrum and subsequently an improvement for the treatment of anxiety, epilepsy, sleep disturbances and, possibly, situations where enhancement of attention and wakefulness is desired.

Table 4. Bidirectional effects of benzodiazepine receptor ligands in humans

Agonists	Partial	Receptor antagonists	Partial	Inverse agonists
Activity				
Anticonvulsive Anxiolytic Muscle relaxant Sedative, hypnotic Anterograde amnestic		Without effect, but reversal of		Convulsive Anxiogenic Increase muscle tone Stimulating Promnestic?
Compounds[a]				
Benzodiazepines	ZK 91 296 ZK 95 962	ZK 93 426 Ro 15-1788 CGS 8216	FG 7142	(DMCM)[b]

[a] For exact chemical nomenclature see text.

[b] 4-Ethyl-6,7-dimethoxy-β-carboline-3-carboxylic acid methylester (not tested in humans).

Acknowledgments. We are grateful Dr. Schmiechen (Schering AG), Dr. Christensen (A/S Ferrosan) and their colleagues for synthesis of the various β-carbolines.

We thank the volunteers for their willingness to participate in the studies and their helpful comments: G. Bodewitz, I. Columbus, R. Herrmann, C. Knittel, and H. Riemer for technical assistance; J. Horkulak for help in preparation of the manuscript and A. Dahrmann for typing it.

References

Bennet DA, Petrack B (1984) CGS 9896: a non-benzodiazepine, non-sedating potential anxiolytic. Drug Dev Res 4:75–82

Bieck PR, Antonin KH, Britzelmeyer C, Cremer C, Gleiter C, Nilsson E, Schoenleber W (1984) Human pharmacology of CGS 8216, a benzodiazepine antagonist. Clin Neuropharmacol 7 [Suppl 1]:674–675

Braestrup C, Nielsen M, Olsen CE (1980) Urinary and brain β-carboline-3-carboxylates as potent inhibitors of brain benzodiazepine receptors. Proc Natl Acad Sci USA 77:2288–2292

Braestrup C, Schmiechen R, Neef G, Nielsen M, Petersen EN (1982) Interaction of convulsive ligands with benzodiazepine receptors. Science 216:1241–1243

Braestrup C, Honoré T, Nielsen M, Petersen EN, Jensen LH (1984) Ligands for benzodiazepine receptors with positive and negative efficacy. Biochem Pharmacol 33:859–862

Cepeda C, Tanaka T, Besselièvre R, Potier P, Naquet R, Rossier J (1981) Proconvulsant effects in baboons of β-carboline, a putative endogenous ligand for benzodiazepine receptors. Neurosci Lett 24:53–57

Cowen PJ, Green AR, Nutt DJ (1981) Ethyl β-carboline carboxylate lowers seizure threshold and antagonizes flurazepam-induced sedation in rats. Nature 290:54–55

Czernik AJ, Kalinsky HJ, Psychoyos S, Cash WD, Tsai C, Rinehart RK, Granat FR, Lovell RA, Brundish DE, Wade R (1982) CGS 8216: receptor binding characteristics of a potent benzodiazepine antagonist. Life Sci 30:363–372

Darragh A, Lambe R, Brick I, Downie WW (1981) Reversal of benzodiazepine induced sedation by intravenous Ro 15-1788. Lancet 2:1042

Darragh A, Lambe R, Kenny M, Brick I, Taaffe W, O'Boyle C (1982) Ro 15-1788 antagonises the effects of diazepam in man without altering diazepam bioavailability. Br J Clin Pharmacol 14:677–682

Darragh A, Lambe R, O'Boyle C, Kenny M, Brick I (1983) Absence of effects in man of the benzodiazepine antagonist Ro 15-1788. Psychopharmacology (Berlin) 80:192–195

Doenicke A, Suttmann H, Kapp W, Kugler J, Ebentheuer H (1984) Zur Wirkung des Benzodiazepin-Antagonisten Ro 15-1788. Anaesthesist 33:343–347

Dorow R (1985) Anxiety and its generation by pharmacological means. In: Iverson SD (ed) Psychopharmacology. Recent advances and future aspects. Oxford University Press, Oxford, pp 100–112

Dorow R, Duka T (1986) Anxiety: its generation by drugs and by their withdrawal. In: Biggio G, Costa E (eds) Gabaergic transmission and anxiety. Advances in neurology, vol 41. Raven, New York (in press)

Dorow R, Horowsky R, Paschelke G, Amin M, Braestrup C (1983) Severe anxiety induced by FG 7142, a β-carboline ligand for benzodiazepine receptors. Lancet 2:98–99

Dorow R, Paschelke G, Horowski R (1984) Clinical pharmacology of FG 7142, an inverse agonist of benzodiazepine receptors. Clin Neuropharmacol 7 [Suppl 1]:676–677

Emmet-Oglesby M, Spencer DG, Lewis M, Elmessalamy F, Lal H (1983) Anxiogenic aspects of diazepam withdrawal can be detected in animals. Eur J Pharmacol 92:127–130

Ferrero A, Guidotti A, Conti-Tronconi B, Costa E (1984) A brain octadecaneuropeptide generated by tryptic digestion of DBI (diazepam-binding inhibitor) functions as a proconflict ligand of benzodiazepine recognition sites. Neuropharmacology 23:1359–1362

Haefely W (1984) Pharmacological profile of two benzodiazepine partial agonists: Ro 16-6028 and Ro 17-1812. Clin Neuropharmacol 7 [Suppl 1]:670–674

Haefely W (1985) Pharmacology of Benzodiazepine antagonists. Pharmacopsychiatria 18:163–166

Hunkeler W, Möhler H, Pieri L, Polc P, Bonetti EP, Cumin R, Schaffner R, Haefly W (1981) Selective antagonists of benzodiazepines. Nature 290:514–516
Jensen LH, Petersen EN, Braestrup C (1983) Audiogenic seizures DBA/2 mice discriminate sensitively between low efficacy benzodizapine receptor agonist and inverse agonists. Life Sci 33:393–399
Jensen LH, Petersen EN, Braestrup C, Honore T, Kehr W, Stephens DN, Schneider HH, Seidelmann D, Schmiechen R (1984) Evaluation of the β-carboline ZK 93426 as a benzodiazepine receptor antagonist. Psychopharmacology (Berlin) 83:249–256
Kapfhammer HP (1984) Ro 17-1812 in the treatment of anxious syndromes. 14th CINP Congress, Florence, Book of Abstract, p 90 (F-88)
Klockgether T, Schwarz M, Lechoslaw T, Sonntag KH (1985) ZK 91296, an anticonvulsant β-carboline which lacks muscle relaxant properties. Eur J Pharmacol 110:309–315
Klotz U, Duka T, Dorow R, Doenicke A (1985) Flunitrazepam and lormetazepam do not affect the pharmacokinetics of the benzodiazepine antagonist Ro 15-1788. Br J Clin Pharmacol 19:95–98
Lukas SE, Griffiths RR (1982) Precipitated withdrawal by a benzodiazepine receptor antagonist (Ro 15-1788) after 7 days of diazepam. Science 217:1161–1163
Lukas SE, Giffiths RR (1984) Precipitated diazepam withdrawal in baboons: Effects of dose and duration of diazepam exposure (1984). Eur J Pharmacol 100:163–171
McNicholas LF, Martin WR (1982) The effect of a benzodiazepine antagonist, Ro 15-1788, in diazepam dependent rats. Life Sci 31:731–737
Merz WA (1984) Partial benzodiazepine agonists: initial results in man. Clin Neuropharmacol 7[Suppl 1]:672–673
Oakley NR, Jones BJ (1980) The proconvulsant and diazepam reversing effects of ethyl β-carboline-3-carboxylate. Eur J Pharmacol 68:381–382
O'Boyle C, Lambe R, Darragh A, Taffe A, Brick I, Kenny M (1983) Ro 15-1788 antagonizes the effects of diazepam in man without affecting its biovailability. Br J Anaesth 55:349–355
Pellow S, File SE (1984) Multiple sites of action for anxiogenic drugs: Behavioural, electrophysiological, and biochemical correlations. Psychopharmacology (Berlin) 83:304–315
Petersen EN, Paschelke G, Kehr W, Nielsen M, Braestrup C (1982) Does the reversal of the anticonflict effect of phenobarbital by β-CCE and FG 7142 indicate benzodiazepine receptor-mediated anxiogenic properties. Eur J Pharmacol 82:217–221
Petersen EN, Jensen LH, Honoré T, Braestrup C, Kehr W, Stephens DN, Wachtel H, Seidelmann D, Schmiechen R (1984) ZK 91296, a partial agonist at benzodiazepine receptors. Psychopharmacology (Berlin) 83:240–248
Petursson H, Lader MH (1981) Withdrawal from longterm benzodiazepine treatment. Br Med J 283:643–645
Polc P, Bonetti PE, Schaffner R, Haefely W (1982) A three-state model of the benzodiazepine receptor explains the interactions between the benzodiazepine tranquilizers, β-carbolines, and phenobarbitone. Naunyn-Schmiedebergs Arch Pharmacol 321:260–264
Rechtschaffen A, Kales A (1968) A manual of standardized terminology techniques and scoring system of sleep stages of human subjects. Brain Research Center, University of California, Los Angeles
Richardson G, Carskadon MA, Flagg W, van den Hoed J, Dementct WC, Mitler MM (1978) Excessive daytime sleepiness in man, multiple sleep latency measurement in narcoleptic and control subjects. Electroencephalogr Clin Neurophysiol 45:621–627
Schöpf J (1983) Withdrawal phenomena after long-term administration of benzodiazepines. A review of recent investigations. Pharmacopsychiatria 16:1–8
Schöpf J, Laurian S, Le PK, Gaillard JM (1984) Intrinsic activity of the benzodiazepine antagonist Ro 15-1788 in man: an electrophysiological investigation. Pharmacopsychiatria 17:79–83
Schoch P, Richards JG, Häring P, Takacs B, Stähli C, Stachelin T, Haefely W, Möhler H (1985) Co-localisation of GABA receptors and benzodiazepine receptors in the brain shown by monoclonal antibodies. Nature 314:168–171
Schubert H, Fleischhacker WW, Hinterhuber H (1984) Preliminary results on Ro 17-1812, a benzodiazepine agonist/antagonist, in the treatment of anxiety. 14th CINP Congress, Florence, Book of Abstracts p 89 (F-87)

Scollo-Lavizarri G (1983) First clinical investigation of the benzodiazepine antagonist Ro 15-1788 in comatose patients. Eur Neurol 22:7–11
Scollo-Lavizarri G (1984) The anticonvulsant effect of the benzodiazepine antagonist Ro 15-1788: an EEG study in 4 cases. Eur Neurol 23:1–6
Squires RF, Casida JE, Richardson M, Saederup E (1983) [^{35}S]t-Butyl-bicyclophosphorothionate binds with high affinity to brain specific sites coupled to γ-aminobutyric acid-A and ion recognition sites. Mol Pharmacol 23:326
Stephens DN, Kehr W (1985) β-Carbolines can enhance or antagonize the effects of punishment in mice. Psychopharmacology (Berlin) 85:143–147
Stephens DN, Kehr W, Schneider HH, Braestrup C (1984a) Bidirectional effects on anxiety of β-carbolines acting as benzodiazepine receptor ligands. Neuropharmacology 23:879–880
Stephens DN, Kehr W, Schneider HH, Schmiechen R (1984b) β-Carbolines with agonistic and inverse agonistic properties at benzodiazepine receptors of the rat. Neurosci Lett 47:333–338
Stephens DN, Kehr W, Wachtel H, Schmiechen R (1985) The anxiolytic activity of β-carboline derivatives in mice, and its separation from ataxic properties. Pharmacopsychiatria 18:167–170
Supavilai P, Karobath M (1983) Differential modulations of [^{35}S]-TBPS binding by the occupancy of benzodiazepine receptors with its ligands. Eur J Pharmacol 91:145–146
Tenen SS, Hirsch JD (1980) β-carboline-3-carboxylic acid ethyl ester antagonizes diazepam activity. Nature 288:609–610
Ziegler G, Ludwig L, Fritz G (1985) Reversal of slow-wave-sleep by benzodiazepine antagonist Ro 15-1788. Lancet 2:510

Pharmacodynamic Approaches to Benzodiazepine Action in Man

D. W. HOMMER[1], V. MATSUO[2], O. M. WOLKOWITZ[1], H. WEINGARTNER[3], and S. M. PAUL[1]

1 Introduction

Since their introduction, the benzodiazepines have become one of the most widely prescribed class of drugs in the world (Baum et al. 1985). Despite the extensive clinical experience with these drugs it is only in the past few years that we have developed any understanding of their underlying molceular mechanisms of action. It is now known that specific receptors for benzodiazepines are present in brain and that these receptors are functionally linked to the receptor for the major inhibitory neurotransmitter, gamma aminobutyric acid (GABA), and its associated chloride ion channel (Skolnick and Paul 1982; Tallman et al. 1980). Furthermore, there is evidence that an endogenous ligand for the benzodiazepine receptor may exist (Guidotti et al. 1983) and that stress modifies various aspects of the benzodiazepine/GABA/Cl ionophore receptor complex (see Skolnick et al., this volume). For these reasons it would be useful to develop techniques to measure benzodiazepine receptor sensitivity in vivo, in order to determine whether psychiatric disorders such as depression or anxiety may be characterized by alterations in benzodiazepine receptor sensitivity.

To measure benzodiazepine receptor sensitivity we have employed a pharmacodynamic approach (Goldstein et al. 1973) which consists in examining changes in a number of physiological responses to increasing concentrations of a selective benzodiazepine receptor agonist. Since benzodiazepines appear to produce most, if not all, of their pharmacological actions via the benzodiazepine receptor [both the sedative and anticonflict actions of the benzodiazepines are mediated through specific receptors and these actions can be reversed by selective benzodiazepine receptor antagonists (Hunkler et al. 1981)], we chose to study the effects of i.v. benzodiazepine infusions on a number of dependent variables as a presumptive measure of human benzodiazepine receptor sensitivity in vivo. For such an approach to be a valid and useful measure of human sensitivity to benzodiazepines, it should meet several criteria. First, the variables to be measured should be quantifiable. Second, benzodiazepine-induced changes in these variables should correlate with the known pharmacological actions of the benzodiazepines (e.g., tranquilization/sedation). Third, these variables should be altered in a dose-depen-

[1] Clinical Neuroscience Branch, National Institute of Mental Health, Bethesda, MD 20892, USA.
[2] Clinical Branch, NEI
[3] Laboratory of Psychology and Psychopathology, National Institute of Mental Health, Bethesda, MD 20892, USA.

Clinical Pharmacology in Psychiatry
Editors: Dahl, Gram, Paul, Potter
(Psychopharmacology Series 3)

dent fashion. We selected diazepam as a benzodiazepine agonist in these studies since it is available for i.v. administration and has high lipid solubility which results in the rapid occurrence of peak blood and brain levels (Greenblatt et al. 1983 a, b). We measured saccadic eye velocity, because it is highly quantifiable and decreases in a dose-dependent fashion with diazepam administration (Gentles and Thomas 1971; Jürgens et al. 1981). A saccade is a rapid ballistic eye movement from one position in the orbit to another. Once a saccade is initiated it is not influenced by motivations as many other psychomotor performance measures are (Becker and Fuchs 1970).

Other variables measured were self-rates sedation and anxiety. Sedation is one of the principal pharmacological effects of the benzodiazepines, and it was therefore important to examine the relationship between the increasing sedation produced by diazepam and the changes in other dependent variables. We also measured the effects of diazepam on growth hormone (GH) and cortisol secretion, since both have been shown to be affected by benzodiazepine administration (Sylvalahti and Kanto 1975; Lackmann et al. 1982; Butler et al. 1968). Because a number of studies (Clark et al. 1970; Ghoneim and Newaldt 1975; Hart et al. 1976) have demonstrated that the benzodiazepines produce antegrade amnesia, we examine the effects of diazepam on several subjective and objective measures of cognitive function, including attention and memory.

If the objective and subjective effects of diazepam occurred in a consistently and significantly dose-dependent fashion, and if such changes were highly intercorrelated, their measurement might be useful in the construction of dose-response curves that would constitute a presumptive measure of human benzodiazepine receptor sensitivity in vivo.

2 Methods

Ten normal volunteers (7 female and 3 male) were used as subjects. Their ages were between 21 and 38 years, and all were drug free and in good health. Diazepam or saline placebo was administered i.v. in a single-blind fashion at 15-min intervals, in increasing doses of 4.4, 8.8, 17.5, 35, and 70 µg/kg. The total cumulative dose was 10.0 mg in a 70-kg subject. At baseline and after each episode of drug administration, saccadic eye velocity, self-rated sedation and anxiety, GH and cortisol, and plasma diazepam concentration were measured. Memory and attention were evaluated at baseline and after every other dose of diazepam. Saccadic eye velocity was measured using an infrared scleral reflection device which monitors changes produced in the horizontal eye position as the subject directs his or her gaze towards lighted diodes in a horizontal array. The eye position signal was differentiated with respect to time, yielding the saccadic eye velocity (Hommer et al. 1986). Anxiety and sedation were measured using 100-mm visual analog line scales. Cortisol and GH were measured using radioimmunassay techniques (Odell et al. 1967; Abraham et al. 1972). The plasma diazepam concentration was measured using electron-capture gas chromatography (Greenblatt et al. 1980). Memory was tested using a previously described method, which produced measures of episodic memory and attention (Weingartner et al. 1982). Data were analyzed using three 3-way analysis of variance (ANOVA) with repeated measures, except in cases where some other technique is noted. Correlations are Pearson product moment correlations between the group means of each variable pair being examined. All data are presented as the means ±standard errors of the mean (SEM).

3 Results

3.1 Effects of Diazepam on Saccadic Eye Velocity

Diazepam produced a significant, dose-dependent slowing of saccadic eye velocities. Saccades of all amplitudes appear to be slowed by diazepam, but larger saccades were reduced to the greatest extent. For this reason only saccades of 16–20° and 24–28° were considered for further analysis (Fig. 1). Analysis of variance demonstrated that the decrease in saccadic eye velocity induced by cumulative diazepam doses of 0.7 and 0.14 mg/kg were significantly lower than those with the corresponding placebo infusion and also than baseline values ($P<0.05$, for all comparisons). There was no significant change in saccadic eye velocity during placebo infusions.

3.2 Effects of Diazepam on GH and Cortisol

Diazepam administration resulted in a significant dose-dependent increase in plasma GH (Fig. 2). This increase was significant ($P<0.01$) following the two highest doses of diazepam. Placebo administration resulted in no change in GH.

The effect of diazepam on plasma cortisol was examined using a a two-way ANOVA with repeated measures. A significant effect of diazepam in reducing plasma cortisol was observed, but placebo had no significant effect (Fig. 3).

3.3 Effect of Diazepam on Self-Ratings of Sedation and Anxiety

Diazepam administration resulted in a dose-dependent increase in self-ratings of sedation (Fig. 4). Following a cumulative dose of 0.07 or 0.14 mg/kg diazepam, subjects rated themselves significantly more sedated than at baseline ($P<0.01$).

In contrast to diazepam's effects on sedation, diazepam did not produce any significant effect on self-ratings of anxiety. However, baseline anxiety ratings were rather low in this group of healthy volunteers.

3.4 Effect of Diazepam on Memory and Attention

Diazepam produced a dose-dependent decrease in attention in a task which involved immediate recognition of repeated words from a list of 12 words, half of which were presented twice. This effect was not significant when the data were analyzed using a three-way ANOVA with repeated measures for both diazepam and placebo infusion, but was highly significant when the attentional data were analyzed using a two-way ANOVA with repeated measures for the diazepam in-

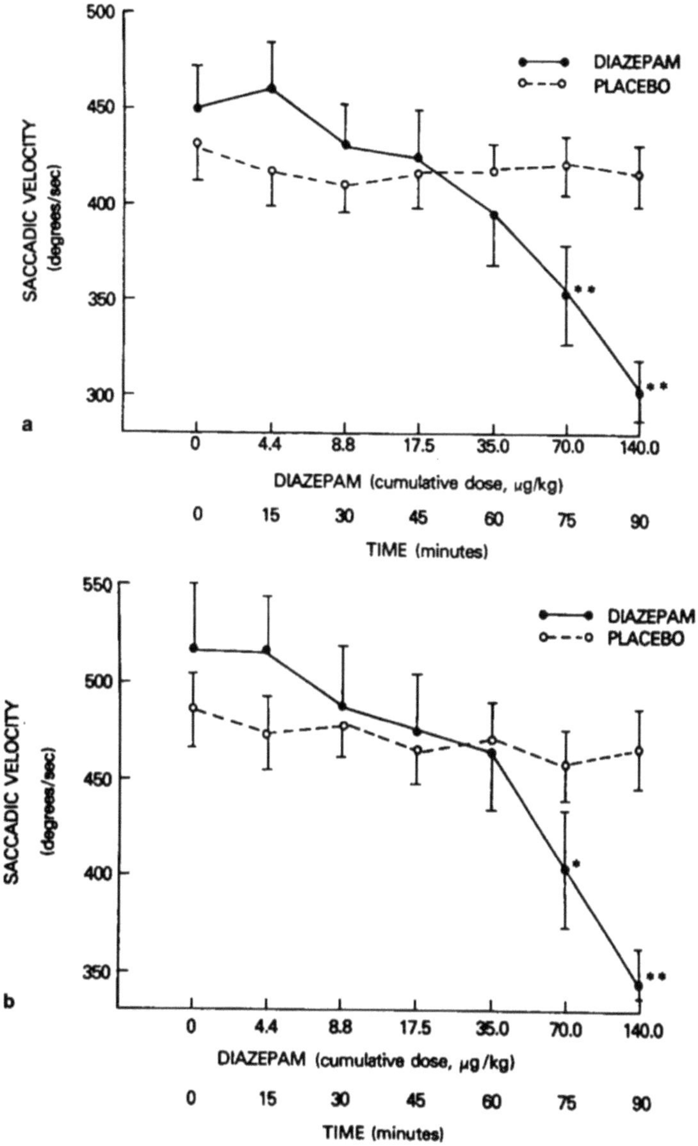

Fig. 1 a, b. Effects of diazepam on saccadic eye velocity. Diazepam administration resulted in a dose-dependent slowing of saccadic velocity for both 16–20° (**a**) and 24–28° (**b**) saccades. $*P<0.05$; $**P<0.01$ (post hoc Tukey test for differences between means of drug effect versus corresponding placebo administration). Data plotted are means ±SEM from ten subjects

fusions. A similar analysis carried out on the data derived from the placebo infusions showed no significant effects of placebo on attention.

Similarly, diazepam produced a significant, dose-dependent increase in two types of recognition memory errors. Following diazepam administration subjects were impaired in their ability to distinguish between words presented once versus

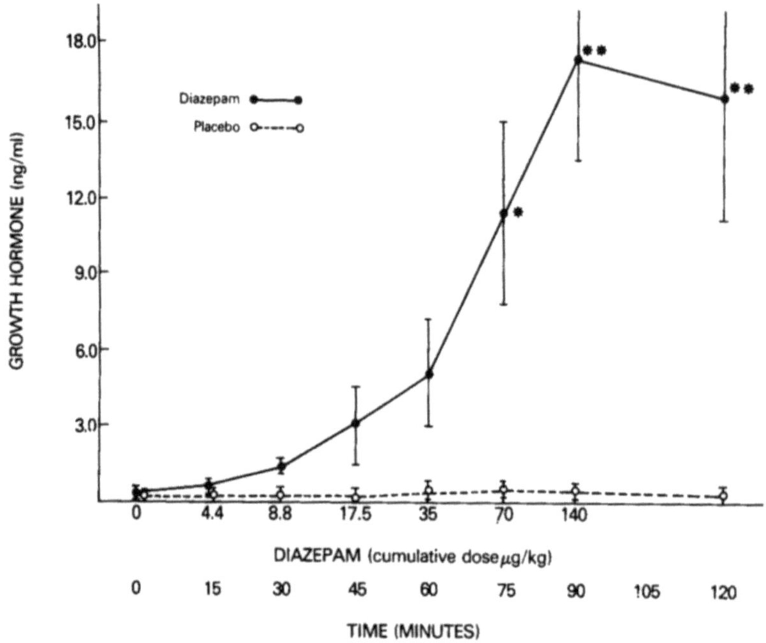

Fig. 2. Effects of diazepam administration on plasma growth hormone. Diazepam administration results in a dose-dependent increase in plasma growth hormone. $^{**}P<0.01$ (post hoc Tukey test, drug versus corresponding placebo infusion). Values plotted are means ±SEM

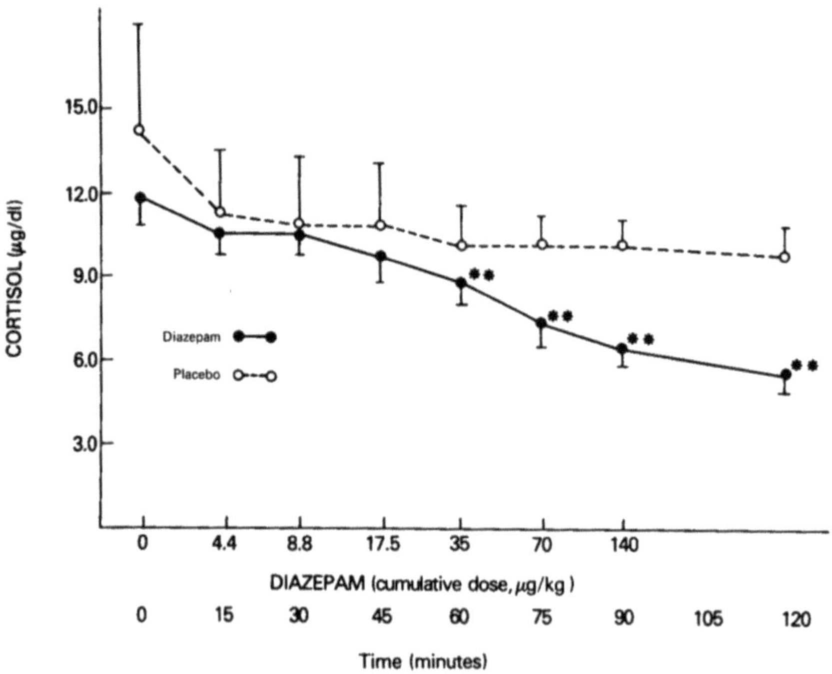

Fig. 3. Effects of diazepam administration on plasma cortisol. Diazepam reduces cortisol in a dose-dependent fashion. $^{**}P<0.01$ (post hoc Tukey test, diazepam dose compared with baseline). Values plotted are means ±SEM

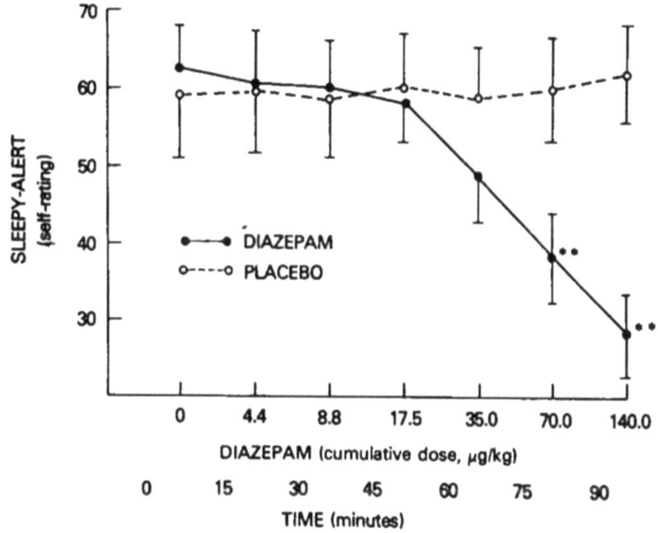

Fig. 4. Effects of diazepam administration on self-ratings of sedation. Diazepam administration results in a dose-dependent increase in self-rated sedation. $**P<0.01$ (post hoc Tukey test, drug compared with corresponding placebo infusion). Values plotted are means $\pm$SEM of ratings from ten subjects. (See text for details)

twice in the original list as well as between originally presented stimuli words and semantically similar distractor words. Diazepam administration also led to an increase in intrusion errors during a free recall task (i.e., subjects "recalled" words which were not part of the original list). None of these effects occurred during placebo administration.

3.5 Diazepam Plasma Concentration

Diazepam administered i.v. at 15-min intervals resulted in a dose-dependent increase in diazepam plasma concentration: 4.4 µg/kg: 33.7$\pm$6.3 ng/ml; 8.8 µg/kg: 47.0$\pm$10.2 ng/ml; 17.5 µg/kg: 87.9$\pm$16.7 ng/ml; 35.0 µg/kg: 161.9$\pm$28.8 ng/ml; 70.0 µg/kg: 296$\pm$28.2 ng/ml; 140.0 µg/kg: 486.8$\pm$40.3 ng/ml. The major metabolite of diazepam (*n*-desmethyldiazepam) was not detected during these infusions, since the time between drug administration and blood sampling was relatively short.

3.6 Relationships Among Variables Affected by Diazepam

The effects of diazepam on saccadic eye velocity, cortisol, GH, and sedation were all significantly correlated with each other (Fig. 5). Thus, as diazepam decreased saccadic eye velocity it also decreased cortisol concentration and increased GH concentration and sedation.

3.7 Diazepam Plasma Levels and Physiological Response

The plasma levels of diazepam were highly correlated with drug-induced changes in saccadic eye velocity, self-rated sedation, GH, cortisol, attention, and memory

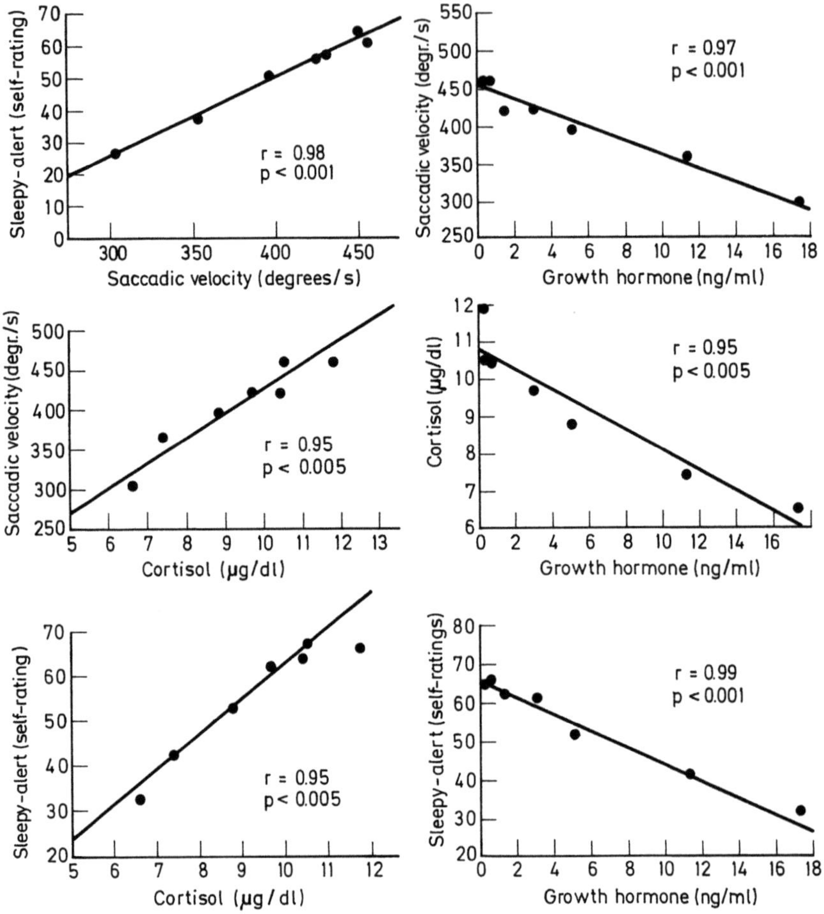

Fig. 5. Correlations between the various affected variables following diazepam administration. Pearson product moment correlations between the group means of variables affected by diazepam show that there are highly significant relationships between diazepam-induced effects on self-ratings of sedation, saccadic eye velocity, plasma cortisol and growth hormone. (See text for details)

(Fig. 6). However, the blood level of diazepam following the highest dose (peak plasma level measured for each subject) correlated significantly only with the maximum change in cortisol and intrusion errors. Thus, although in any given subject increasing plasma levels of diazepam predict an increasing response in all variables examined, the absolute plasma level itself did not always predict the magnitude of response in different individuals.

4 Comment

Intravenous administration of increasing doses of diazepam produced dose-dependent changes in self-rated sedation, peak saccadic eye velocity, GH, cortisol,

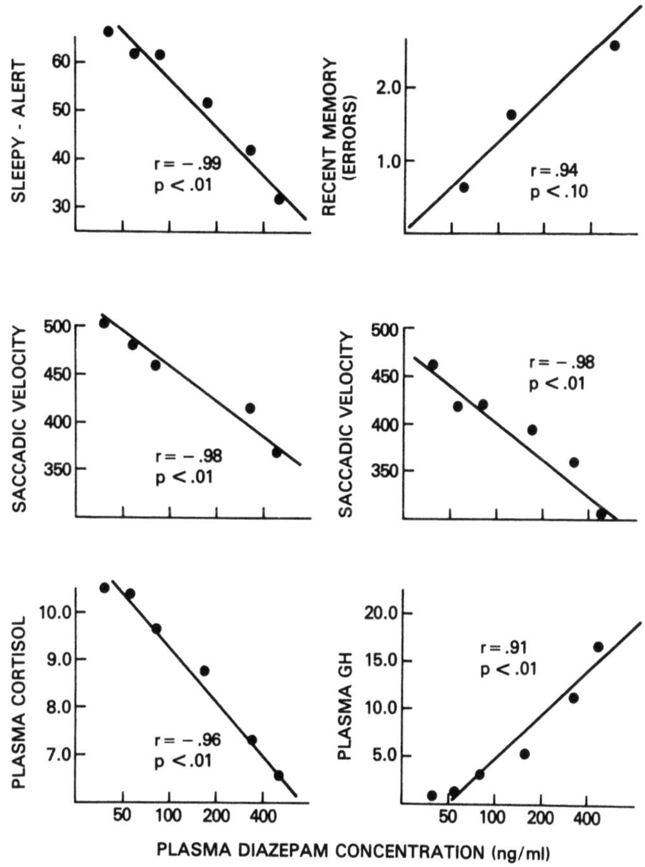

Fig. 6. Pearson product moment correlations among the group means for plasma cortisol and GH, saccadic eye velocity (for 16–20° and 29–28° saccades), sedation, and recent memory following each dose of diazepam and the corresponding plasma diazepam concentration demonstrate highly significant relationships between diazepam plasma levels and pharmacodynamic effects

attention and recent memory. The majority of these changes occurred at a plasma drug concentration of approximately 300 ng/ml. Significantly, this is approximately the blood level of diazepam and its metabolites that has been reported to be associated with diazepam's anxiolytic action during chronic administration (Bowden and Fisher 1982). Our finding that the diazepam-induced changes in sedation, saccadic eye velocity, GH, cortisol, attention and memory are all highly intercorrelated suggests that these changes may result from a common mechanism (presumably involving the benzodiazepine-GABA receptor complex) and that they might be used as a valid in vivo measure of benzodiazepine receptor sensitivity. Diazepam-induced changes in peak saccadic eye velocity may constitute the best measure of benzodiazepine receptor sensitivity, since this parameter is highly quantifiable and not influenced by attentional or motivational factors.

We observed good correlations between the increase in plasma concentration of diazepam and changes in the all affected variables. Thus, increasing plasma concentrations of diazepam were highly predictive of an increasing pharmacological effect of diazepam. The clear relationship between plasma diazepam concentration and the pharmacodynamic response which we observed contrasts with several reports of failure to find a significant correlation between drug levels and the psychomotor effects of diazepam in normal volunteers (Linnoila and Mattila 1973; Linnoila et al. 1983). In these studies, however, the benzodiazepine was administered p.o. We administered the drug i.v. and examined its pharmacological effects close to the expected time of peak plasma concentration. This may have reduced the impact of intervening variables (e.g., drug absorption, metabolism), which may obscure the relationship between plasma level and pharmacodynamic response as well as reducing the impact of acute tolerance or tachyphylaxis.

Our findings that diazepam administered to healthy subjects produces dose-dependent changes in saccadic eye velocity, sedation, GH, cortisol, attention and memory, and that these changes are all highly correlated, are consistent with the hypothesis that these effects are mediated through the benzodiazepine receptor and that their measurement could be used to estimate human benzodiazepine receptor sensitivity. We have recently examined the effects of the specific benzodiazepine receptor antagonist, Ro 15-1788 (Darragh et al. 1981) on the diazepam-induced changes in saccadic eye velocity and sedation in healthy volunteers. In six subjects we found that Ro 15-1788 clearly shifts the diazepam dose-effect curve to the right without changing its slope. These results suggest that the technique we have reported here constitutes a valid measure of the sensitivity of human benzodiazepine receptors. It should thus be possible to use benzodiazepine-induced slowing of saccadic eye velocity to examine benzodiazepine receptor sensitivity in a variety of neuropsychiatric disorders which may be characterized by alterations in the benzodiazepine/GABA/chloride ionophore complex.

Acknowledgement. We thank Dr. David Greenblatt for measuring plasma levels of diazepam.

References

Abraham GE, Buster JE, Teller TC (1972) Radioimmunossary of plasma cortisol. Anal Lett 5:757–766

Baum C, Kennedy DL, Forbes MB, Jones JK (1985) Drug use and expenditures in 1982. JAMA 253:382–386

Becker W, Fuchs AF (1970) Further properties of the human saccadic system: eye movements and correction saccades with and without visual fixation points. Vision Res 9:1247–1258

Bowden CL, Fisher JG (1982) Relationship of diazepam serum level to antianxiety effects. J Clin Psychopharmacol 2:110–114

Butler PW, Bersser GM, Steinberg H (1968) Changes in plasma cortisol induced by dexamphetamine and chlordiazepoxide given alone and in combination in man. J Endocrinol 40:391–392

Clark P, Eccersley P, Frisby J, Thornton J (1970) The amnestic effect of diazepam (Valium). Br J Anaesth 42:690–696

Darragh A, Lambe R, Scully M, Brick I, O'Boyle C, Downie WW (1981) Investigation in man of the efficacy of a benzodiazepine antagonist, Ro 15-1788. Lancet 2:8–10

Gentles W, Thomas EL (1971) Effect of benzodiazepines upon saccadic eye movements in man. Clin Pharmacol Ther 12:563–574

Ghoneim MM, Newaldt SP (1975) Effects of diazepam and scopolamine on storage, retrieval, and organizational processes in memory. Psychopharmacologia (Berlin) 44:257–262

Goldstein A, Aronow L, Kalman SM (1973) Principles of drug action, 2nd edn. Wiley, New York
Greenblatt DJ, Ochs HR, Lloyd BL (1980) Entry of diazepam and its major metabolite into cerebrospinal fluid. Psychopharmacology (Berlin) 70:89–93
Greenblatt DJ, Shader RI, Aberrnethy DR (1983a) Current status of benzodiazepines: 1. N Engl J Med 309:354–358
Greenblatt DJ, Shader RI, Aberrnethy DR (1983b) Current status of benzodiazepines: 2. N Engl J Med 309:410–416
Guidotti A, Forchetti CM, Corda MG, Konkel D, Bennett CD and Costa E (1983) Isolation, characterisation, and priufication to homogeneity of endogenous polypeptide with agonistic action on benzodiazepine receptors. Proc Natl Akad Sci USA 80:3531–3535
Hart J, Hill HM, Carol EB, Wilkinson RT, Peck SW (1976) The effect of low doses of amylobarbitone sodium and diazepam on human performance. Br J Clin Pharmacol 3:289–298
Hommer DW, Matsuo V, Wolkowitz O, Chrousos G, Greenblatt D, Weingartner H, Paul SM (1986) Benzodiazepine sensitivity in normal human subjects. Arch Gen Psychiatry 43:542–551
Hunkeler W, Möhler H, Pieri L, Polc P, Bonetti EP, Cumin R, Schaffner R, Haefely W (1981) Selective antagonists of benzodiazepines. Nature 290:514–516
Jürgens R, Becker W, Kornhuber HH (1981) Natural and drug-induced variations of velocity and duration of human saccadic eye movements: evidence for a control of the neural pulse generator by local feedback. Biol Cybern 39:87–96
Lackmann G, Treusch J, Schmouss M, Schmitt E, Trensch U (1982) Comparison of growth hormone stimulation induced by desimipramine, diazepam and metaclazepan in man. Psychoneuroendocrinology 7:141–146
Linnoila M, Mattila MJ (1973) Drug interaction on psychomotor skills related to driving: diazepam and alcohol. Eur J Clin Pharmacol 5:186–194
Linnoila M, Erwin CW, Brendle A, Simpson D (1983) Psychomotor effects of diazepam in anxious patients and healthy volunteers. J Clin Psychopharmacol 3:88–96
Odell WD, Rayford PL, Ross GT (1967) Simple partially automated method for radioimmunoassay of human thyroid stimulation, growth, lutenizing and follicle-stimulating hormones. J Lab Clin Med 70:973–980
Skolnick P, Paul SM (1982) Benzodiazepine receptors in the central nervous system. In: Smythies JR, Bradley R (eds) International revue of neurobiology. Academic, New York, pp 103–104
Sylvalahti E, Kanto J (1975) Serum growth hormone, serum immunoreactive insulin and blood glucose responses to oral and intravenous diazepam in man. Int J Clin Pharmacol 12:74–82
Tallman JF, Paul SM, Skolnick P, Gallager DW (1980) Receptors for the age of anxiety: pharmacology of the benzodiazepines. Science 207:274–281
Weingartner H, Langer D, Grice J, Rapoport J (1982) Acquisition and retrieval of information in amphetamine-treated hyperactive children. Psychiatry Res 6:21–29
Weingartner H, Bushsbaum M, Linnoila M (1984) Zimelidine effects on memory impairments produced by ethanol. Life Sci 33:2159–2163
Young LR, Sheena D (1975) Eye-movement measurement techniques. Am Psychologist 30:315–330

Correlating Pharmacokinetics and Pharmacodynamics of Benzodiazepines: Problems and Assumptions

D. J. GREENBLATT, H. L. FRIEDMAN, and R. I. SHADER

1 Introduction

The development of reliable and specific methods for quantitation of benzodiazepine derivatives in body fluids has led to the accumulation of considerable knowledge of their pharmacokinetic properties in humans and in other species (Klotz et al. 1980; Guentert 1984; Greenblatt et al. 1983a, b; Greenblatt and Shader 1985a). These data include the kinetic properties in healthy individuals, the influence of physiologic states and disease processes on benzodiazepine disposition, and alterations in kinetics due to drug interactions. The study of benzodiazepine pharmacokinetics has elucidated much about the general mechanisms controlling the biotransformation of foreign chemicals, and factors influencing drug disposition.

An understanding of the kinetic properties of benzodiazepines assumes even greater medical and scientific interest when the data are of value for the understanding of individual variability in clinical response to these drugs. Unfortunately, the relation of benzodiazepine plasma concentrations and pharmacokinetics to clinical pharmacodynamic response is less well understood. This is partly attributable to the intrinsic difficulties of quantitating the clinical response to centrally acting compounds such as benzodiazepines. Such responses include reduction in anxiety, alteration in sleep pattern, alterations in alertness (fatigue, drowsiness), changes in motor function and reaction time, impairment (or improvement) in intellectual function, and alterations in memory and recall. These variables may be difficult to quantitate reliably and replicably, thereby complicating attempts to relate kinetic variables or plasma drug concentrations to clinical response. Other problems complicating the interpretation of the kinetic-dynamic relationship arise from some pharmacokinetic principles that are not intuitively obvious. This paper reviews some basic and clinical pharmacokinetic properties of the benzodiazepines that are pertinent to the methodology and interpretation of studies relating benzodiazepine disposition to the time-course of central effects in the living organism.

Division of Clinical Pharmacology, Departments of Psychiatry and Medicine, Tufts University School of Medicine and New England Medical Center Hospital, Boston, MA 0211, USA.

Clinical Pharmacology in Psychiatry
Editors: Dahl, Gram, Paul, Potter
(Psychopharmacology Series 3)

2 Primary Assumptions

For plasma concentrations and/or pharmacokinetic properties of benzodiazepines to be useful for our understanding of pharmacodynamics, a series of fundamental conditions must be satisfied (Friedman and Greenblatt 1985; Koch-Weser 1972). These conditions are similar to those needed for plasma concentrations or kinetic properties of other classes of drugs – such as digitalis glycosides, antiarrhythmics, anticonvulsants, aminoglycoside antibiotics, analgesics, or lithium salts – for them to have clinical utility. First, the free (unbound) concentration of drug in plasma must diffuse freely and reversibly to the extravascular tissue which contains the functional receptor site mediating the drug's pharmacologic action. The receptor site concentration must also be proportional to the unbound concentration in plasma so that a rise or fall in free plasma concentration will cause a proportionate rise or fall in the concentration at the receptor site. Second, the drug concentration at the site of action must parallel its clinical effect. As the receptor site concentration rises from low to intermediate to high, so the intensity of clinical action changes proportionally. Finally, there must be a reasonably close time relationship between the receptor site concentration and the clinical effect of the drug. That is, the occurrence of changes in the intensity of clinical action caused by changes in drug concentration must be approximately parallel in time. The benzodiazepines appear to fulfill some but not all of these fundamental requisites.

3 Pharmacokinetic Facts

3.1 Tissue Uptake of Benzodiazepines

The brain is the principal pharmacologic site of benzodiazepine activity, and its pharmacodynamic effects are necessarily mediated by interaction with one or more molecular recognition sites located in brain tissue. This recognition site will be referred to as the functional benzodiazepine receptor. This functional receptor site is widely assumed to correspond to the specific benzodiazepine binding site reported to be present in brain tissue of animals and humans (Skolnick and Paul 1982; Müller 1981). While this specific binding site may be identical to the functional benzodiazepine receptor that actually mediates benzodiazepine action, this correspondence has not yet been proven. Therefore, we caution that all subsequent references to a benzodiazepine receptor require this qualification.

Because this receptor site is in any case located within brain tissue, the extent of benzodiazepine uptake into brain must be an important determinant of the amount of drug available to interact with the receptor. The extent of entry of benzodiazepines into brain tissue appears to be a process governed mainly by passive diffusion, with the partitioning between brain and systemic plasma related at least in part to the lipophilicity or lipid solubility of the particular benzodiazepine. Two methods used for in vitro quantitation of benzodiazepine lipophilicity are: (a) the partitioning of drugs between an aqueous buffer at physiologic pH and an organic solvent (usually octanol); and (b) the evaluation of retention on a reverse-phase high-pressure liquid chromatographic (HPLC) system. One or both of these in vitro indexes can explain a significant portion of the variability among the benzodiazepines as to the extent of their uptake into brain tissue relative to any given unbound plasma concentration (Arendt et al. 1983; Greenblatt et al. 1983c; Friedman et al. 1985a; Greenblatt and Arendt 1985). Similar relationships may be found when benzodiazepine uptake into other tissues is examined, whether in experimental studies or in human autopsy studies (Friedman et al. 1985a, b). In interpretation of the extent of drug uptake into tissue considerable importance attaches to the extent of serum or plasma protein binding, since it is only the unbound fraction that is available for uptake and distribution into peripheral tissues such as brain (Greenblatt et al. 1982).

Thus, the findings currently available indicate that benzodiazepine availability to the target tissue occurs as a result of passive diffusion and that the unbound drug concentration in plasma is proportional to the amount present in brain (Friedman et al. 1985c).

3.2 Rate of Equilibration

Not only is the extent of benzodiazepine uptake into brain determined by predictable physicochemical properties, but the rate of uptake and equilibration is very rapid. The rapidity of this equilibration has been demonstrated in a number of studies directed at quantitation of: (a) actual measurement of the relative time-course of benzodiazepine concentrations in brain and plasma following single doses in animals (Friedman et al. 1985c; Hironaka et al. 1984; Igari et al. 1982); (b) the entry of drug and subsequent equilibration with the cerebrospinal fluid (Greenblatt et al. 1980; Arendt et al. 1983; Ramsay et al. 1979) (Fig. 1); and (c) the

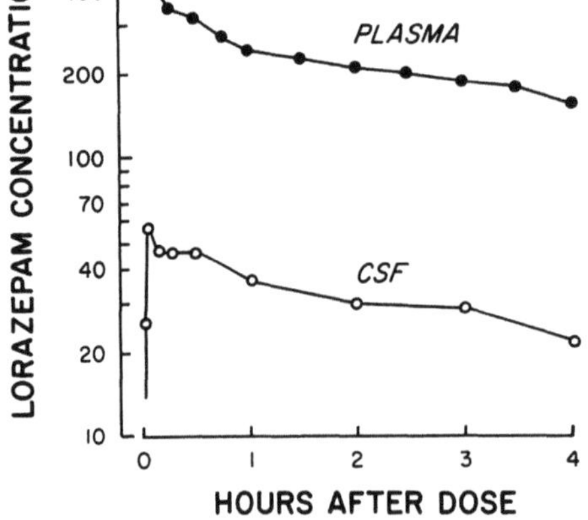

Fig. 1. Plasma and cerebrospinal fluid (CSF) concentrations of lorazepam in an experimental animal following a single dose of 0.5 mg/kg i.v. The study demonstrates the rapid entry of drug into CSF. (See Arendt et al. 1983)

rapidity of onset of pharmacodynamic activity of benzodiazepines when measured by objective techniques such as the appearance of characteristic electroencephalographic activity (Arendt et al. 1983) or alterations in saccadic eye movement velocity (Tedeschi et al. 1983). Some studies suggest that, although the onset of activity of all benzodiazepines is rapid following single i.v. injections, the small variability in time of onset of action may be explained by differences in their lipophilicity (Tedeschi et al. 1983).

Thus benzodiazepine equilibration between systemic plasma and brain tissue is rapid.

3.3 Disappearance of Drug from Blood and Brain

Disparities between benzodiazepine plasma concentration and clinical effect have sometimes been attributed to a possible differential time-course of drug disappearance from these two sites (Müller and Stillbauer 1983; Paul et al. 1979). However, there is virtually no experimental data to support this suggestion. A carefully controlled study evaluating the rate of benzodiazepine disappearance from systemic plasma in relation to the disappearance rate from brain tissue demonstrated no difference in the rate of drug disappearance from these sites (Friedman et al. 1985c). Once distribution equilibrium is attained, the drug disappears from all body compartments in parallel. This is consistent with accepted pharmacokinetic theory, based on the assumption that processes of drug distribution and clearance are first-order phenomena. Thus, currently available data do not support the idea that any tissue, including the brain, preferentially "retains" benzodiazepines. In fact, the rate of drug disappearance from plasma equals the rate of disappearance from all tissues after the attainment of distribution equilibrium.

4 Pharmacokinetics and Pharmacodynamics

4.1 The Pharmacodynamic Role of Drug Distribution

Derived kinetic variables rather than actual plasma concentrations are often used in an attempt to explain the pharmacodynamic profile of a given benzodiazepine derivative. The most common of these is the elimination half-life determined from the plasma concentration curve (Ansseau et al. 1984). An apparent "paradox" is that the elimination half-life of a benzodiazepine derivative may bear no relationship to the time course of decrement of its clinical effect following single doses (George and Dundee 1977; Conner et al. 1978; Arendt et al. 1983). This observation, while generally correct, is not really a paradox, but rather is consistent with the pharmacokinetic profile of many benzodiazepines. Because all these drugs are lipophilic substances, their plasma concentration profile following single doses – particularly single rapid i.v. injections – has a biphasic profile (Greenblatt and Shader 1985b). The initial rapid and precipitous phase of drug distribution from plasma is attributed to drug distribution from the central compartment (including brain) to peripheral compartments. The extent of peripheral distribution of unbound drug (as determined by volume of distribution) increases as benzodiazepines become increasingly lipophilic (Greenblatt et al. 1983c; Arendt et al. 1983). For a highly lipid-soluble benzodiazepine, such as diazepam, the initial decrement in plasma concentrations following a single i.v. dose may actually cause a five- to tenfold decline in plasma concentrations over the first 30 min to 3 h after dosage, as the drug egresses from the "central compartment" into peripheral tissues, particularly fat, skeletal muscle, and liver (Fig. 2 and 3). This phase of drug distribution can lead to termination of clinical effects, depending on which pharmacodynamic variable is under evaluation and how it is being quantitated. The drug's apparent elimination half-life is a much slower phase, which is determinable only after the distribution phase is complete (Greenblatt 1985). Diazepam distribution rather than elimination is the major determinant of its pharmacodynamic profile following a single dose (Conner et al. 1978). It is not surprising, therefore, that diazepam's elimination half-life is not related to the time-course of its effects following single doses. Drugs with long half-lives may actually have very short durations of action after single doses, because of their very extensive distribution.

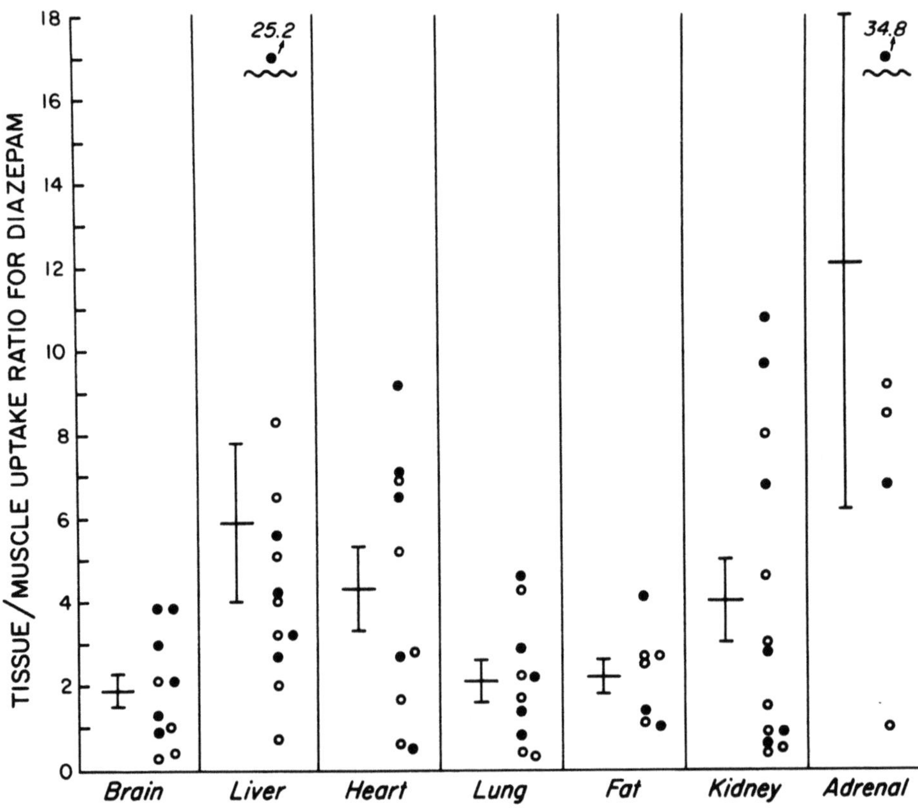

Fig. 2. Ratio of tissue to skeletal muscle concentrations of diazepam in a human autopsy study of diazepam distribution. For each tissue, individual and mean (±SE) ratio values are shown. *Closed circles* are values for male patients; *open circles* are those for female patients. (See Friedman et al. 1985b)

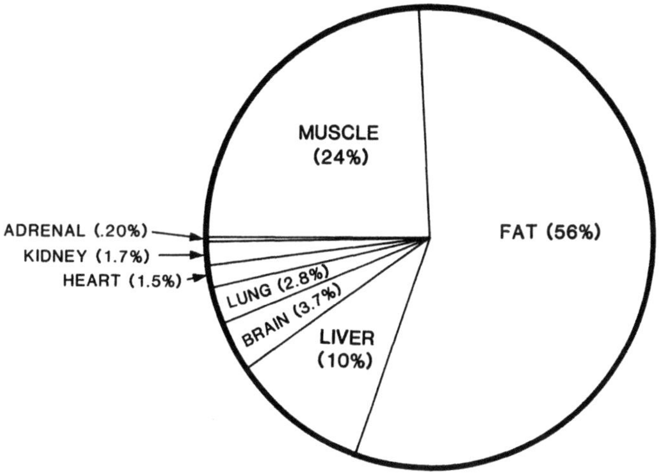

Fig. 3. The mean distribution patterns documented in Fig. 2 were used to estimate the relative fraction of total-body stores of diazepam present in various tissues for a normal human woman in whom 30% of her body weight was accounted for by adipose tissue. The findings demonstrate that the largest fractions of the total-body store of diazepam are present in adipose tissue and skeletal muscle

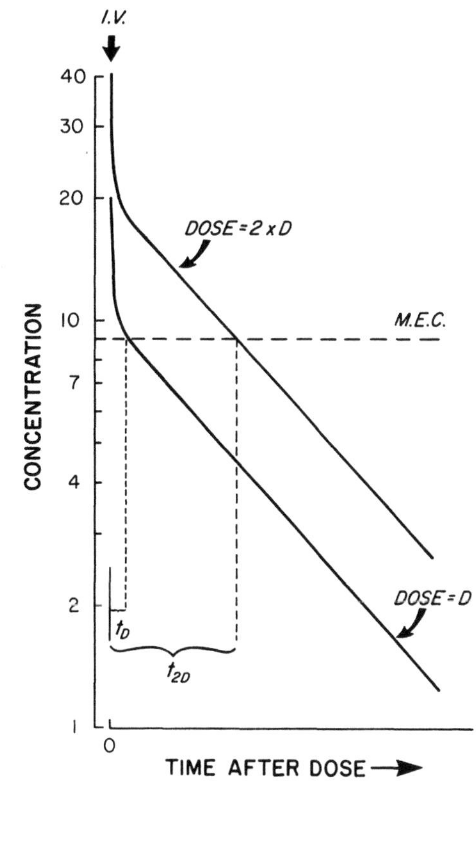

Fig. 4. Influence of dose on the duration of pharmacodynamic action of a drug following i.v. injection. It is assumed that the pattern of drug disappearance following i.v. administration is consistent with a two-compartment model, leading to a "bi-phasic" plasma concentration profile. The minimum effective concentration (MEC) necessary to produce pharmacodynamic activity is assumed to be 9 concentration units. After the lower dose (D) the duration of action is short (T_D), because the initial phase of drug distribution causes the concentration to fall below the MEC. Increasing the dose by a factor of two (2 x D) causes a disproportionate increase in the duration of action (t_{2D}), because the distribution phase is completed before concentrations fall below the MEC. This scheme demonstrates that duration of pharmacodynamic action is not necessarily proportional to dose for a drug that undergoes substantial tissue distribution

From this pharmacokinetic model it follows that proportional increments or decrements in dosage may not cause a corresponding proportional change in the duration of pharmacodynamic activity. Since the clearance of benzodiazepines within the therapeutic dosage range is concentration-independent, pharmacokinetic parameters such as the area under the plasma concentration curve and peak level are directly proportional to dosage, and highly predictable for a given individual. However, because of the important role played by distribution in the termination of drug action, an upward increment of dosage may lead to a disproportionate prolongation of clinical effects (Fig. 4).

4.2 The Tolerance Factor

The benzodiazepines as a class of drugs are notorious for their capacity to produce adaptation or tolerance to a number of their central actions (File 1985; Smith et al. 1984; Ellinwood et al. 1985; Greenblatt and Shader 1978). The precise molecular mechanisms of tolerance are not fully understood, but the phenomenon can be operationally described as a reduction in the intensity of pharmacologic effect of a drug resulting from a prior exposure to that drug or to a related drug.

Many studies demonstrate tolerance to benzodiazepines following chronic dosage, as well as acute tolerance following single doses (Smith et al. 1984; Ochs et al. 1983; Greenblatt et al. 1979, 1981). It is likely that tolerance develops to different central actions of benzodiazepines at different rates, and that for any given central effect different benzodiazepines may show different rates of inducing tolerance (Ellinwood et al. 1985). Tolerance phenomena complicate attempts to relate benzodiazepine concentrations to effect, and indicate that duration of drug exposure must clearly be considered in studies of this type.

4.3 Within- Versus Between-Individual Variation

Evaluation of the relationship of plasma concentration to clinical effect of benzodiazepines within the same individual, as opposed to among different individuals, poses different methodologic problems. For any given individual, one can assess the concentration-response relationship following single doses by concurrent measurement at multiple time points of plasma concentration and response, both of which will change with time. A second approach is to administer different doses of the same benzodiazepine to the same individual on different occasions. At a fixed point in time following each dose, both concentration and response can be evaluated. The first approach has the advantage that between-trial variability in response is minimized. On the other hand, acute tolerance usually will have a significant influence on the concentration-response relationship. Typically, drug effects such as sedation, impairment of performance, or alteration in saccadic eye movement velocity are altered shortly after administration of the dose, but they recover to baseline long before plasma (and presumably brain) concentrations fall to zero (Smith et al. 1984; Greenblatt et al. 1979; Ellinwood et al. 1985; Bittencourt et al. 1981). The second methodologic approach minimizes effects of acute tolerance, in that effects are consistently measured at a fixed time point after each dose. Using this design, the relative contribution of acute tolerance should be similar from trial to trial. The effect of chronic tolerance, however, is unknown. In addition, there may be inherent between-trial variability in the pattern of response, as well as practice or learning effects on some or all of the clinical tasks evaluated. Thus, both approaches have their benefits and disadvantages, and each study design may yield a different concentration-response relationship.

Evaluation of concentration-effect relationships among different individuals is an exceedingly difficult problem, even after single doses of benzodiazepines. Under rigorously controlled study conditions, different individuals may have inherently different benzodiazepine "sensitivity," yielding markedly different slopes of a hypothetical concentration-effect relationship. Furthermore, tolerance may develop at different rates in different individuals.

Space limitations preclude discussion of the numerous factors known to influence benzodiazepine pharmacokinetics and/or clinical response. A few of these are: old age, other disease states, drug interactions, obesity, and cigarette smoking (Greenblatt et al. 1983 a, b; Greenblatt and Shader 1985 b).

5 Comment

Despite the inherent problems in relating benzodiazepine plasma concentrations and pharmacokinetics to measures of clinical outcome, important methodologic advances have been made in recent years. Improved methodologic approaches, combining principles of clinical pharmacokinetics with more sophisticated approaches to quantitating clinical outcome and increasing understanding of molecular receptor phenomena, should yield meaningful answers to these difficult problems.

Acknowledgements. The work described in this paper was supported in part by grants MH-34223 and AG-00106 from the US Public Health Service.

We are grateful for the collaboration and assistance of D. R. Abernethy, H. R. Ochs, R. M. Arendt, J. M. Scavone, M. K. Divoll, J. S. Harmatz, and A. Locniskar.

References

Annseau M, Doumont A, von Frenckell R, Collard J (1984) Duration of benzodiazepine clinical activity: Lack of direct relationship with plasma half-life. Psychopharmacology (Berlin) 84:293–298

Arendt RM, Greenblatt DJ, deJong RH et al. (1983) In vitro correlates of benzodiazepine cerebrospinal fluid uptake, pharmacodynamic action, and peripheral distribution. J Pharmacol Exp Ther 227:95–106

Bittencourt PRM, Wade P, Smith AT, Richens A (1981) The relationship between peak velocity of saccadic eye movements and serum benzodiazepine concentration. Br J Clin Pharmacol 12:523–533

Conner JT, Katz RL, Bellville JW, Graham C, Pagano R, Dorey F (1978) Diazepam and lorazepam for intravenous surgical premedication. J Clin Pharmacol 18:285–292

Ellinwood EH, Heatherly DG, Nikaido AM, Bjornsson TD, Kilts C (1985) Comparative pharmacokinetics and pharmacodynamics of lorazepam, alprazolam and diazepam. Psychopharmacology (Berlin) 86:392–399

File SE (1985) Tolerance to the behavioral actions of benzodiazepines. Neurosci Biobehav Rev 9:113–121
Friedman HL, Greenblatt DJ (1985) Rational therapeutic drug monitoring (submitted for publication)
Friedman HL, Scavone JM, Greenblatt DJ, Shader RI (1985a) Effect of age and body composition on benzodiazepine distribution in rats. Pharmacologist 27:207
Friedman H, Ochs HR, Greenblatt DJ, Shader RI (1985b) Tissue distribution of diazepam and its metabolite desmethyldiazepam: a human autopsy study. J Clin Pharmacol (in press)
Friedman H, Abernethy DR, Greenblatt DJ, Shader RI (1985c) The pharmacokinetics of diazepam and desmethyldiazepam in rat brain and plasma. Psychopharmacology (Berlin), (in press)
George KA, Dundee JW (1977) Relative amnesic actions of diazepam, flunitrazepam and lorazepam in man. Br J Clin Pharmacol 4:45–50
Greenblatt DJ (1985) Elimination half-life of drugs: value and limitations. Ann Rev Med 36:421–427
Greenblatt DJ, Arendt RM (1985) Lipid solubility and brain uptake of benzodiazepines. Pharmacologist 27:207
Greenblatt DJ, Shader RI (1978) Dependence, tolerance, and addiction to benzodiazepines: clinical and pharmacokinetic considerations. Drug Metab Rev 8:13–28
Greenblatt DJ, Shader RI (1985a) Clinical pharmacokinetics of the benzodiazepines. In: Smith DE, Wesson DR (eds) The Benzodiazepines: current standards for medical practice. MTP Press, Lancaster, p 43–58
Greenblatt DJ, Shader RI (1985b) Pharmacokinetics in clinical practice. Saunders, Philadelphia
Greenblatt DJ, Shader RI, Harmatz JS, Georgotas A (1979) Self-rated sedation and plasma concentrations of desmethyldiazepam following single doses of clorazepate. Psychopharmacology (Berlin) 66:289–290
Greenblatt DJ, Ochs HR, Lloyd BL (1980) Entry of diazepam and its major metabolite into cerebrospinal fluid. Psychopharmacology (Berlin) 70:89–93
Greenblatt DJ, Divoll M, Harmatz JS, MacLaughlin DS, Shader RI (1981) Kinetics and clinical effects of flurazepam in young and elderly noninsomniacs. Clin Pharmacol Ther 30:475–486
Greenblatt DJ, Sellers EM, Koch-Weser J (1982) Importance of protein binding for the interpretation of serum or plasma drug concentration. J Clin Pharmacol 22:259–263
Greenblatt DJ, Shader RI, Abernethy DR (1983a) Current status of benzodiazepines. N Engl J Med 309:354–358, 410–416
Greenblatt DJ, Divoll M, Abernethy DR, Ochs HR, Shader RI (1983b) Benzodiazepine kinetics: implications for therapeutics and pharmacogeriatrics. Drug Metab Rev 14:251–292
Greenblatt DJ, Arendt RM, Abernethy DR et al. (1983c) In vitro quantitation of benzodiazepine lipophilicity: relation to in vivo distribution. Br J Anaesth 55:985–989
Guentert TW (1984) Pharmacokinetics of benzodiazepines and of their metabolites. Prog Drug Metab 8:241–386
Hironaka T, Fuchino K, Fujii T (1984) Absorption of diazepam and its transfer through the blood brain barrier after intraperitoneal administration in the rat. J Pharmacol Exp Ther 229:809–815
Igari Y, Sugiyama Y, Sawada Y et al. (1982) Tissue distribution of ^{14}C-Diazepam and its metabolites in rats. Drug Metab Dispos 10:676–679
Klotz U, Kangas L, Kanto J (1980) Clinical pharmacokinetics of benzodiazepines. Prog Pharmacol 3:1–72
Koch-Weser J (1972) Serum drug concentrations as therapeutic guides. N Engl J Med 287:227–231
Müller WE (1981) The benzodiazepine receptor: an update. Pharmacology 22:153–161
Müller WE, Stillbauer AE (1983) Benzodiazepine hypnotics: time course and potency of benzodiazepine receptor occupation after oral application. Pharmacol Biochem Behav 18:545–549
Ochs HR, Greenblatt DJ, Eckardt B, Harmatz JS, Shader RI (1983) Repeated diazepam dosing in cirrhotic patients: cumulation and sedation. Clin Pharmacol Ther 33:471–476

Paul SM, Syapin PJ, Paugh BA et al. (1979) Correlation between benzodiazepine receptor occupation and anticonvulsant effects of diazepam. Nature 281:688–689
Ramsay RE, Hammond EJ, Perchalski RJ et al. (1979) Brain uptake of phenytoin, phenobarbital, and diazepam. Arch Neurol 36:535–539
Skolnick P, Paul SM (1982) Benzodiazepine receptors in the central nervous system. Int Rev Neurobiol 23:103–140
Smith RB, Kroboth PD, Vanderlugt JT, Phillips JP, Juhl RP (1984) Pharmacokinetics and pharmacodynamics of alprazolam after oral and IV administration. Psychopharmacology (Berlin) 84:452–456
Tedeschi G, Smith AT, Dhillon S, Richens A (1983) Rate of entrance of benzodiazepines into the brain determined by eye movement recording. Br J Clin Pharmacol 15:103–107

Benzodiazepine-Serotonin Interactions in Man

D. J. NUTT[1] and P. J. COWEN[2]

1 Introduction

It is well established that the benzodiazepines (BDZs) act at specific receptor sites in the CNS and modulate the inhibitory effects of GABA (see Olsen 1981). Which other neurotransmitters are secondarily affected is less clear, though changes in monoamine function have been demonstrated in numerous animal studies (Fuxe et al. 1975; Rostogi et al. 1976). These studies used high doses of BDZs, although some more recent investigations have used doses that are more relevant to the clinical, anxiolytic/anticonvulsant effects than the sedative/anesthetic ones. For instance, Collinge et al. (1983) showed that low doses of BDZ reduced 5HT turnover in the rat. This effect persisted for at least 3 weeks.

In view of these claims that BDZs may exert some of their effect via alterations of 5HT transmission, we have attempted to demonstrate whether BDZs alter 5HT function in man. To this end we used the L-tryptophan (LTP) infusion challenge test. LTP given i.v. has been shown to release prolactin in man (Charney et al. 1982), and in our studies it also reliably stimulates growth hormone (GH) release (Cowen et al. 1985). In addition, it produces sedation or sleepiness, which is easily assessed on self-rating scales. Although it is not yet certain that these responses are mediated by a direct increase in 5HT function by LTP (see Cowen and Anderson 1986), the test is the most convenient presently available.

2 Methods

Seven fit drug-free males (20–35 years) were tested. They gave informed consent and were low consumers of alcohol. All were given three LTP tests according to the method of Cowen et al. (1985). Briefly, 110 mg/kg^{-1} LTP was administered as a 10 g/liter solution in 0.5% saline over 25 min. Subjects had bloodsamples taken via butterfly cannula at 15-min intervals for 1 h before and 2 h after the infusion. Visual analogue sedation scores were assessed at 15 min before the infusion and at +30, +60, +90 after the infusion. Prolactin and GH levels were determined by radioimmunoassay. All tests were done between 09.00 and 12.00 h. Subjects had fasted from midnight. They were recumbent throughout the test.

[1] Department of Psychiatry, Warneford Hospital, Oxford, England.
[2] MRC Clinical Pharmacology Unit, Littlemore Hospital, Oxford, England.

Clinical Pharmacology in Psychiatry
Editors: Dahl, Gram, Paul, Potter
(Psychopharmacology Series 3)

LTP tests were performed before any treatment (pre) and then both after a single dose of 15 mg diazepam taken the night before (acute) and after about 3 weeks of administration of 25 mg diazepam/day in divided doses (chronic).

3 Results

Prediazepam LTP-induced neuroendocrine responses in these subjects were essentially the same as for the normal population studied previously (Cowen et al. 1985). Acute diazepam treatment markedly attenuated both GH and prolactin responses (Fig. 1 a, b). Both AUC and peak responses were reduced for both hormones. Although after acute diazepam pre-LTP sedation scores were slightly elevated, this was not significant. The increase in sedation (Δ sedation) produced by LTP was unaltered compared with pre-LTP sedation (Table 1).

After chronic administration of diazepam different findings emerged. Neither prolactin nor GH responses were different from values before the tests (Fig. 1).

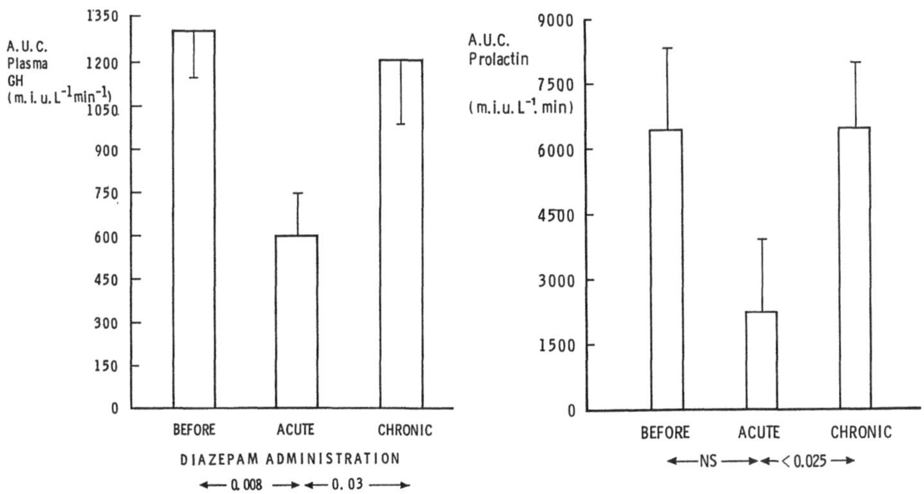

Fig. 1. Effects of acute and chronic diazepam administration on growth hormone (GH) and prolactin responses to LTP. Histograms show means ($\pm$SEM) for AUCs. Comparisons by paired *t*-test

Table 1. Effect of diazepam on LTP sedation

Diazepam	Before LTP[a]	Peak response[a]	Δ Sedation[a]
Pretreatment	25 (0– 6)	65 (50– 80)	40 (20–50)
Acute	42 (0–70)	82 (60–100)	40 (0–70)
Chronic	31 (0–60)	76 (50– 95)	45 (20–70)

[a] Numbers are mean scores (mm) on a 100-mm line marked from 0 – "I feel not at all sleepy" – to 100 – "I feel extremly sleepy". (Numbers in brackets are ranges of individual scores.)

Table 2. Plasma diazepam and desmethyldiazepam levels

	Diazepam treatment		
	Acute	Chronic	*P* value
Diazepam	110 ± 9	355 ± 30	<0.001
Desmethyldiazepam	60 ± 20	655 ± 102	<0.001

Means ± SEM of total plasma drug.

Both hormones showed significantly increased AUC and peak responses compared with those after acute medication. At no time point before the LTP infusion were basal prolactin or GH levels significantly elevated above the pre-test levels after either the acute or the chronic treatment.

Chronic diazepam did not alter basal sedation scores (Table 1). Similarly, the LTP-induced increase in sedation was unaltered.

Plasma diazepam and desmethyl diazepam levels were measured by HPLC. As can be seen from Table 2 they were significantly greater in the chronic phase.

4 Discussion

Four main findings emerge from this study:
1. Acute diazepam attenuates LTP neuroendocrine responses.
2. Chronic administration of diazepam does not attenuate LTP neuroendocrine responses despite much higher levels of drug. This suggests tolerance has developed with the acute treatment.
3. These quite high doses of diazepam do not significantly alter subjective levels of sedation measured prior to LTP infusion.
4. Neither acute nor chronic diazepam affects LTP sedation.

The effect of acute diazepam is perhaps a little unexpected, given that benzodiazepines have been reported to release GH (Kannan 1981). However, with diazepam this is only seen when the drug is given i.v., and it is a fairly unpredictable phenomenon even then (Hommer et al. 1986; R. Dorow 1985, personal communication).

The acute findings are consistent with the animal data showing a reduction of 5HT turnover with acute benzodiazepines, since LTP is presumably metabolised to 5HT. They contrast with the claims that tolerance to this effect does not occur (Collinge et al. 1983). The mechanism of this tolerance development is unclear, but may include changes in 5HT function. For instance, Green et al. (1985) have shown that 14 days of diazepam treatment in mice enhances 5HT-induced head twitch and increases $5HT_2$ receptor numbers. An alternative explanation is offered by our findings that in these subjects chronic diazepam reduced platelet [^{3}H]imipramine binding Bmax (Nutt et al. 1985). If such a change occurred in the brain then it would have to magnify the effects of reduced 5HT and so would tend to offset a presynaptic shutdown of production. Perhaps the most likely explanation is that tolerance has occurred at the BDZ receptor complex, perhaps by way of a change in drug efficacy (Little et al. 1984) or compensatory alterations in GABA function (see Cowen and Nutt 1982; Gallager et al. 1984).

The lack of effect of either acute or chronic diazepam on either sedation or LTP sedation is interesting. The fact that basal sedation was unaltered shows tolerance development to the effect, as has been reported by others (Greenblatt et al. 1978) and is well recognised clinically. The failure of diazepam to alter LTP-induced sedation may argue against this being 5HT-mediated. It is interesting that in vitro LTP is a weak ligand for BDZ receptors (Marangos et al. 1981). If its sedative effects in vivo were similarly mediated they might be expected to be attenuated by the much higher affinity ligand diazepam. Since LTP sedation was not altered, this strongly argues against BDZ receptor involvement in this effect of LTP.

Acknowledgements. This work was supported by the Wellcome Trust and Masons Trust. Roche (UK) gave additional help. We thank M. Franklin, S. Fraser, P. Murdock, and B. Gosden for technical help, and Di Disley for expert nursing care. D. J. N. is a Wellcome Senior Fellow in Clinical Science.

References

Charney DS, Heninger GR, Renhard JF, Sternberg DE, Hafstead KM (1982) Effect of intravenous L-tryptophan on prolactin and growth hormone and mood in healthy subjects. Psychopharmacology (Berlin) 77:217–222

Collinge J, Pycock CJ, Taberner PV (1983) Studies on the interaction between cerebral 5-hydroxytryptamine and gammaaminobutyric acid in the mode of action of diazepam in the rat. Br J Pharmacol 79:637–643

Cowen PJ, Anderson IM (1986) 5-HT neuroendocrinology: changes during depressive illness and antidepressant drug treatment. Br J Psychiatry (in press)

Cowen PJ, Nutt DJ (1982) Abstinence symptoms after withdrawal of tranquillizing drugs: is there a common neurochemical mechanism? Lancet 2:360–362

Cowen PJ, Gadhvi H, Gosden B, Kolakowska T (1985) Responses of prolactin and growth hormone to L-tryptophan infusion: effects in normal subjects and schizophrenic patients receiving neuroleptics. Psychopharmacology (Berlin) 86:164–169

Fuxe K, Agnati LF, Bolme P, Hokfelt T, Lidbrink P, Ljungdahl A, Perez-de-la-Mora M, Ogren S (1975) The possible involvement of GABA mechanisms in the action of benzodiazepines on central catecholamine neurons. Adv Biochem Psychopharmacol 14:45–61

Gallager DW, Lakoski JM, Gonsalves SF, Rauch SL (1984) Chronic benzodiazepine treatment decreases postsynaptic GABA sensitivity. Nature 308:74–77

Green AR, Johnson P, Mountford JA, Nimgoankar VC (1985) Some anticonvulsant drugs alter monoamine-mediated behaviours in mice in ways similar to electroconvulsive shock: implications for antidepressant therapy. Br J Pharmacol 84:337–346

Greenblatt DJ, Woo E, Allen MD, Orsulak PJ, Shader RI (1978) Rapid recovery from massive diazepam overdose. JAMA 240:1872–1874

Hommer DW, Matsuo V, Wolkowitz O, Chrousos G, Greenblatt DJ, Weingartner H, Paul SM (1986) Benzodiazepine sensitivity in normal human subjects. Arch Gen Psychiatry 43:542–551

Kannan V (1981) Diazepam test of growth hormone secretion. Horm Metab Res 13:390–393

Little HJ, Nutt DJ, Taylor SC (1984) Selective potentiation of the effects of a benzodiazepine contragonist after chronic flurazepam treatment in mice. Br J Pharmacol 83:360

Marangos PJ, Patel J, Hirata F, Sondheim D, Paul SM, Skolnich P, Goodwin FK (1981) Inhibition of diazepam binding by tryptophan derivatives including melatonin and its brain metabolite N-acetyl-5-methoxy kynureamine. Life Sci 29:259–267
Nutt DJ, Fraser S, Gosden B, Stump K, Elliott JM (1985) Benzodiazepines and human platelet receptor binding. Br J Clin Pharmacol 19:554–555
Olsen RW (1981) GABA-benzodiazepine-barbiturate receptor interactions. J Neurochem 37:1–13
Rastogi RB, Lapierre YD, Singhal RL (1976) Evidence for the role of brain norepinephrine and dopamine in "rebound" phenomena seen during withdrawal after repeated exposure to benzodiazepines. J Psychiatr Res 13:65–75

Comparative Pharmacodynamics of Benzodiazepines

E. H. ELLINWOOD, Jr., A. M. NIKAIDO, and D. G. HEATHERLY

1 Introduction

Dispositional pharmacokinetics have been shown to have little relationship to drug effects after acute doses of certain benzodiazepines (Ellinwood et al. 1983, 1985; Lader 1979; Ziegler et al. 1983). For diazepam the rapid onset of acute tolerance follows the peak behavioral effect; that is, impairment of performance in cognitive-neuromotor tests declines considerably faster than the corresponding serum drug concentration (Ellinwood et al. 1983, 1985). Other studies have described a relatively short period of impairment for high single doses of diazepam (George and Dundee 1977) and a more prolonged period of impairment for lorazepam (Seppala et al. 1976), although the elimination half-lives ($t_{1/2}$) of diazepam and its active metabolite *N*-desmethyldiazepam (Mandelli et al. 1978) are over twice as long as that of lorazepam, which has no active metabolites.

Potential sources of variability in drug-induced impairment include (a) acute peak effects in part secondary to lipid solubility; (b) acute tolerance; (c) drug distribution and elimination kinetics; (d) benzodiazepine receptor kinetics reflecting differential binding and adaptation; and (e) individual differences in sensitivity associated with age, sex, and menstrual cycle. In a series of studies recently completed in our laboratory we were primarily concerned with elucidating the relationship of pharmacokinetic and receptor kinetic processes to impairment. Specifically, we compared the effects of five benzodiazepines on cognitive-neuromotor tasks. These drugs differed in pharmacological characteristics, including lipid solubility, elimination half-life, plasma binding and receptor-binding affinity.

2 Methods

The subjects were healthy males with height-to-weight ratios within 10% of ideal, aged 21–26 years in the first two studies and 21–30 years in the third study. A single oral dose of lorazepam, alprazolam, diazepam, or placebo was administered every 2 weeks at dosages of 0.057, 0.028, 0.286, or 0.000 mg/kg body weight, respectively, in the first study and at lower doses of 0.028, 0.014, 0.143, or 0.000 mg/kg, respectively, in the second study. Placebo and two doses each of triazolam (0.5 and 1.0 mg) and quazepam (15 and 30 mg) were given at 3-week intervals in the

Behavioral Neuropharmacology Section, Department of Psychiatry, Box 3870, Duke University Medical Center, Durham, NC 27710, USA.

Clinical Pharmacology in Psychiatry
Editors: Dahl, Gram, Paul, Potter
(Psychopharmacology Series 3)

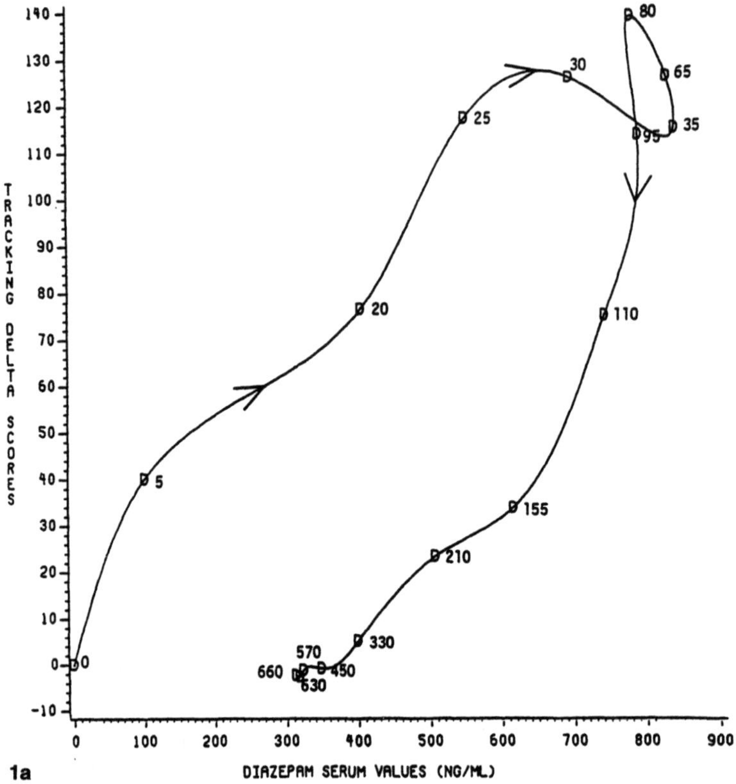
TRACKING DELTA SCORES
DIAZEPAM SERUM VALUES (NG/ML)
0
5
20
25
30
80
65
35
95
110
155
210
330
570
450
660
630

1a

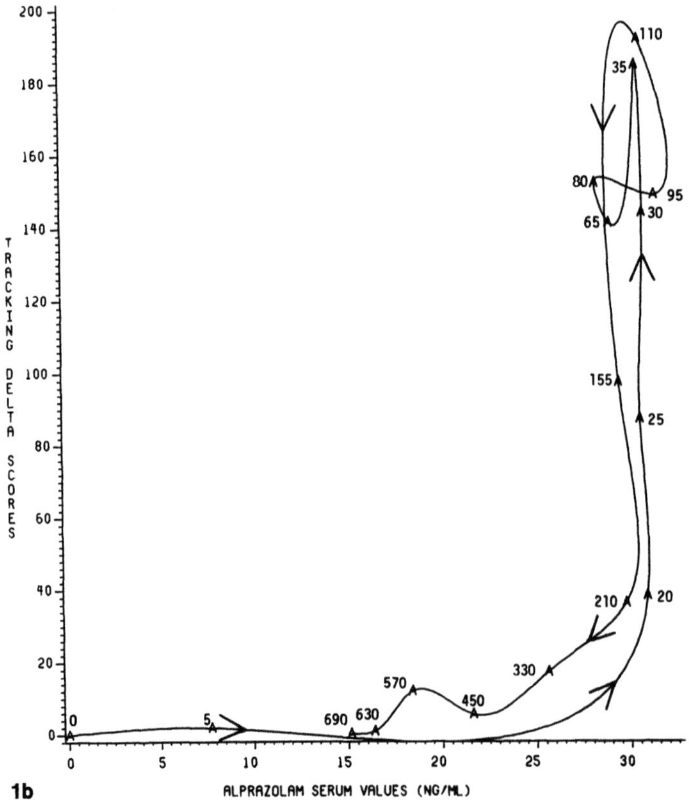
TRACKING DELTA SCORES
ALPRAZOLAM SERUM VALUES (NG/ML)
0
5
690
630
570
450
330
210
20
25
155
30
95
80
65
35
110

1b

third study. Each drug session included a predrug baseline trial followed by drug ingestion and postdrug performance testing at various time intervals over 690-, 330-, and 415-min periods in the first, second, and third studies, respectively. The experimental procedure, test room, apparatus, tasks, and drug assay techniques for diazepam, alprazolam, and lorazepam have been described previously in greater detail by Ellinwood et al. (1985). Drug levels are currently being determined for quazepam and triazolam.

3 Results and Discussion

There was a similar time-course of the drug effect for the lower and higher doses of each drug (Ellinwood et al., unpublished data). However, differences between drugs were also clearly evident when we compared the nature of the relationship

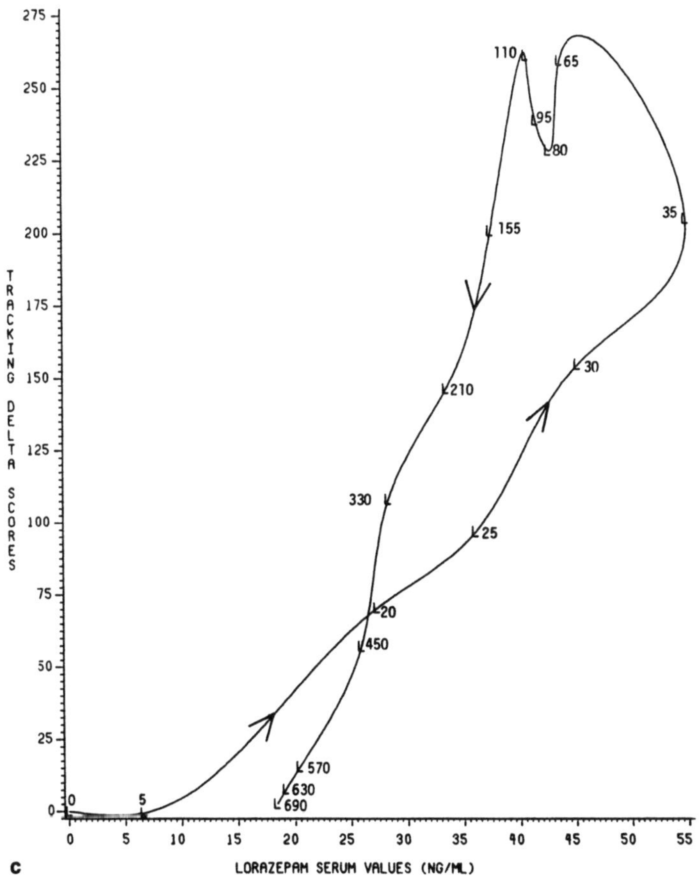

Fig. 1 a–c. Hysteresis curves illustrating the relationship across time between SCT performance and drug serum levels for diazepam (**a**), alprazolam (**b**) and lorazepam (**c**). Performance is expressed as delta scores. *Points* correspond to successive testing time periods, which are indicated as minutes after drug ingestion. *Arrows* show sequence of the observations across time between subcritical tracking (SCT) performance and serum drug concentration during both distribution and elimination phases for the high doses of diazepam, alprazolam, and lorazepam [see Ellinwood et al. (1985) for a more detailed presentation of these results.]

Specifically, acute tolerance was demonstrated with diazepam; greater impairment was manifested at much lower serum concentrations during the onset than during the offset impairment period (Fig. 1 a). On the other hand, with lorazepam there was an impairment onset that lagged behind serum drug rise; in addition, lorazepam had a slower offset of impairment relative to falling serum levels than diazepam (Fig. 1 c). Compared with diazepam and lorazepam, alprazolam had a unique hysteresis profile. Impairment increased steeply between 20 and 35 min and was followed by a very precipitous improvement in performance from 110–210 min, while serum levels remained within a narrow range from 28–31 ng/ml (Fig. 1 b).

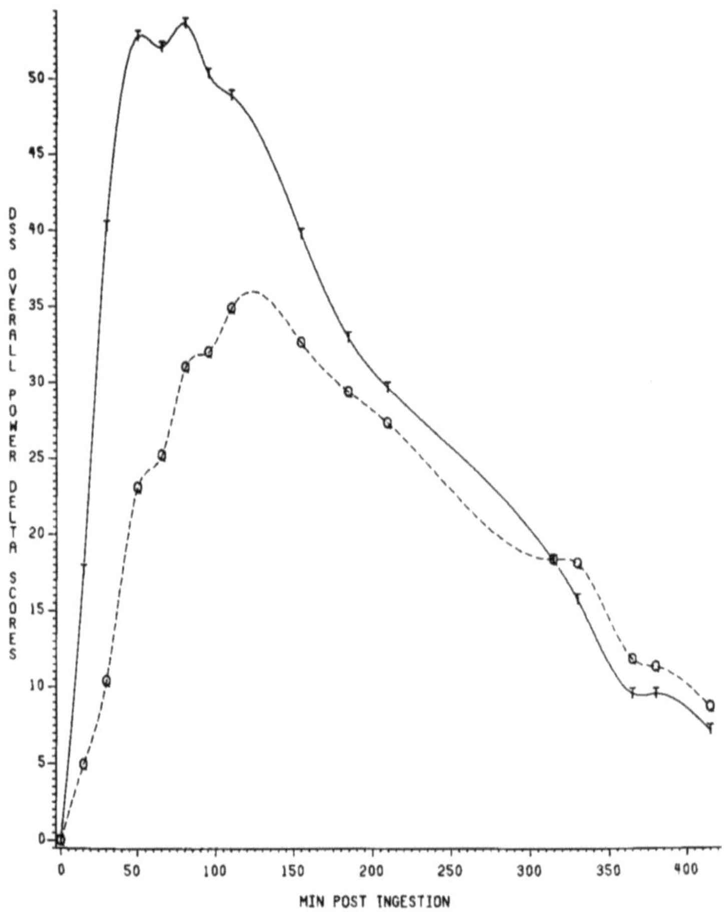

Fig. 2. DSS impairment over time for quazepam (*Q*) and triazolam (*T*). Doses for quazepam and triazolam were 30 mg and 0.5 mg, respectively. Performance is represented as unit changes from the predrug score. A smooth spline-fitting procedure was used to connect all time points.

Preliminary analyses have been completed for the third study examining the behavioral effects of (a) triazolam, an ultrashort $t_{1/2}$ benzodiazepine, and (b) quazepam, a long $t_{1/2}$-benzodiazepine with BZ_1 receptor specificity for the parent compound and intermediate metabolites (Iorio et al. 1984; Sieghart 1983). Like diazepam, alprazolam, and lorazepam, triazolam induced a very rapid onset of impairment on both the SCT and digit symbol substitution (DSS) tasks, while the onset of the quazepam effect was much slower. The SCT is primarily a motor coordination task, and the DSS is a complex reaction time task that involves both cognitive and motor components.

The DSS impairment profiles for quazepam (30 mg) and triazolam (0.5 mg) are shown in Fig. 2. Of particular interest is the observation that performance for both triazolam and quazepam demonstrated a similarly slow rate of recovery on the cognitive DSS task although the two drugs and acitve metabolites differ widely in $t_{1/2}$. As for diazepam and alprazolam, the subjects had impaired performance for a shorter period of time on the SCT than on the DSS task after either quazepam or triazolam.

In conclusion, the lack of correspondence between impairment of performance in cognitive tests and drug level in plasma suggests the involvement of other rate-limiting mechanisms in the drug effect, besides distribution and elimination kinetics. The hypothesis has been proposed that receptor kinetics or adaptation is a more important determinant of the time-course of the drug effect, independently of serum concentration, even when equilibrium between brain and serum levels has been reached within the first few minutes after drug administration. A truly integrative pharmacokinetic-pharmacodynamic model should consider estimates of the adaptation of receptor-ligand interaction over time as well as receptor internalization and life cycle. The clinical implication for single-dose prescribing is that a short duration of action needs to be anticipated even for long pharmacokinetic half-life drugs. The effects of these mechanisms under conditions of chronic dosing awaits further study.

Acknowledgement. The research reported in this paper was supported by N.I.D.A. grant DA 01883.

References

Ellinwood EH Jr, Linnoila M, Easler ME, Molter DW (1983) Profile of acute tolerance to three sedative anxiolytics. Psychopharmacology (Berlin) 80:376–379

Ellinwood EH Jr, Heatherly DG, Nikaido AM, Bjornsson TD, Kilts C (1985) Comparative pharmacokinetics and pharmacodynamics of lorazepam, alprazolam and diazepam. Psychopharmacology (Berlin) 86:392–399

George KA, Dundee JW (1977) Relative amnesic actions of diazepam, flunitrazepam and lorazepam in man. Br J Clin Pharmacol 4:45–50

Greenblatt DJ, Divoll M, Moschitta LJ, Shader RI (1981) Electron-capture gas chromatographic analysis of the triazolobenzodiazepines alprazolam and triazolam. J Chromatogr 225:202–207

Greenblatt DJ, Divoll M, Abernethy DR, Ochs HR, Shader RI (1983) Clinical pharmacokinetics of the newer benzodiazepines. Clin Pharmacokinet 8:233–252

Iorio LC, Barnett A, Billard W (1984) Selective affinity of 1-*N*-trifluoroethyl benzodiazepines for cerebellum type 1 receptor sites. Life Sci 35:105–113
Lader M (1979) Correlation of plasma concentrations of benzodiazepines with clinical effect. In: Priest RG, Pletscher A, Ward J (eds) Sleep research. MTP Press, Lancaster
Mandelli M, Tognoni G, Garattini S (1978) Clinical pharmacokinetics of diazepam. Clin Pharmacokinet 3:72–91
Seppala T, Leino T, Linnoila M, Huttunen M, Ylikahri R (1976) Effects of hangover on psychomotor skills related to driving: modification by fructose and glucose. Acta Pharmacol Toxicol 38:209–218
Sieghart W (1983) Several new benzodiazepines selectively interact with a benzodiazepine receptor subtype. Neurosci Lett 38:73–78
Sieghart W, Karobarth M (1980) Molceular heterogeneity of benzodiazepine receptors. Nature 286:285–287
Ziegler WH, Schalch E, Leishman B, Eckert M (1983) Comparison of the effect of intravenously administered midazolam and triazolam and their hydroxymetabolites. Br J Clin Pharmacol 16:63s–69s

Abuse Liability of Triazolam: Experimental Measurements in Animals and Humans

R. R. Griffiths[1,2] N. A. Ator[1], J. D. Roache[1], and R. J. Lamb[1]

1 Definition of Abuse Liability

Drug abuse liability refers to: (a) the liability for abuse (i.e., the likelihood that a drug will be abused) and/or (b) the liability of abuse (i.e., the untoward effects of abusing the drug). These two senses of abuse liability correspond directly to two major characteristics of drugs of abuse: (a) they have *reinforcing properties* (they have the capacity to maintain drug self-administration) and (b) they produce *adverse effects* (they have the capacity to harm the individual and/or society). The presence of both characteristics is necessary to define a drug of abuse. A drug devoid of reinforcing effects but producing significant adverse effects should be considered a poison, not a drug of abuse (e.g., cyanide). Similarly, a drug having some reinforcing properties but producing no adverse effects is not meaningfully considered a drug of abuse (e.g., a nontoxic, non-nutritive sweetener). The relative abuse liability of a compound is a positive interactive function of the degree of reinforcing properties and adverse effect. Thus, compounds with high abuse liability could be: (a) highly efficacious reinforcers producing highly significant adverse effects (e.g., phencyclidine); (b) equivocal reinforcers producing highly significant adverse effects (e.g., lysergic acid diethylamide); or (c) highly efficacious reinforcers producing modest adverse effects (e.g., moderate cocaine doses). Compounds with low abuse liability must necessarily be those which are marginal reinforcers and produce marginal adverse effects (e.g., caffeine). It should be recognized that reinforcing properties and adverse effects are not necessarily independent dimensions. For example, a highly efficacious drug reinforcer may produce adverse effects solely by virtue of maintaining high levels of drug-seeking and self-administration behaviors to the exclusion of more socially desirable behavior. A further illustration of the nonindependence of reinforcing properties and adverse effects is that some adverse effects (e.g., physiological dependence) can modulate the reinforcing properties of drugs. Experimental approaches to the assessment of the abuse liability of benzodiazepine anxiolytic and hypnotic compounds have been reviewed previously (Griffiths and Ator 1981; Griffiths and Roache 1985).

[1] Department of Psychiatry and Behavioral Sciences and
[2] Department of Neuroscience, The Johns Hopkins University School of Medicine, Baltimore, MD 21205, USA.

Clinical Pharmacology in Psychiatry
Editors: Dahl, Gram, Paul, Potter
(Psychopharmacology Series 3)

2 Experimental Assessment of Triazolam Abuse Liability

Of all the benzodiazepine anxiolytics and hypnotics on the market, triazolam has been the most controversial with respect to abuse liability (Griffiths et al. 1985). Triazolam is a triazolobenzodiazepine, which is marketed as an ultrashort-acting hypnotic (mean half-life 2–3 h) under the product name Halcion. The present set of multidisciplinary studies concerning the abuse liability of triazolam was undertaken in our preclinical and clinical behavioral pharmacology laboratories at Johns Hopkins to help resolve some of this controversy.

2.1 Intravenous Drug Self-Injection in Baboons

Triazolam (0.0001–0.32 mg/kg) was evaluated in a standard drug self-injection substitution paradigm in which each drug dose was substituted for cocaine (0.32 mg/kg) for 15 days under a continuously available fixed-ratio (FR 160) schedule with a 3-h timeout following each injection. Comparison of the peak rates of self-injection (i.e., no. of injections per day for different drugs) revealed that triazolam maintained lower rates of self-injection than those maintained by the barbiturates amobarbital, pentobarbital and secobarbital, but consistently higher rates than those maintained by benzodiazepines that are slowly eliminated or have active metabolites which are eliminated slowly (e.g., diazepam and flurazepam). It is possible that elimination rate is a determinant of self-injection rate under this paradigm. However, the possibility remains that triazolam is a more efficacious reinforcer than other benzodiazepines.

2.2 Oral Drug Self-Administration in Baboons

Triazolam (0.01–1.28 mg/ml) was studied under conditions in which drug and/or vehicle suspensions were available to baboons for oral consumption during daily 3-h sessions. The baboons consumed behaviorally active amounts of drug, with peak intake exceeding 10 mg/kg for all baboons. Animals had free access to water except during daily sessions. At each drug concentration, over a wide range, a two-bottle choice situation was offered, in which the baboons had simultaneous access to vehicle and drug suspensions, with side positions of vehicle and drug alternating daily. In contrast to methohexital, triazolam and diazepam generally were not preferred to vehicle. Thus, under these conditions, triazolam is less efficacious as a reinforcer than methohexital, but indistinguishable from diazepam.

2.3 Drug Discrimination in Baboons

Triazolam (0.0032–0.32 mg/kg, p.o.) was evaluated in baboons trained to discriminate lorazepam (1.0 mg/kg) in a two-lever drug vs no drug food reinforcement drug discrimination procedure. In contrast to pentobarbital and methaqualone, triazolam and a variety of other benzodiazepines (alprazolam, bromazepam, diazepam, halazepam, temazepam) occasioned drug lever responding. These data suggest that the abuse liability of triazolam may be similar to that of other benzodiazepines and dissimilar to that of classically abused sedatives such as pentobarbital.

2.4 Physical Dependence in Baboons

The physical-dependence-producing properties of triazolam were evaluated in three different procedures. In the *substitution procedure*, baboons were maintained on pentobarbital via a continuous intragastric infusion. Twenty-four hour substitution of vehicle in baboons that have been maintained on 100 mg kg^{-1} day^{-1} pentobarbital resulted in suppressed food intake, while a similar vehicle substitution for 180–200 mg kg^{-1} day^{-1} pentobarbital resulted in suppressed food intake, tremor, and convulsion. Triazolam, lorazepam and pentobarbital attenuated the suppression of food intake at the pentobarbital dose of 100 mg kg^{-1} day^{-1}, in contrast to chlorpromazine, which did not. Triazolam has not yet been evaluated at the high pentobarbital dose.

A second procedure for providing information about the physical dependence-producing capabilities of benzodiazepine-like compounds is to administer a test drug chronically and determine the presence and extent of withdrawal signs precipitated (e.g., scratching, nose-rubbing, vomiting, tremor) upon administration of a benzodiazepine antagonist (i.e., *precipitated withdrawal test*). Baboons chronically exposed to triazolam (3.0–8.9 mg kg^{-1} day^{-1}) or diazepam (2.6–20.0 mg kg^{-1} day^{-1}) received i.m. injections of the benzodiazepine antagonist Ro 15-1788 (5.0 mg/kg). The profile and severity of withdrawal signs at these somewhat arbitrary but high doses of triazolam and diazepam were identical.

Some limited observations of *spontaneous withdrawal* have been made by observing baboons for withdrawal signs after abruptly terminating drug after a period of chronic administration. After termination of triazolam (2.7–21.8 mg kg^{-1} day^{-1}) tremor and scratching/nose-rubbing increased over previous baseline levels, returning to the baseline levels when triazolam was reinstated. These relatively mild withdrawal signs were similar to those observed in baboons undergoing diazepam spontaneous withdrawal, and contrast with the severe signs (e. g., convulsion) observed during spontaneous withdrawal from 200 mg kg^{-1} day^{-1} pentobarbital. As would be expected on the basis of the known pharmacokinetic differences between triazolam and diazepam in humans, onset of spontaneous withdrawal signs tended to occur sooner after triazolam than after diazepam.

2.5 Comparison of Acute Effects of Triazolam and Pentobarbital in Drug Abusers

The acute effects and time course of oral doses of placebo, triazolam (0.5–3.0 mg), and pentobarbital (100–600 mg) were examined using a within-subject, double-blind design in male volunteers with histories of drug abuse, who resided in a research ward (Roache and Griffiths 1985). Triazolam and pentobarbital produced comparable dose-related impairment on staff-rated and objective performance measures. With these measures, triazolam was 159–274 times more potent than pentobarbital. With subject-rated measures of drug effect, sleepiness, and drunkenness, in contrast, triazolam produced smaller effects than pentobarbital or was only 135–163 times more potent than pentobarbital. Similarly, with subject ratings of drug liking and estimated street value, triazolam produced smaller effects than pentobarbital and was only 91–122 times more potent than pentobarbital. Thus, these data indicate that at triazolam and pentobarbital doses which produced similar degrees of impairment, triazolam was less well liked than pentobarbital. Other results showed that higher doses of triazolam were categorized by the subjects as being predominantly benzodiazepine-like, in contrast to higher doses of pentobarbital, which were categorized as being predominantly barbiturate-like. Triazolam produced greater amnestic effects than pentobarbital on both immediate and delayed item recognition tasks. When subjects were required to rate how well they thought they had done on two performance tasks, subjects under the influence of triazolam more consistently underestimated the degree of their impairment. Overall, these results suggest that triazolam has a lower liability *for* abuse (likelihood) than pentobarbital, but a greater liability *of* abuse (hazard) with regard to performance impairment on certain kinds of tasks.

2.6 Tolerance Development to Triazolam and Diazepam in Drug Abusers

The effects of repeated administration of triazolam and diazepam on psychomotor performance and subject-rated liking were studied under double-blind conditions in male volunteers with histories of drug abuse, who resided in a research ward. Six subjects received triazolam (2.0 or 3.0 mg) every 2nd day (4 subjects) or every 3rd day (2 subjects) for a total of three to five dosing occasions, and six subjects received 80 mg diazepam every 3rd day (3 subjects) or every 6th day (3 subjects) for a total of three to six dosing occasions. The results showed that on the first dosing occasion the two drugs produced generally similar degrees of psychomotor impairment and subject-rated drug liking. Following the first diazepam dose, subsequent doses produced less of an effect (i.e., single-dose tolerance). Progressive tolerance development was observed across at least the first three dose occasions with diazepam, but no tolerance was observed with triazolam. It is possible that pharmacokinetic differences between diazepam and triazolam may account for the difference in the development of tolerance.

The implication of these results for the relative abuse liability of triazolam and diazepam is unclear. It could be suggested that the development of tolerance to diazepam but not to triazolam may indicate a greater propensity for diazepam to produce dose escalation and physical dependence. On the other hand, it could be suggested that tolerance to subject-rated drug liking with diazepam but not with triazolam may make triazolam the preferred drug of abuse.

2.7 Self-Administration of Triazolam and Diazepam in Drug Abusers

Oral self-administration of triazolam (1.0 or 2.0 mg), diazepam (40 or 80 mg), and placebo was studied under double-blind conditions in each of eight male subjects with histories of drug abuse, who resided in a research ward. Each drug condition (triazolam, diazepam, and placebo) lasted a week. On the first day of a condition the drug dose or placebo was administered. On each of the next 6 days the same drug dose (or placebo) was available for self-administration once daily. In order to receive the drug on self-administration days, subjects were required to ride a stationary exercise bicycle; the riding requirement was progressively increased across the 6 days (from 0.5–3 h). To minimize carryover effects between the two active drug conditions these were scheduled in counterbalanced order, with 3 weeks between the end of one and the beginning of the other; the placebo condition was scheduled during the middle week of the 3-week period. The results showed that triazolam and diazepam were self-administered more frequently than placebo, but there were no significant differences between the compounds in self-administration. Subjects tended to cite reduced/weak effects and drug-produced sluggishness as being undesirable attributes of the diazepam condition, while subjects did not cite such effects for the triazolam condition. Subjects tended to cite memory impairment as an adverse effect of the triazolam condition and indicated that this effect would make the drug undesirable for street use. Subjects tended not to make such comments about diazepam.

3 Conclusion

On the basis of studies of baboon i.v. and p.o. drug self-administration, baboon drug discrimination, baboon spontaneous drug withdrawal, and human acute dosing, it is concluded that triazolam has less abuse liability than barbiturates such as pentobarbital, which are generally considered to have significant abuse liability. However, the greater impairments of memory and judgement with triazolam than with pentobarbital demonstrated in the human acute effects study represent domains of concern that warrant future research.

These studies of baboon i.v. and p.o. drug self-administration, baboon drug discrimination, baboon physical dependence (substitution, precipitated withdrawal, and spontaneous withdrawal), and human drug self-administration suggest that the abuse liability of triazolam is quite comparable to that of diazepam, the prototypic benzodiazepine. Limited data from the human drug self-administration study suggest that memory impairment may be greater with triazolam than with diazepam and underscore the need for future research concerning this potential adverse effect of triazolam.

Acknowledgements. This research was supported in part by USPHS research grants R 01 DA 03889 and R 01 DA 01147.

References

Griffiths RR, Ator NA (1981) Benzodiazepine self-administration in animals and humans: a comprehensive literature review. In: Ludford J, Szara S (eds) Benzodiazepines. U.S. Government Printing Office, Washington, pp 22–36 [National Institute on Drug Abuse Monograph no 33, DHHS publication no (ADM) 81-1052], pp 22–36

Griffiths RR, Roache JD (1985) Abuse liability of benzodiazepines: a review of human studies evaluating subjective and/or reinforcing effects. In: Smith DE, Wesson DR (eds) The benzodiazepines: current standards for medical practice. MTP Press, Lancaster, pp 209–225

Griffiths RR, Lamb RJ, Ator NA, Roache JD, Brady JV (1985) Relative abuse liability of triazolam: experimental assessment in animals and humans. Neurosci Biobehav Rev 9:133–151

Roache JD, Griffiths RR (1985) Comparison of triazolam and pentobarbital: Performance impairment, subjective effects, and abuse liability. J Pharmacol Exp Ther 234:120–133

Clinical Studies of "Specific" Anxiolytics as Therapeutic Agents

K. Rickels

1 Introduction

Anxiety disorder is the most frequent psychiatric diagnosis made in America. A recent NIMH catchment area household survey (Shapiro et al. 1984), which involved almost 10000 persons, estimated that 8.3% of the adult U.S. population had suffered from anxiety disorders during the past 6 months. The two next highest diagnostic categories were alcohol and drug abuse (6.4%) and depression (6.0%), followed by schizophrenia (1.0%). Interestingly, however, only 23% of those patients suffering from anxiety actually received treatment. These data are in agreement with those obtained in the 1979 National Household Survey conducted by Balter's group (Mellinger and Balter 1981; Uhlenhuth et al. 1983), who found the following psychiatric illness prevalences for the past year: agoraphobic-panic disorder (1.2%), other phobic disorders (2.3%), generalized anxiety disorder (6.4%), and depressive disorders (5.1%). In this household survey it was again observed that only a relatively small percentage of those suffering from psychic distress and given a DSM III diagnosis as derived from the Hopkins Symptom Checklist criteria actually were treated for anxiety (Uhlenhuth et al. 1983).

The major indications for the use of anxiolytics according to the DSM III are given in Table 1. It should be noted that panic disorder without agoraphobia is included as an appropriate treatment indication. Drugs used for the treatment of anxiety in the past included herbal preparations, opiates and bromides. Alcohol is still used as a tranquilizer today, as are, to a limited extent, such nonbenzodiazepines as the barbiturates, meprobamate, the antihistamine hydroxyzine, tricyclic antidepressants, MAO inhibitors, and neuroleptics. Tricyclic antidepressants and

Department of Psychiatry, University of Pennsylvania, University Hospital, 203 Piersol Building/Gl, Philadelphia, PA 19104, USA.

Table 1. Major indications for benzodiazepine use (DSM-III)

Generalized anxiety disorder
Atypical anxiety disorder
Panic disorder
Post-traumatic anxiety
Adjustment disorder with anxious mood
Somatization disorders

Clinical Pharmacology in Psychiatry
Editors: Dahl, Gram, Paul, Potter
(Psychopharmacology Series 3)

MAO inhibitors have been found to be particularly effective in patients suffering from panic disorder with or without agoraphobia (Sheehan et al. 1984). More recently, Lipman et al. (1981) reported that imipramine was found to be as effective as chlordiazepoxide in treating patients suffering from anxiety disorder as long as patients could be persuaded to take the drug for at least 2 weeks and to cope with its rather disturbing anticholinergic side effects.

2 Specific Anxiolytic Drug Treatment

The major drugs used today in the symptomatic treatment of anxiety disorders are the benzodiazepines (Table 2). Benzodiazepines have consistently been found to produce significantly more symptom relief in anxious patients than placebo, and also significantly more improvement than phenobarbital and meprobamate (Rickels 1978). It is of great clinical interest that the major amount of improvement is produced within the first week of treatment; if patients do not respond within several weeks at the most (Rickels 1981), benzodiazepine therapy should therefore be discontinued and the patient shifted to other treatment methods. This swift onset of action is probably the reason for the wide use of benzodiazepines as p.r.n. medications. In fact, in several recent studies 50%–70% of chronically anxious patients who had improved after only 4–6 weeks of benzodiazepine therapy, maintained such improvement for weeks or months when shifted either to placebo or to no treatment condition (Rickels et al. 1983; Rickels 1985).

Yet, not all patients treated with benzodiazepines do improve, and in fact many patients rating themselves as moderately improved are indeed still rather anxious (Rickels 1978).

In the treatment of anxiety, probably more than in any other psychiatric illness, nonspecific factors play an important role (Rickels 1978). In general it has been found that benzodiazepines are most effective in nonpsychotic anxiety and in patients suffering from emotional and somatic symptoms of anxiety, but that they are less effective in those suffering from symptoms of depression and inter-

Table 2. Benzodiazepines marketed as anxiolytics in the U.S.

Drugs	Dosage (mg)	Half-life (h)	Active metabolites
Moderately long-acting			
Diazepam	4 – 40	26– 53	*N*-Desmethyldiazepam
Chlordiazepoxide	15 –100	8– 28	Several
Long-acting			
Clorazepate	7.5– 60	30–100	*N*-Desmethyldiazepam
Prazepam	10 – 60	30–100	*N*-Desmethyldiazepam
Halazepam	20 –160	30–100	*N*-Desmethyldiazepam
Short-/intermediate-acting			
Oxazepam	30 –120	5– 15	None
Lorazepam	1 – 8	10– 20	None
Alprazolam	0.5– 4.0	12– 15	Not clinically significant

personal problems. In fact, until a few years ago it was felt that all benzodiazepines were ineffective or only mildly effective in depressive states. This view must now be partially revised, since the triazolobenzodiazepine alprazolam has been shown to exert clear-cut antidepressive effects (Feighner et al. 1983; Rickels et al. 1985a). One may speculate that alprazolam's triazolo ring structure might contribute to its antidepressant effect, and the fact that in a recently completed study it indeed produced a significantly larger antidepressant effect than diazepam lends support to such speculation (Rickels 1986a). A finding recorded by the same author about 10 years ago with the hypnotic triazolam (Rickels et al. 1975) lends support to this speculation. Before and after a 1-week study of the hypnotic effect of triazolam, patients completed the Hopkins Symptom Checklist (HSCL-35); patients improved significantly on its depression factor.

3 Panic Disorders and Agoraphobia

Ever since Klein and co-workers showed that the tricyclic antidepressant imipramine was useful in the treatment of agoraphobic patients suffering from panic disorder (Klein 1964), it has been more or less assumed that benzodiazepines are ineffective in the treatment of panic disorder. This does not seem to be the case at all, and particularly not if one separates out those patients who suffer very little from agoraphobia and avoidance behavior and only from panic attacks. In fact, prior to 1980, i.e., before the DSM III was introduced, no differentiation was made in the nomenclature between panic disorder and generalized anxiety disorder, as panic attacks are very much a picture of the symptomatology of the typical anxious patient; and most of these patients never develop avoidance behavior and agoraphobia (Rickels and Schweizer 1986).

Alprazolam prescribed in dosages up to 6–10 mg/day has been demonstrated to be effective in patients suffering from both panic disorder and agoraphobia. Sheehan (1984), for example, demonstrated that alprazolam, phenelzine, and imipramine were all significantly more effective than placebo in reducing panic attacks and associated phobic avoidance behavior, and a large multicenter study sponsored by The Upjohn Company showed highly significant differences in favor of alprazolam over placebo in panic disorder patients, most of whom were also suffering from agoraphobia (Ballenger et al. 1985). The problem with many of the studies conducted in panic disorder is that authors do not differentiate between those patients who suffer from panic disorder with agoraphobia and those without agoraphobia. It may well be possible that most benzodiazepines are effective in alleviating panic symptoms as long as no agoraphobia is present (Noyes et al. 1984), while alprazolam may produce more reliable results than older benzodiazepines in agoraphobic patients. Whether or not benzodiazepines other than alprazolam in higher than the recommended dosages may also be effective in agoraphobic-panic patients cannot be said at this time. Only controlled clinical research comparing alprazolam with other benzodiazepines prescribed in equipotent dosages for patients suffering from panic disorder with and without agoraphobia will answer this question.

4 Buspirone, a Nonbenzodiazepine Anxiolytic

Recently a nonbenzodiazepine, buspirone, has received particular interest, as it is the first nonbenzodiazepine anxiolytic for which a new drug application has been filed in the United States. Results given in Fig. 1 may be viewed as representative of a large proportion of the data collected in the U.S. It gives results of a controlled trial conducted by Rickels et al. (1982). Both buspirone and diazepam produced significantly more improvement than placebo at weeks 1, 2, 3, and 4 in a study of 4 weeks' duration at a mean dosage intake of about 20 mg/day for both drugs. There was an insignificant but rather consistent tendency for diazepam to produce slightly more improvement during the first week or two of treatment than buspirone, pointing towards a possibly slightly slower onset of action for buspirone. In a 1-week study conducted recently, again a trend was observed for buspirone to produce slightly less improvement than diazepam while at the same time producing significantly fewer side effects (Rickels, Lucki, Giesecke, unpublished data). Two other interesting findings are that diazepam was found to be slightly more effective than buspirone in alleviating somatic symptoms of anxiety, while buspirone was found to be slightly more effective than diazepam in relieving symptoms of anger and hostility (Rickels et al. 1982). In all studies, side effects, and particularly sedation, were significantly less with buspirone than with benzodiazepines (Rickels 1986b). More recently, this author's group conducted an open trial with 30 patients suffering from major depressive episodes, prescribing buspirone in a daily dosage range of 20–90 mg/day (Schweizer et al. 1986). While buspirone was found to be ineffective in major depressives belonging to the melancholia subtype, it did produce significant improvement in those depressed patients who were suffering from the nonmelancholic subtype. These data, if con-

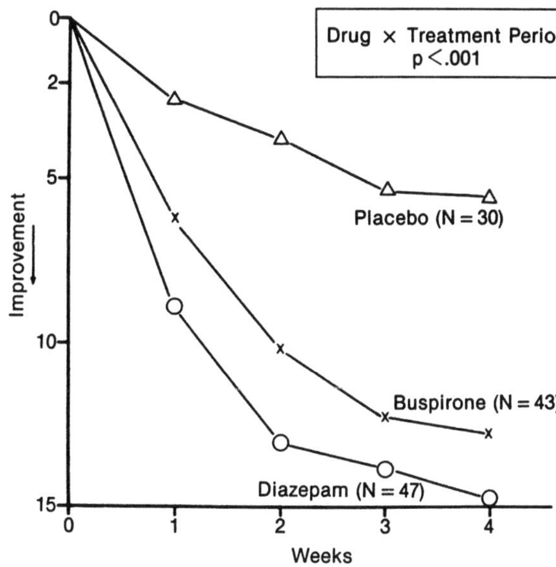

Fig. 1. Cumulative change scores on repeated measurement analysis: Hamilton Anxiety Scale (total score)

firmed by controlled studies, suggest that patients with mixed symptoms of anxiety and depression, or patients suffering from generalized anxiety as well as dysthymic reactions, or possibly even patients suffering from major depression of the nonmelancholic subtype, may respond well to buspirone. Finally, during abrupt placebo substitution after 24 weeks of treatment with either clorazepate or buspirone, more rebound anxiety and/or withdrawal symptoms were observed with clorazepate than with buspirone, and these differences were highly significant (Rickels et al. 1985b).

5 Physical Dependence

It has been known for a long time that physical dependence to benzodiazepines can be produced with excessive dosages given for a prolonged period of time (Hollister et al. 1961). What has been known only for a much shorter period of time is that even in low therapeutic dosages, benzodiazepines, when prescribed for prolonged periods of time, may produce physical dependence as evidenced by the appearance of withdrawal symptoms after abrupt drug discontinuation (Rickels et al. 1983; Shoepf 1983; Marks 1983; Petursson and Lader 1981; Tyrer et al. 1983). The time-course of withdrawal symptoms has been clearly defined in that symptoms of withdrawal occur within a few days of abrupt drug discontinuation, peak within 5–7 days, and then slowly decrease with time. Some mild rebound anxiety may already be present in some patients treated for only 4–6 weeks (Fontaine et al. 1984). These rebound symptoms usually last for only a few days and are usually not as severe as the initial anxiety. In contrast, the original symptoms recur more gradually. Recurrence is frequently not noticeable until 1–2 weeks after discontinuation of treatment; its symptoms are similar to those the patient had originally and they do not decrease with time (Rickels 1980).

In the only prospective study of maintenance benzodiazepine therapy published so far, Rickels et al. (1983) showed that 43% of patients who had been taking a benzodiazepine for a year or longer suffered from clear-cut withdrawal responses, and another 14% from transient responses or anxiety rebound. More recently, in patients who visited a benzodiazepine withdrawal clinic after having taken benzodiazepines for many years, the incidence of definite withdrawal was found to be 62% (Rickels et al. 1984). Thus, what Winokur et al. (1980) said in the first placebo-controlled case report is still true: withdrawal responses can be abated by a single dose of a benzodiazepine, and patients in whom these drugs are abruptly withdrawn will lose their withdrawal symptoms with time. Withdrawal symptoms are usually less marked or nonexistent when patients are being gradually discontinued from benzodiazepine therapy, a procedure now considered to be the treatment of choice; yet, even during gradual withdrawal, patients frequently experience disturbing withdrawal symptoms, which, while of a milder nature, may last for prolonged periods of time. Therefore, some patients prefer to withdraw "cold turkey," thus assuring that the withdrawal period will most probably be over within several weeks. Sometimes authors blame long-lasting psychiatric symptoms occurring after the discontinuation of long-term chronic benzodiazepine therapy onto either the benzodiazepine or its discontinuation. I suggest that these prolonged symptoms may not be related to the benzodiazepine at all in most instances, but most probably represent an emergence of old or new symptoms related to the patient's loss of support via benzodiazepines.

6 Conclusions

In summary, anxiety is indeed an important public health issue, and benefit/risk as well as benefit/cost issues have to be considered in selection of a benzodiazepine for the symptomatic mangement of the anxious patient. While in many cases the passage of time is a sufficient healer, even here drugs may help the patient through such difficult time-limited periods by alleviating disturbing and distressing symtpoms. Anxiety symptoms of a generalized nature and panic symptoms are clearly improved by benzodiazepines. The role of benzodiazepines, with the exception of alprazolam, in the treatment of patients suffering from marked agoraphobia has still to be determined. More recent findings have indicated that besides its antipanic effect, alprazolam clearly also possesses antidepressant properties. For the clinician, it should be of interest that buspirone, a non-benzodiazepine anxiolytic, will now soon be available. While possibly not acting quite as quickly as benzodiazepines, which makes it less helpful as a p.r.n. medication, buspirone has the advantage of causing little sedation and probably possessing either no potential or only very little for production of physical dependence. However, since physicians have begun to realize during recent years that for the symptomatic treatment of anxious patients, anxiolytics should be prescribed only for short periods of time or, at the most, intermittently rather than continuously, even for severely and chronically anxious patients, the occurrence of physical dependence with benzodiazepine therapy can be largely prevented. Thus, the lack of potential for production of such physical dependency with buspirone could be of only limited clinical importance. Alternatives to drug therapy, such as various psychotherapies (Zilbergeld 1983; Langs 1985), may not always be the preferred or safest treatment methods, at least for the short term. And certainly excessive smoking, heavy intake of alcohol, overeating, or the use of street drugs are not appropriate alternatives to the use of anxiolytics.

Anxiolytics prescribed appropriately and cautiously by a caring physician providing emotional support and guidance is probably the most acceptable treatment currently available for many patients, besides being the most cost-effective and the least hazardous way of managing various anxiety conditions.

Acknowledgements. Presentation of this paper was supported in part by research grant MH-08957.

References

Ballenger JC, Burrows GD, Noyes R, Lydiard RB, Norman T, Chaudhry DR, Zitrin CM (1985) Alprazolam treatment of agoraphobia/panic disorder. Presented at the 138th annual meeting of the American Psychiatric Association, May 1985, Dallas

Feighner JP, Aden GC, Fabre LF, Rickels R (1983) Comparison of alprazolam, imipramine, and placebo in the treatment of depression. JAMA 249:3057–3064
Fontaine R, Chouinard G, Annable L (1984) Rebound anxiety in anxious patients after abrupt withdrawal of benzodiazepine treatment. Am J Psychiatry 141:848–852
Hollister LE, Motzenbecker FP, Degan RO (1961) Withdrawal reactions from chlordiazepoxide. Psychopharmacologia (Berlin) 2:63–68
Klein DE (1964) Delineation of two drug-responsive anxiety syndromes. Psychopharmacologia (Berlin) 5:397–408
Langs R (1985) Madness and cure. Newcompt, New York
Lipman RS, Covi L, Downing RW, Fisher S, Kahn RJ, McNair DM, Rickels K, Smith VK (1981) Pharmacotherapy of anxiety and depression. Psychopharmacol Bull 17(3):91–103
Marks J (1983) The benzodiazepines – for good or evil. Neuropsychobiology 10:115–126
Mellinger GD, Balter MB (1981) Prevalence and patterns of use of psychotherapeutic drugs: results from a 1979 national survey of American adults. In: Tognoni G, Bellantuono C, Lader M (eds) Epidemiologic impact of psychotropic drugs. Elsevier/North Holland, Amsterdam, pp 117–135
Noyes R, Anderson DJ, Clancy J, Crowe RR, Slymen DJ, Ghoneim MM, Hinrichs JV (1984) Diazepam and propranolol in panic disorder and agoraphobia. Arch Gen Psychiatry 41:287–292
Petursson H, Lader MH (1981) Withdrawal from long-term benzodiazepine treatment. Br Med J 283:643–645
Rickels K (1978) Use of antianxiety agents in anxious outpatients. Psychopharmacology (Berlin) 58:1–17
Rickels K (1980) Clinical comparisons. Psychosomatics [Suppl] 21:15–20
Rickels K (1981) Benzodiazepines: use and misuse. In: Klein DF, Rabkin J (eds) Anxiety: new research and changing concepts. Raven, New York, pp 1–26
Rickels K (1985) Alprazolam in the management of anxiety. In: Lader MH, Davies HC (eds) Drug treatment of neurotic disorders – focus on alprazolan. Churchill Livingstone, Edinburgh, pp 84–93
Rickels K (1986a) Benzodiazepines in the treatment of anxiety syndromes (anxiety, panic, phobias). In: Hippius H, Laakmann G, Engel R (eds) Benzodiazepines, Rückblick und Ausblick. Proceedings of a meeting in Bad Reichenhall, Germany, 1–2 February, 1985. Springer, Berlin Heidelberg New York Tokyo
Rickels K (1986b) Buspirone: clinical profile. In: Anxiety disorders: an international update. Proceedings of an international symposium in Düsseldorf, Germany, 18–19 April 1985. Academy Professional Information Systems, New York
Rickels K, Schweizer EE (1986) Benzodiazepines for treatment of panic attacks: a new look. Presented at the 25th annual meeting of the NCDEU, 2 May 1985, Key Biscayne, Florida. Psychopharmacol Bull (in press)
Rickels K, Gingrich RL, Morris RJ, Rosenfeld H, Perlott MM, Clark EL, Schilling A (1975) Triazolam in insomniac family practice patients. Clin Pharmacol Ther 18:315–324
Rickels K, Wiseman K, Norstad N, Singer M, Stoltz D, Brown A, Danton J (1982) Buspirone and diazepam in anxiety: A controlled study. J Clin Psychiatry 43(12):81–86
Rickels K, Case WG, Downing RW, Winokur A (1983) Long-term diazepam therapy and clinical outcome. JAMA 250:767–771
Rickels K, Case WG, Winokur A, Swenson C (1984) Long-term benzodiazepine therapy: benefits and risks. Psychopharmacol Bull 20:608–615
Rickels K, Feighner JP, Smith WT (1985a) Alprazolam, amitriptyline, doxepin, and placebo in the treatment of depression. Arch Gen Psychiatry 42:134–141
Rickels K, Csanalosi I, Chung H, Case WG, Schweizer EE (1985b) Buspirone, clorazepate and withdrawal. Presented at the annual APA Meeting, 18–24 May 1985, Dallas
Schweizer EE, Amsterdam JA, Rickels K, Kaplan M, Droba M (1986) Open trial of buspirone in the treatment of major depressive disorder. Psychopharmacol Bull (in press)
Schoepf J (1983) Withdrawal phenomena after long-term administration of benzodiazepines: a review of recent investigations. Pharmacopsychiatria (Berlin) 16:1–8
Shapiro S, Skinner EA, Kessler LG, Von Korff M, German PS, Tischler GL, Leaf PJ, Benham L, Cottler L, Regier DA (1984) Utilization of health and mental health services – Three epidemiologic catchment area sites. Arch Gen Psychiatry 41:971–978

Sheehan DV, Coleman JH, Greenblatt DJ, Jones KJ, Levine PH, Orsulak PJ, Peterson M, Schildkraut JJ, Uzogara E, Watkins D (1984) Some biochemical correlates of panic attacks with agoraphobia and their response to a new treatment. J Clin Psychopharmacol 4:66–75

Tyrer P, Owen R, Dawling S (1983) Gradual withdrawal of diazepam after long-term therapy. Lancet 1:1402–1406

Uhlenhuth EH, Balter MB, Mellinger GD, Cisin IH, Clinthorne J (1983) Symptom checklist syndromes in the general population. Arch Gen Psychiatry 40:1167–1173

Winokur A, Rickels K, Greenblatt DJ, Snyder PJ, Schatz NJ (1980) Withdrawal reaction from long-term low-dosage administration of diazepam – A double-blind, placebo-controlled case study. Arch Gen Psychiatry 37:101–105

Zilbergeld B (1983) The shrinking of America – Myths of psychological change. Little, Brown, Boston

Antidepressants

Regulation of Beta Adrenergic and Serotonin-S_2 Receptors in Brain by Electroconvulsive Shock and Serotonin

K. J. KELLAR, C. A. STOCKMEIER, and A. M. MARTINO

1 Introduction

Two of the most consistent changes in brain that have been found following repeated administration of antidepressant drugs are decreases in the numbers of beta adrenergic receptors (Banerjee et al. 1977; Wolfe et al. 1978; Sarai et al. 1978; Bergstrom and Kellar 1979 a) and decreases in the number of serotonin-S_2 (5-HT-2) receptors (Peroutka and Snyder 1980; Kellar et al. 1981 a). The decrease in the density of beta adrenergic receptors is associated with a decrease in the receptor-mediated production of cAMP (Vetulani and Sulser 1975; Vetulani et al. 1976). The functional consequences of the decrease in serotonin-S_2 receptor density is less clear at this time. These receptors appear to mediate serotonin-stimulated phosphatidylinositol hydrolysis (Conn and Sanders-Bush 1984), but the effect of antidepressant drug treatment on this response is just beginning to be explored (Kendall and Nahorski 1985). The decrease in serotonin-S_2 receptors may be linked to decreases in serotonin-mediated behavioral responses, but the high affinity of most of the antidepressants tested for the serotonin-S_2-binding site in vitro and the possibility that the drugs block these receptors clouds this issue.

Electroconvulsive shock (ECS) affects both these receptors. The effect of ECS on beta adrenergic receptors and the attendant cAMP response appears to be very similar to that of antidepressant drugs (Vetulani et al. 1976; Bergstrom and Kellar 1979 b; Kellar and Bergstrom 1983). However, the effect of ECS on serotonin-S_2 receptors is opposite to that of antidepressant drugs (Kellar et al. 1981 a; Vetulani et al. 1981).

2 Effects of ECS on Beta Adrenergic Receptors

Repeated administration of ECS (once a day) decreases the binding of [^{3}H]dihydroalprenolol ([^{3}H]DHA) to beta adrenergic receptors in homogenates of rat brain (Bergstrom and Kellar 1979 b; Pandey et al. 1979; Kellar et al. 1981 b). Time-course studies show that the decrease in the cerebral cortex is detectable by the fourth day of treatment and is maximal (to about 40% below control values) by 10–12 days of treatment (Kellar et al. 1981 b). The decrease in binding is due entirely to a decrease in the number of measurable receptors (down-regulation)

Department of Pharmacology, Georgetown University Schools of Medicine and Dentistry, Washington, DC 20007, USA.

Clinical Pharmacology in Psychiatry
Editors: Dahl, Gram, Paul, Potter
(Psychopharmacology Series 3)

Table 1. Effects of repeated ECS (once a day, 12–14 days) on beta adrenergic receptors in homogenates from different rat brain regions. (From Kellar 1981b)

Brain region	[^{3}H]DHA specifically bound (pmol/g tissue)	
	Control	ECS
Cortex	6.2±0.4	3.9±0.4*
Hippocampus	5.9±0.3	4.5±0.3*
Striatum	10.1±0.8	9.1±0.1
Hypothalamus	6.2±0.6	5.7±0.6
Cerebellum	5.5±0.4	4.8±0.2

Rats were sacrificed 1 day after the last ECS. Beta adrenergic receptor binding sites were measured using 3.5–4.5 n*M* [^{3}H]dihydroalprenolol ([^{3}H]DHA). Values are means ± SEM for 5–9 rats.
* $P<0.01$ against control.

and appears to be a cellular adaptive mechanism for regulating incoming signals carried by noradrenaline. Beta adrenergic receptors in the cerebral cortex are still decreased 1 week after the last ECS, but they return to control levels within 4 weeks after the last ECS.

The decrease in beta adrenergic receptors by ECS is brain-region-specific. In studies measuring [^{3}H]DHA binding to rat brain homogenates, receptors were found to be decreased in the cerebral cortex and in the hippocampus but not in the striatum, cerebellum or hypothalamus (Table 1). In the hippocampus, as in the cortex, the decrease in beta adrenergic receptors coincides with a decrease in

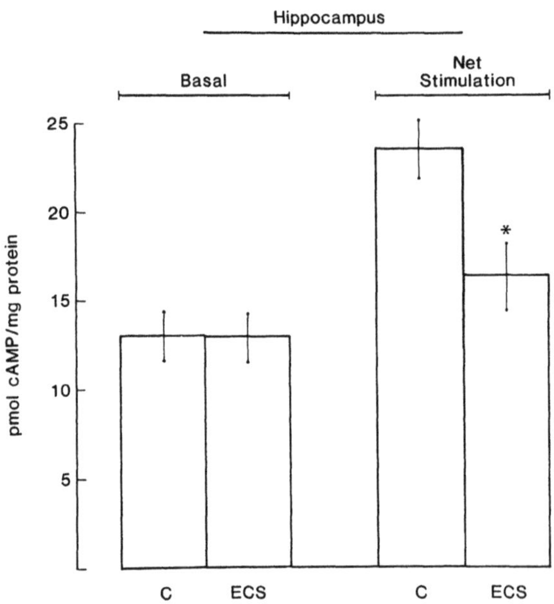

Fig. 1. Effect of ECS (12 days) on beta adrenergic receptor-mediated cAMP production in the hippocampus. The basal and the isoproterenol-stimulated production of cAMP was measured in fresh slices of hippocampus from control and ECS-treated rats sacrificed 1 day after the last treatment. The cAMP was measured by radioimmunoassay after a 10-min incubation in the absence (basal values) or presence of 10 μ*M* isoproterenol. The net stimulated values are the total cAMP produced in the presence of isoproterenol minus the basal values. Values are the means ± SEM from 9 control (*C*) and 9 ECS-treated rats *$P<0.01$ against control

isoproterenol-stimulated production of cAMP mediated by these receptors (Fig. 1).

[^{3}H]DHA binds to both beta-1 and beta-2 adrenergic receptors, but the brain region specificity of the decreased binding suggests that it is only the beta-1 receptor subtype that is decreased by ECS, and only in those brain areas in which ECS activates the tyrosine hydroxylase enzyme of noradrenaline axons (Kellar et al. 1981 b). However, ligand-binding studies in homogenates are usually limited to examination of the relatively gross brain structures that can be dissected easily, and both subtypes of beta adrenergic receptor are found in varying proportions in most regions of brain (Rainbow et al. 1984).

Therefore, we have recently used a selective quantitative autoradiography method published by Rainbow et al. (1984) to measure [^{125}I]iodopindolol ([^{125}I]P) binding to beta adrenergic receptors in cryostat-cut thin sections of rat brain. This has allowed examination of the effect of ECS on beta adrenergic receptors in some anatomical detail. Furthermore, the binding of [^{125}I]P was carried out in the presence of a selective beta-2 receptor antagonist (ICI 118,551) or a selective beta-1 receptor antagonist (ICI 89,406), which allows independent quantitation of beta-1 or beta-2 adrenergic receptors, respectively (Rainbow et al. 1984). Quantitative analysis of the autoradiograms from brains of control and ECS-treated rats confirmed that ECS decreased the density of beta adrenergic receptors in the cerebral cortex and hippocampus; and in addition, it revealed that these receptors were also decreased in the amygdala and in the thalamus (Kellar et al. 1985 a). In each of these areas, ECS decreased the binding of [^{125}I]P to beta-1 adrenergic receptors only; binding to beta-2 receptors was not affected in any area (Kellar et al. 1985 a). Thus, this autoradiographic study clearly indicates that only the beta-1 adrenergic receptor is decreased by ECS, and only in selected brain areas. In addition, the autoradiographic analysis has allowed detailed localization of the receptor changes in specific layers of the cerebral cortex, specific layers and regions of the hippocampus, and specific nuclei of the amygdala and the thalamus (Kellar et al. 1985 a; Stockmeier et al. 1985). Anatomical localization and comparisons of the effects of ECS and antidepressant drugs on receptors may ultimately aid in determination of the brain structures involved in antidepressant mechanisms.

3 Effects of ECS on Serotonin-S_2 Receptors

Serotonin-S_2 receptors in the cerebral cortex can be labeled with either [^{3}H]spiperone (Peroutka and Snyder 1979) or [^{3}H]ketanserin (Leysen et al. 1982). Antidepressant drugs decrease the apparent density of these receptors in rat cerebral cortex (Peroutka and Snyder 1980; Kellar et al. 1981 a). In contrast, ECS increases binding to these receptors (Kellar et al. 1981 a).

Time-course studies indicate that the increase in serotonin-S_2 receptor binding in the cerebral cortex is evident after 3 days of ECS; that it is maximal after approximately 12 days of ECS; and that binding returns to control values within 7 days after the last ECS (Kellar et al. 1981 a).

Table 2. Effect of repeated electroconvulsive shock (12 days) on binding constants for serotonin S_2 receptors in rat frontal cortex. (From Stockmeier and Kellar 1986)

	B_{max} (fmol/mg tissue)	K_d (n*M*)	n_H
Control	12.6 ± 0.4	0.58 ± 0.09	0.98 ± 0.04
ECS	19.8 ± 0.4*	0.69 ± 0.09	0.99 ± 0.02

Values are the means ± SEM for 3 handled and 3 ECS-treated rats. [^{3}H]Ketanserin binding was measured over a concentration range of 0.1–3.0 n*M*.
* $P < 0.001$ against controls.

The increased binding of [^{3}H]spiperone and [^{3}H]ketanserin is due to an increase in the apparent density of serotonin-S_2 receptor binding sites (Kellar et al. 1981 a; Table 2). Neither the affinity (K_d) of the receptors nor the Hill coefficient of binding (n_H) is altered by ECS (Stockmeier and Kellar 1985; Table 2). Furthermore, neither the IC_{50} nor the Hill coefficient of unlabeled serotonin competing for serotonin-S_2 receptors is altered by ECS (Stockmeier and Kellar 1985). These data indicate that the increase in binding sites is due to up-regulation of a homogeneous population of receptors, suggesting that the more numerous serotonin-S_2 receptors retain the properties of the native receptor. There is convincing evidence from the studies of Green and Grahame-Smith and their colleagues that ECS increases certain serotonin-mediated behaviors in rats (Evans et al. 1976; Green et al. 1977). It is likely that the increases in behavioral responses to serotonin agonists following ECS are a reflection of the increase in serotonin-S_2 receptors (Kellar et al. 1981 a); Green et al. 1983).

The underlying mechanisms which lead to the ECS-induced increase in serotonin-S_2 receptors are not known. It is probably not a simple compensatory adaptation to decreased availability of serotonin. ECS does not appear to affect serotonin synthesis or turnover (Modigh 1976) or its release from brain slices (Minchin et al. 1983); nor does the high-affinity uptake of serotonin into brain homogenates or the binding of [^{3}H]imipramine to sites on serotonin axons appear to be altered by ECS (Kellar et al. 1985 b; Stockmeier and Kellar 1986). Furthermore, even elimination of nearly all forebrain serotonin axons does not increase the density of serotonin-S_2 receptors in the cerebral cortex (Leysen et al. 1983; Stockmeier and Kellar 1986). However, the presence of functional serotonin axons appears to be required for ECS to increase the density of serotonin-S_2 receptors. In rats in which forebrain serotonin axons are selectively lesioned by injection of the neurotoxin 5,7-dihydroxytryptamine (5,7-DHT) into the cerebral ventricles or directly into the dorsal and median raphe nuclei, ECS does not increase serotonin-S_2 receptor density (Kellar et al. 1985 b; Stockmeier and Kellar 1986).

4 Effects of Serotonin Axons on Beta Adrenergic Receptors

Regulation of noradrenaline and serotonin receptors has usually been studied independently, but recently the influence of serotonin on the regulation of beta adrenergic receptors by antidepressant drugs has been considered. Costa's group (Brunello et al. 1982) and Sulser's group (Janowsky et al. 1982) have reported that in rats in which the serotonin axons have been lesioned by intraventricular injection of 5,7-DHT, repeated administration of the antidepressant drugs desipramine or imipramine no longer down-regulates beta adrenergic receptors, which suggests an important role for serotonin in the regulation of these receptors by these antidepressant drugs. Interestingly, mianserin and iprindole, two "atypical" antidepressants, still decreased noradrenaline-stimulated cAMP production after these lesions (Gandolfi et al. 1984). Thus, the apparent influence of serotonin axons on the regulation of beta adrenergic receptors by desipramine and imipramine might not be common to all antidepressants. This could indicate that antidepressant treatments can induce beta adrenergic receptor down-regulation by different mechanisms – some apparently requiring the presence of serotonin axons and some not.

The importance of serotonin axons to beta adrenergic receptor regulatory mechanisms may extend beyond their influence on the down-regulation of these receptors by some antidepressant drugs. Injections of 5,7-DHT directly into the dorsal and median raphe nuclei, which contain the cell bodies of the ascending serotonin axons, result in nearly complete (>90%) elimination of the serotonin axons innervating the frontal cerebral cortex and hippocampus, without producing any apparent damage to noradrenaline axons (Table 3; see also Stockmeier et al. 1985). By 4 weeks after infliction of these lesions there is a marked increase in the density of the beta adrenergic receptors in the frontal cortex and in the hippocampus (Table 4; see also Stockmeier et al. 1985). Similarly, following selective

Table 3. Effects of 5,7-dihydroxytryptamine lesions of the serotonin cell bodies in the dorsal and median raphe nuclei on the uptake of [^{3}H]serotonin and [^{3}H]noradrenaline and noradrenaline content in frontal cortex and hippocampus

	Frontal cortex		Hippocampus	
	Control	Lesioned	Control	Lesioned
[^{3}H]Serotonin uptake (fmol/mg protein/4 min)	2727±129	186±19*	3015±218	225±225*
[^{3}H]Noradrenaline uptake (fmol/mg protein/4 min)	606± 50	577±53	989± 96	866± 60
Noradrenaline content (ng/mg protein)	3.2±0.3	2.7±0.2	3.6±0.3	4.0±0.3

Rats were anesthetized with pentobarbital and pretreated with one injection of desipramine (20 mg/kg) 45 min before injection of 5,7-DHT or vehicle into the raphe nuclei. The rats were sacrificed 4 weeks later, and [^{3}H]serotonin (25 nM) uptake and [^{3}H]noradrenalin (50 nM) uptake were measured in fresh homogenates. The content of noradrenalin was measured by HPLC. Values are the means ± SEM from 12–24 rats.
$P<0.001$ against control.

Table 4. Effect of 5,7-dihydroxytryptamine lesions of the serotonin cell bodies in the dorsal and median raphe nuclei on beta adrenergic receptors in the frontal cortex and hippocampus

	Frontal cortex		Hippocampus	
	Control	Lesioned	Control	Lesioned
B_{max} (fmol/mg protein)	154.6±7.0	201.6±8.1*	154.2±9.9	291.4±25.0*
K_d (n*M*)	1.3±0.1	1.6±0.2	6.0±0.9	6.4±0.3

Rats were sacrificed 4 weeks after injections of 5,7-dihydroxytryptamine or vehicle. Beta adrenergic receptors were measured using 0.2–12 n*M* [^{3}H]dihydroalprenolol. Values are means ± SEM obtained from 5–9 Scatchard analyses.
* $P < 0.001$ against control.

serotonin axon lesions produced by i.p. injections of *p*-chloramphetamine, beta adrenergic receptor density and isoproterenol-stimulated production of cAMP are increased in the hippocampus (Stockmeier et al. 1985). The effects of the serotonin axon lesions appear to be specific to the beta adrenergic receptors, since the lesions do not alter the number of alpha-1 or alpha-2 adrenergic receptors (Stockmeier et al. 1985). This effect of these axon lesions appears to be due to the loss of serotonin itself rather than some other component of the serotonin axon, since long-term inhibition of serotonin synthesis with *p*-chlorophenylalanine produces similar results (Stockmeier and Kellar 1985).

The mechanism underlying this effect of serotonin on beta adrenergic receptors is not yet known. But if the regulation of noradrenaline and serotonin neurotransmission is important in the pathophysiology and/or treatment of depression, the influence of serotonin on beta adrenergic receptors might be a critical link between these two neurotransmission systems.

5 Conclusions

Following ECS, two of the most prominent and consistent changes in neurotransmitter receptors in rat brain are the decreased density of beta adrenergic receptors and the increased density of serotonin-S_2 receptors. The decrease in the density of beta adrenergic receptors brought about by ECS appears to be similar to the effects produced by antidepressant drugs, and thus it is consistent with the concept that these receptors are involved in the treatment of depression and possibly in the pathophysiological process itself.

In contrast to the effects of antidepressant drugs, ECS increases the density of serotonin-S_2 receptors. This difference could be related to the mechanisms of action of drugs and ECS in different types of depression with fundamentally different underlying pathologies; or it might be important to the mechanism of action of ECS in disorders other than depression, such as mania, for which it is an effective treatment.

It is probable that both norepinephrine and serotonin neurotransmission are important in the pathophysiology and treatment of depression. And it is clear that serotonin, via its effects on beta receptors, can have an important influence on noradrenergic neurotransmission. This allows testable models of receptor changes in mood disorders to be built around the interaction of these two neurotransmission systems.

Acknowledgements. The autoradiography project was carried out in collaboration with Drs. Barry B. Wolfe and Thomas C. Rainbow of the University of Pennsylvania School of Medicine. Supported by USPHS grants NS12566 and by the Scottish Rite Schizophrenia Research Program, NMJ, USA. C.A. Stockmeier was supported by NIMH Postdoctoral Fellowship MH08982.

References

Banerjee LP, Kung LS, Rigg ST, Chanda SK (1977) Development of beta-adrenergic receptor subsensitivity by antidepressants. Nature 268:455–456

Bergstom DA, Kellar KJ (1979a) Adrenergic and serotonergic receptor binding in rat brain after chronic desmethylimipramine treatment. J Pharmacol Exp Ther 209:256–261

Bergstrom DA, Kellar KJ (1979b) Effect of electroconvulsive shock on monoaminergic receptor binding sites in rat brain. Nature 278:464–466

Brunello N, Barbaccia ML, Chuang DM, Costa E (1982) Down-regulation of beta-adrenergic receptors following repeated injections of desmethylimipramine: permissive role of serotonergic axons. Neuropharmacology 21:1145–1149

Conn PJ, Sanders-Bush E (1984) Selective 5HT-2 antagonists inhibit serotonin stimulated phosphatidylinositol metabolism in cerebral cortex. Neuropharmacology 23:993–996

Evans JPM, Grahame-Smith DG, Green AR, Tordoff AFC (1976) Electroconvulsive shock increases the behavioral responses of rats to brain 5-hydroxytryptamine accumulation and central nervous system stimulant drugs. Br J Pharmacol 56:193–199

Gandolfi O, Barbaccia ML, Costa E (1984) Comparison of iprindole, imipramine and mianserin action on brain serotonergic and beta-adrenergic receptors. J Pharmacol Exp Ther 299:782–786

Green AR, Heal DJ, Grahame-Smith DG (1977) Further observations on the effect of repeated electroconvulsive shock on the behavioral responses of rats produced by increases in the functional activity of brain 5-hydroxytryptamine and dopamine. Psychopharmacology (Berlin) 52:195–200

Green AR, Johnson P, Nimgaonkar V (1983) Increased 5-HT-2 receptor number in brain as a probable explanation for the enhanced 5-hydroxytryptamine-mediated behavior following repeated electroconvulsive shock administration to rats. Br J Pharmacol 80:173–177

Janowsky A, Okada F, Manier DH, Applegate CD, Sulser F, Steranka LR (1982) Role of serotonergic input in the regulation of the beta-adrenergic receptor-coupled adenylate cyclase system. Science 218:900–901

Kellar KJ, Bergstrom DA (1983) Electroconvulsive shock: effects on biochemical correlates of neurotransmitter receptors in rat brain. Neuropharmacology 22:401–406

Kellar KJ, Cascio CS, Butler JA, Kurtzke RN (1981a) Differential effects of electroconvulsive shock and antidepressant drugs on serotonin-2 receptors in rat brain. Eur J Pharmacol 69:515–518

Kellar KJ, Cascio CS, Bergstrom DA, Butler JA, Iadarola P (1981b) Electroconvulsive shock and reserpine: effects on beta-adrenergic receptors in rat brain. J Neurochem 37:830–836

Kellar KJ, Stockmeier CA, Rainbow TC, Wolfe BB (1985a) Electroconvulsive shock selectively down-regulates beta-1-adrenergic receptors in specific areas of rat brain. Soc Neurosci 11:812 (Abstract)

Kellar KJ, Stockmeier CA, Gomez J (1985b) Regulation of serotonin neurotransmission by antidepressant drugs and electroconvulsive shock: the fall and rise of serotonin receptors. Acta Pharmacol Toxicol 56[Suppl 1]:145–183

Kendall DA, Nahorski SR (1985) 5-Hydroxytryptamine-stimulated inositol phospholipid hydrolysis in rat cerebral cortex slices: pharmacological characterization and effects of antidepressants. J Pharmacol Exp Ther 233:473–479

Leysen JE, Niemegeers CJE, Van Nueten JM, Laduron P (1982) [^{3}H]Ketanserin a selective ligand for serotonin-2 receptor binding sites. Binding properties, brain distribution and functional role. Mol Pharmacol 21:301–314

Leysen JE, Van Gompel P, Verwimp M, Niemegeers CJE (1983) Role and localization of serotonin (S_2)-receptor binding sites: effects of neuronal lesions. In: Mandel P, DeFeudis FV (eds) CNS receptors – From molecular pharmacology to behavior. Raven, New York, pp 373–383

Minchin MCW, Williams J, Bowdler JM, Green Ar (1983) Effect of electroconvulsive shock on the uptake and release of noradrenalin and 5-hydroxytryptamine in rat brain slices. J Neurochem 40:765–768

Modigh K (1976) Long-term effects of electroconvulsive shock therapy on synthesis, turnover and uptake of brain monoamines. Psychopharmacology (Berlin) 49:179–185

Pandey GN, Heinze WJ, Brown BD, Davis JM (1979) Electroconvulsive shock treatment decreases beta adrenergic receptor sensitivity in rat brain. Nature 280:234–235

Peroutka SJ, Snyder SH (1979) Multiple serotonin receptors: Differential binding of [^{3}H]5-hydroxytryptamine, [3H]lysergic acid diethylamide and [^{3}H]spiroperidol. Mol Pharmacol 16:687–699

Peroutka SJ, Snyder SH (1980) Long-term antidepressant treatment decreases spiroperidol-labeled serotonin receptor binding. Science 210:88–90

Rainbow TC, Parsons B, Wolfe BB (1984) Quantitative autoradiography of β_1- and β_2-adrenergic receptors in rat brain. Proc Natl Acad Sci USA 81:1585–1589

Sarai K, Frazer A, Brunswick D, Mendels J (1978) Desmethylimipramine-induced decrease in beta-adrenergic receptor binding in rat cerebral cortex. Biochem Pharmacol 27:2179–2181

Stockmeier CA, Kellar KJ (1986) In vivo regulation of the serotonin-2 receptor in rat brain. Life Sci 38:117–127

Stockmeier CA, Martino AM, Kellar KJ (1985) A strong influence of serotonin axons on beta adrenergic receptors in rat brain. Science 230:323–325

Vetulani J, Sulser F (1975) Action of various antidepressant treatments reduces reactivity of noradrenergic cyclic AMP-generating system in limbic forebrain. Nature 257:495–496

Vetulani J, Stawarz RJ, Dingell JV, Sulser F (1976) A possible common mechanism of action of antidepressant treatments. Naunyn Schmiedebergs Arch Pharmacol 293:109–114

Vetulani J, Lebrecht U, Pilc A (1981) Enhancement of responsiveness of the central serotonergic system and serotonin-2 receptor density in rat frontal cortex by electroconvulsive treatment. Eur J Pharmacol 76:81–85

Wolfe BB, Harden TK, Sporn Jr, Molinoff PB (1978) Presynaptic modulation of beta adrenergic receptor in rat cerebral cortex after treatment with antidepressants. J Pharmacol Exp Ther 207:446–457

α_2-Adrenoceptor Antagonists as Antidepressants: The Search for Selectivity

R. M. PINDER and J. M. A. SITSEN

Introduction

Tricyclic antidepressants and monoamine oxidase inhibitors are presumed to act rapidly to elevate synaptic levels of norepinephrine (NE) and serotonin (5-HT) by inhibiting uptake and metabolism, respectively. Synaptic levels of NE, however, are not controlled entirely by reuptake and metabolic processes, but are under the additional influence of a negative feedback inhibition mediated by an agonist action of NE itself upon α_2-adrenoceptors located presynaptically on the noradrenergic nerve terminal (Timmermans and van Zwieten 1982). Antagonism of these so-called autoreceptors leads to enhancement of the release of NE from its storage sites in the nerve terminal and thereby to a situation akin to that following uptake inhibition. α_2-Autoreceptors have been demonstrated to exist at almost all noradrenergic axons where postsynaptic α-adrenoceptors are known to occur, and they are widely distributed in the brain, particularly in the cortex. The possibility that α_2-autoreceptor antagonism might lead to antidepressant properties has stimulated the development of a number of putative therapeutic agents, which vary widely in their potency and selectivity (Pinder 1985a, b).

2 Is α-Antagonism Involved in Antidepressant Action?

The first indication that antidepressant drugs might block α_2-autoreceptors was provided by Baumann and Maitre (1977), who demonstrated that mianserin not only potentiated the electrically stimulated efflux of ^{3}H-NE from rat brain slices previously incubated with labeled transmitter but also reversed the inhibiting effect of the α_2-agonist clonidine upon NE release. Subsequent in vitro studies in peripheral tissues, such as rat and mouse vas deferens, rat anococcygeus muscle and rat atria, and in such central preparations as rat cortical slices and synaptosomes have confirmed the enhancing effect of mianserin upon NE release (see references in Pinder 1985b). Mianserin has also been shown to raise rat brain levels of NE metabolites after acute administration in vivo, and to reverse the effects of clonidine upon autonomic, cardiovascular, neurochemical, behavioral, and electrophysiological responses. Most studies have suggested that mianserin is about equipotent at α_2- and α_1-adrenoceptors, but that it is the only clinically ef-

Scientific Development Group, Organon International, NL-5340 Oss, The Netherlands.

Clinical Pharmacology in Psychiatry
Editors: Dahl, Gram, Paul, Potter
(Psychopharmacology Series 3)

fective antidepressant that is not highly selective for α_1-adrenoceptors (Pinder 1985 b). Mianserin displays stereoselective antagonism at α_2-autoreceptors with activity residing in the S(+)-enantiomer, while at least two of the racemic metabolites, the desmethyl and 8-hydroxy derivatives, are also α_2-antagonists (Pinder 1985 c). Similar stereoselectivity extends to antagonism at α_1-adrenoceptors and 5-HT_2 receptors, and to inhibition of NE uptake in vitro and to antidepressant-like behavioral activity in vivo, but desmethylmianserin is the only metabolite that inhibits NE uptake and is behaviorally active. It seems likely, therefore, that the S(+)-enantiomer and the desmethyl and the 8-hydroxy metabolites contribute substantially to the antidepressant effects, but efficacy studies have not been performed with those compounds.

Studies of the effect of mianserin upon α_2-adrenoceptor function in humans are limited. Charney et al. (1984) observed that treatment of depressed patients for 4–6 weeks failed to alter either the presynaptic (lowered MHPG plasma levels) or the postsynaptic (increased plasma growth hormone levels) α_2-adrenoceptor effects of clonidine. Pre-mianserin measures of α_2-adrenoceptor sensitivity were normal, and it did not appear that chronic mianserin administration produced presynaptic α_2-supersensitivity, as had been previously observed in rat brain (Cerrito and Raiteri 1981). Furthermore, subacute mianserin did not affect the α_2-mediated effects of acute clonidine in healthy humans, and neither acute nor chronic administration of mianserin affected the postsynaptically mediated antihypertensive effect of clonidine in hypertensive patients (see Elliott et al. 1983).

3 Tetracyclic Analogues of Mianserin

Structure-activity requirements for α_2-autoreceptor antagonism in the mianserin series have been extensively studied (Nickolson and Wieringa 1981; Pinder 1985 b), and three tetracylic analogues of mianserin are currently undergoing clinical evaluation as antidepressants (Fig. 1). Both Org 3770, which has enantiomers and shows similar stereoselectivity in its α_2-antagonism and antidepressant-like behavioral activity to mianserin, and teciptiline, which lacks chirality, are clinically effective antidepressants (Pinder 1985 a). Aptazapine, which has enantiomers but for which no chiral pharmacology has been published, has only been studied in uncontrolled studies. Org 3770 is almost as potent as mianserin in blocking α_2-autoreceptors, but lacks the ability to inhibit NE uptake. The therapeutic efficacy of Org 3770 at daily dose levels of 15–60 mg suggests that α_2-antagonism may be more important to the antidepressant action of mianserin than inhibition of NE uptake. Any differences in the therapeutic efficacy of the enantiomers of Org 3770, which is currently under study, could provide a clue to the relevance of α_2-antagonism to antidepressant activity in the tetracyclic series (Pinder 1985 b).

Teciptiline has lesser potency than mianserin as an α_2-antagonist and inhibitor of NE uptake, although its clinical potency (daily dosage 6–9 mg) is somewhat higher. Whether this is a consequence of the greater 5-HT_2 antagonist potency of teciptiline contributing to the antidepressant action and more than compensating for diminished effects on noradrenergic systems is presently unclear. How-

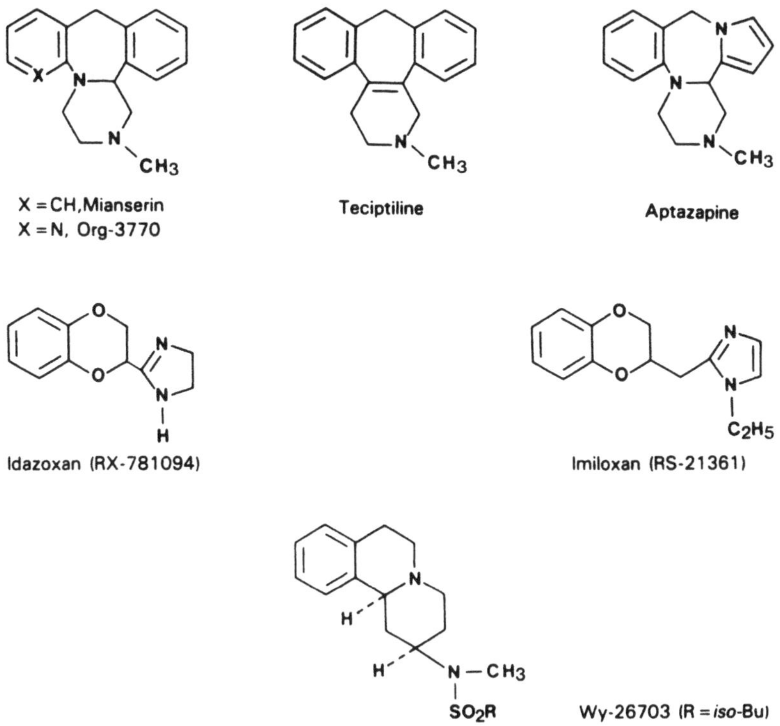

Fig. 1. Chemical structures of tetracyclic antidepressants and of the highly selective α_2-antagonists idazoxan, imiloxan, and Wy 26703

ever, the fourth tetracyclic analogue, aptazapine, has lesser 5-HT_2 antagonist potency than teciptiline or mianserin, retains something of the inhibitory effects on NE uptake, and has enhanced α_2-antagonist potency. Comparison of the relative antidepressant potencies and pharmacological profiles of these four tetracyclic substances may help to dissociate the respective contributions of NE uptake inhibition, 5-HT_2 antagonism, and α_2-autoreceptor antagonism.

4 The Search for Selectivity

The search for α-antagonists with greater selectivity for α_2-adrenoceptors and higher potency than mianserin and its analogues has focused upon modifications of the structures of the nonselective α-antagonists phentolamine and piperoxan. Two compounds, idazoxan and imiloxan, are currently being evaluated for their antidepressant effects, among other things. A third substance, Wy 26703 (Fig. 1), appears to be somewhat more lipophilic than the two benzodioxan derivatives, and may therefore penetrate better to, and remain longer in, the brain than its short-acting fellows. In peripheral tissues idazoxan is more α-selective than imiloxan and Wy 26703, while the α_2-antagonist potency of both idazoxan and Wy 26703 is markedly greater than that of imiloxan (Table 1). In radioligand-

Table 1. Comparative central and peripheral potency and selectivity of some α_2-antagonists. (Pinder 1985b)

Compound	Rat cortical binding, K_i, n*M*		Selectivity ratio	Calf cortical binding, K_i, n*M*		Selectivity ratio	Antagonism of α-agonists in vitro, pA_2		Selectivity
	^{3}H-Idazoxan (α_2)	^{3}H-Prazosin (α_1)	α_2/α_1	^{3}H-Clonidine (α_2)	^{3}H-Prazosin (α_1)	α_2/α_1	Rat vas deferens, clonidine (α_2)	Rat anococcygeus, noradrenaline (α_1)	α_2/α_1
Mianserin	35[a]	86[a]	2.5	17	43	2.5	7.27	7.24[b]	1.1
Yohimbine	40	230	6	49	220	4.5	8.14	6.49	45
Phentolamine	2.5[a]	3.6[a]	1.4	0.93	2.1	2.1	8.38	7.70	5
Piperoxan	140[c]	720[c]	5.1	–	–	–	7.72	6.61	13
Idazoxan	3.1	91	29	1.5	500	333	8.56	6.10	288
Imiloxan	80[d]	3000	375	–	–	–	6.98	4.85	135
Wy 26703	18	833	46	–	–	–	8.46	6.49[e]	93

[a] Using ^{3}H-clonidine (α_2) and ^{3}H-WB-4101 (α_1) as ligands.
[b] Using methoxamine as α_1-agonist in rat vas deferens.
[c] IC_{50} values using ^{3}H-clonidine and ^{3}H-prazosin binding.
[d] Using ^{3}H-yohimbine as α_2 ligand.
[e] Using methoxamine as α_1 agonist.

binding studies of cortical tissue, however, imiloxan is by far the most selective for α_2-sites, followed by Wy 26703, but idazoxan remains the most potent α_2-antagonist. All three compounds are markedly more selective for central α_2-adrenoceptors than the classic α_1/α_2 antagonists phentolamine and piperoxan, the α_2-antagonist yohimbine, and the antidepressant mianserin (Table 1). The affinity of idazoxan for α_2-sites is also much greater than that of mianserin, and that of Wy 26703 less so, while imiloxan has a lower affinity than mianserin. If α_2-antagonism is entirely responsible for, or is a major contributing factor to, the antidepressant action of mianserin and its tetracyclic analogues, these more selective and potent compounds should possess antidepressant effects. If they do not, the source of the antidepressant effects of mianserin must be sought in other features of its pharmacological profile. Controlled clinical studies so far reported with the more selective α_2-antagonists are limited to the effects of single doses of idazoxan and imiloxan in healthy volunteers. Oral imiloxan appears to be much less potent than idazoxan in reversing the effects of i.v. clonidine 0.2 mg, as expected from the pharmacological data (Table 1). A dose of 5 mg/kg produced partial blockade, with 10 mg/kg giving full blockade when given concurrently with clonidine, while partial and full blockade was produced by oral idazoxan 0.3 and 0.6 mg/kg, respectively (see Pinder 1985 b). However, in an open study in 24 patients with major depressive disorder who completed at least 3 weeks of active treatment, idazoxan 20 and 40 mg daily was effective in reducing mean Hamilton scores by about 50% (Crossley 1984).

5 Discussion

Some established antidepressants are α_2-adrenoceptor antagonists and are able to enhance NE release via blockade of the α_2-autoreceptor. The most potent in this respect is mianserin, which is the only one that is not selective for α_1-adrenoceptors. Several mianserin analogues, such as Org 3770, teciptiline, and aptazapine, have similar effects, and at least the first two of these have established antidepressant efficacy. The availability of highly selective and more potent α_2-adrenoceptor antagonists which can preferentially block presynaptic autoreceptors will be helpful in the assessment of the contribution made by α_2-blockade to the antidepressant action of tetracylic antidepressants. Yohimbine, which has several other pharmacological activities in addition to α_2-antagonism, is not known to be an antidepressant, however, and controlled clinical trials have not yet been reported for the relatively pure α-blockers idazoxan, imiloxan, and Wy 26703. α_2-Adrenoceptor sensitivity in depression appears to be normal with regard to postsynaptic receptors in the hindbrain controlling blood pressure responses to α_2-agonists, but can be reduced by long-term antidepressant treatment (Pinder 1983). However, depressed patients consistently display a blunted response to the stimulatory effects of clonidine upon growth hormone release, a forebrain event mediated by postynaptic α_2-adrenoceptors, which is unchanged during long-term antidepressant treatment (Checkley et al. 1982). Human blood platelet radioligand-binding studies have given equivocal results on α_2-adrenoceptor sensitivity; no difference is apparent between depressed patients and normal subjects with α_2-

antagonist ligands, but the use of clonidine has suggested increased α_2-binding in depression (Elliott 1984).

It is not yet clear whether α_2-autoreceptor sensitivity is abnormal in depression, and the influence of antidepressant treatment is far from established. It is likely that antagonism of α_2-autoreceptors plays a contributory role in the antidepressant action of mianserin and its close analogues. Clinical evaluation of more selective α_2-antagonists is necessary for further assessment of the contribution made by such properties, and will allow better study of changes in α_2-adrenoceptor sensitivity during treatment.

References

Baumann PA, Maitre L (1977) Blockade of the presynaptic α-receptors and of amine uptake in the rat brain by the antidepressant mianserin. Naunyn-Schmiedebergs Arch Pharmacol 300:31–37

Cerrito F, Raiteri M (1981) Supersensitivity of central noradrenergic presynaptic autoreceptors following chronic treatment with the antidepressant mianserin. Eur J Pharmacol 70:425–426

Charney DS, Heninger GR, Sternberg DE (1984) The effect of mianserin on α_2-adrenergic receptor function in depressed patients. Br J Psychiatry 144:407–416

Checkley SA, Glass IB, Shaw E (1982) Central α_2-adrenoceptor function in depression. Lancet 1:1359

Crossley DI (1984) The effects of idazoxan, an α_2-adrenoceptor antagonist in depression – a preliminary investigation. Abstract of the 9th IUPHAR congress, London, 1984 (Abstract 1724P)

Elliott JM (1984) Platelet receptor binding studies in affective disorders. J Affective Disord 6:219–239

Elliott HL, McLean K, Sumner DJ, Reid JL (1983) Absence of an effect of mianserin on the action of clonidine or methyldopa in hypertensive patients. Eur J Clin Pharmacol 24:15–19

Nickolson VJ, Wieringa JH (1981) Presynaptic α-block and inhibition of noradrenaline and 5-hydroxytryptamine reuptake by a series of compounds related to mianserin. J Pharm Pharmacol 33:760–766

Pinder RM (1983) Antidepressants and α-adrenoceptors. In: Gram LF, Usdin E, Dahl SG, Kragh-Sørensen P, Sjöqvist F, Morselli PL (eds) Clinical pharmacology in psychiatry: bridging the experimental-therapeutic gap. MacMillan, London, pp 268–287

Pinder RM (1985a) Antidepressant drugs of the future. In: Iversen SE (ed) Psychopharmacology: recent advances and future prospects. Oxford University Press, London, pp 44–62

Pinder RM (1985b) α_2-Adrenoceptor antagonists as antidepressants. Drugs of the Future 10:841–857

Pinder RM (1985c) Adrenoceptor interactions of the enantiomers and metabolites of mianserin. Are they responsible for the antidepressant effect? Acta Psychiatr Scand 72 [Suppl 320]:1–9

Timmermans PBMWM, van Zwieten PA (1982) α_2-Adrenoceptors. Classification, localisation, mechanisms and targets for drugs. J Med Chem 25:1389–1401

GABA Synapses, Depression, and Antidepressant Drugs

K. G. Lloyd and P. Pichat

1 Limitations of the Monoamine Hypotheses of Depression and Antidepressant Drug Action

In the quest for the pathological basis of depression and an understanding of the mechanisms of the clinical action of antidepressant drugs (ADs), multiple hypotheses have been proposed, invoking many central synaptic mechanisms. Of these, the monoaminergic hypotheses have been the most persistent, and propose to link both the etiology of depression and the mechanism of action of ADs. However, during the intense study which these hypotheses have received, several anomalies and paradoxes have come to light which indicate that these monoaminergic theories are insufficient per se to account for the pathogenesis of affective disorders or to provide a common mechanism of AD action. Briefly, the problems are that:

1. No consistent changes in central noradrenergic or serotonergic function have been demonstrated in depressed patients.
2. Inhibition of monoamine uptake or monoamine oxidase activity is rapid (probably <24 h), whereas the onset of clinical action is delayed (10–20 days).
3. Not all compounds whose effects include inhibition of monoamine uptake are antidepressant (e.g., amphetamine), and the converse is also true.
4. Some putative ADs do not inhibit either monoamine uptake or monoamine oxidase activity (e.g., progabide, fengabine, iprindole).
5. There is no evident correlation between specificity for different monoamine synapses and different types of clinical depression (Montgomery, this volume).
6. Even for beta adrenoceptor down-regulation, perhaps the most consistent change observed for different AD classes, there is no correlation between biological and clinical activities (Willner 1984).

From these observations, several alternatives seem possible. First, that manipulation of different monoamine systems more or less independently will have the same net result on affect. Secondly, that the actions of ADs on monoaminergic synapses are epiphenomena not essential to the clinical effect. Thirdly, that the different monoaminergic mechanisms have a common effect on another neuronal system which is the key system for the pathogenesis of depression and the clinical action of ADs. We have investigated the latter possibility.

Laboratoires d'Etudes et de Recherches Synthelabo, 31, Av. P. V. Couturier, F-92220 Bagneux, France.

Clinical Pharmacology in Psychiatry
Editors: Dahl, Gram, Paul, Potter
(Psychopharmacology Series 3)

2 GABA Synapses and Depression

2.1 Clinical Data

Of the different neuronal mechanisms operative in the CNS, one of the most ubiquitous is that using GABA as the neurotransmitter. However, a possible role of GABA in depression has been generally ignored. There is in fact a body of evidence which, although less voluminous than that for the monoamine hypotheses, strongly supports a GABAergic dysfunction in depression. GABA synthesis (GAD activity) is reported to be low in the frontal cortex and striatum of depressed patients (Perry et al. 1977), and GABA levels are consistently lower in the CSF (four of six studies) and plasma (six of six studies) of depressed patients than in that of controls (Table 1). It has recently been reported that factorial analysis between the different neurotransmitters and their metabolites in the CSF demonstrates that the greatest correlation occurs between GABA levels and depressive symptoms (Gerner and Fairbanks 1985).

The clinical psychopharmacology of GABAergic agents in affective disorders strongly supports a GABA hypothesis of depression. Cycloserine, an antituberculosis drug which is a GAD inhibitor (the only one used clinically to the author's knowledge), is associated with mood changes which remit on drug withdrawal, and depression (even resulting in suicide) is reputedly the most serious side effect of cycloserine (Lewis et al. 1957; Walker and Murdock 1957; Ruiz 1964). Specific augmentation of $GABA_A$ receptor activity by either diazepam or THIP has not been effective in manic disorders, whereas a generalized increase in GABA at all GABAergic synapses (by means of valproate therapy) is reported to have an antimanic action (Emrich et al. 1983, 1985). In unipolar affective disorders GABA

Table 1. Neurochemical evidence for a deficit in GABAergic function in depression

GAD activity			
Decreased in:	Frontal cortex	(60%)	Perry et al. (1977)
	Occipital cortex	(53%)	
	Caudate nerve	(74%)	
	Substantia nigra	(44%)	
CSF GABA levels			
Decreased		55%	Gold et al. (1980)
		25%	Kasa et al. (1982)
		22%	Gerner et al. (1984)
		20%–25%	Gerner and Fairbanks (1985)
Unchanged			Post et al. (1980)
			Joffee et al. (1986)
Plasma GABA levels			
Decreased		70%	Petty and Schlesser (1981)
		45%	Petty and Sherman (1984)
		40%	Coffmann and Petty (1986)
		35%	Petty and Sherman (1982)
		30%	Berrettini et al. (1985)
		28%	Berrettini et al. (1982)

mimetics such as progabide (Lloyd et al. 1983; Morselli et al. 1986) or fengabine (Musch 1986) are effective antidepressant agents, as shown in double-blind clinical trials, with 60%–70% of patients showing a marked response.

2.2 Experimental Data

Studies in animal models for depression also indicate a role for GABA synapses in the understanding of affective disorders and their treatment (Table 2). In the learned helplessness model, a decrease in GABA release parallels the onset of the behavioral deficit and both alterations are reversed by imipramine. Furthermore, intracerebral bicuculline provokes a learned-helplessness-like state (Sherman and Petty 1982; Petty 1986) and reverses the action of tricyclic ADs in this model (Zivkovic et al. 1986). GABA mimetics such as progabide and fengabine, (Lloyd et al. 1983; Zivkovic et al. 1986; Sanger et al. 1986) or GABA itself administered intracerebrally (Petty 1966) antagonize the behavioral deficits in this model. However, manipulation of the $GABA_A$-linked macromolecular complex by benzodiazepine or barbiturates is apparently ineffective (Sherman et al. 1982).

GABA mimetics are also active in another behavioral model of depression, the olfactory bulbectomized rat. Both $GABA_A$ and $GABA_B$ receptors are probably involved, as the $GABA_A$ agonist muscimol reverses the passive avoidance deficit (but not muricidal behavior; Delina-Stula and Vassout 1978) and the $GABA_B$ agonist baclofen reverses both the muricidal behavior (Delina-Stula and Vassout 1979) and the open-field activation (14-day treatment; Leonard 1984). Activation of both $GABA_A$ and $GABA_B$ receptors by progabide (Lloyd et al. 1983; Sanger et al. 1986) or fengabine (Zivkovic et al. 1986) reverses the passive avoidance deficit in olfactory-bulbectomized rats in a bicuculline-sensitive man-

Table 2. Activity of GABA mimetics in behavioral models of depression

Learned helplessness	
Active: Progabide	Lloyd et al. (1983)
Fengabine	Zivkovic et al. (1986)
Olfactory bulbectomy	
Passive avoidance deficit	
Active: Progabide	Lloyd et al. (1983)
Muscimol	Lloyd et al. 1983)
Fengabine	Zivkovic et al. (1986)
Muricidal behavior	Delina-Stula and Vassout (1978)
Active: Baclofen	
Inactive: Muscimol	
Open field activation	Leonard (1984)
Active: Baclofen	
Gamma vinyl-GABA	
Exacerbation: Diazepam	
Decrease in paradoxical sleep	
Progabide	Lloyd et al. (1983)
Fengabine	Depoortere and Riou-Merle (1986)

ner. Inhibition of GABA metabolism by gamma vinyl-GABA reverses the open-field activation, whereas diazepam exacerbates this effect of olfactory bulbectomy (14-day treatment; Leonard 1984).

A further confirmation of an antidepressant activity of GABA mimetics is demonstrated in the sleep-wakefulness cycle, for which clinically active ADs decrease the content and prolong the onset of paradoxical sleep. In the rat progabide and fengabine both reduce the paradoxical sleep content and delay the onset to the first phase of paradoxical sleep, as do other ADs (Lloyd et al. 1983; Depoortere and Riou-Merle 1986).

3 GABA and the Mechanism of Action of Antidepressant Drugs

3.1 Presynaptic Aspects

From the above it appears that there is sufficient evidence to support the hypothesis that a deficit in GABAergic synaptic function occurs in some brain regions in depression (the learned helplessness model implicates the frontal cortex and/or hippocampus; Petty 1986) and that GABA mimetics are potential ADs. If this is the case, do the clinically effective ADs in current use exert an action at GABA

Table 3. Published data on the interaction of antidepressant drugs and GABA synapses

GAD activity	
In vitro:	IMI inactive at 100 μ*M*
Ex vivo:	Little or variable effect (↑) (5–10 mg kg^{-1} day^{-1}, 14–21 days) IMI, DMI, CIT, NOR, VIL, NOM.
GABA levels	
Low doses (5 mg kg^{-1} day^{-1}, 1–18 days):	DMI, VIL, AMI: no effect
High doses (50–100 mg/kg):	DMI, PARG, ECT (10× in 10 days): ↑25%–50%
GABA uptake	
IC_{50}:	10–100 μ*M*: DMI, IPR
	120 μ*M*: IMI
	<200 μ*M*: AMI, NOR
In vivo:	5–10 mg kg^{-1} day^{-1}, 15 days: DMI, VIL, AMI, CIT: increase
GABA release	
IC_{50}:	DMI = 8 μ*M*
$GABA_A$ receptors	
Neurophysiology, chronic DMI, AMI, CMI, IPR:	no effect on GABA responses
GABA binding in vitro, 100 μ*M*:	DMI, AMI, IMI: no effect
ex vivo	5–10 mg kg^{-1} day^{-1}: DMI, VIL, CIT, AMI: no effect;
	32 mg kg^{-1} day^{-1} IMI: decrease
Benzodiazepine binding, chronic DMI, ZIM, BUPR:	decrease;
	ECT (×10): no effect
Chloride ion channel, 100 μ*M* IMI:	no effect

Abbreviations: AMI, amytryptyline; BUPR, buproprion; CMI, chlorimipramine; CIT, citalopram; DMI, desipramine; ECT, electroconvulsive treatment; IMI, imipramine; IPR, iprindole; NOM, nomifensine; NOR, nortryptiline; PARG, pargyline; VIL, viloxazine; ZIM, zimelidine. See text for references.

synapses? The literature does not provide a clear answer to this question, especially as most studies have been performed with acute rather than repeated administration. There is no consistent action of ADs on presynaptic aspects of GABA neurons (Table 3). GAD activity is generally unaltered either in vitro or after a single or repeated administration in vivo (Olsen et al. 1978; Pilc and Lloyd 1984; Lloyd and Pilc 1984; Rampello et al. 1982). Behaviorally relevant doses of ADs do not alter GABA levels after either single or repeated administrations (Lloyd and Pilc 1984), although very high doses (Patel et al. 1975; Tunnicliff 1976) and ten daily ECT treatments (Bowdler et al. 1983) increase GABA levels by 25% –50%. On initial observation it appears that the concentrations of ADs needed to inhibit GABA uptake (10–200 μM; Gottesfeld and Elliott 1971; Snodgrass et al. 1973; Harris et al. 1973; Olsen et al. 1978) are too high to be clinically relevant. However, at a daily therapeutic dose of 2–4 mg/kg and with therapeutic blood concentrations of 0.54–4 μM (Hollister 1978; Winek 1976) and a blood: brain partition coefficient of 20–22 (Hrdina et al. 1978), a brain DMI concentration of 10–80 μM would be present. Such levels may result in at least a partial inhibition of uptake with resultant increases in synaptic GABA availability. However, countering this is the report that desipramine decreases Ca^{2+}-dependent GABA release in vitro at 8 μM (Olsen et al. 1978), although an enhanced GABA release is observed in vivo (Korf and Venema 1983). Thus, of the presynaptic aspects of GABA neuron function studied, none appears consistent or sensitive enough to be a likely candidate for a common mechanism of AD action.

3.2 $GABA_A$ Receptor Complex

$GABA_A$ receptor function and its associated benzodiazepine-chloride ionophore macromolecular complex do not seem to be altered in a consistent manner by behaviorally relevant doses of ADs (Table 3). Thus, after repeated administration of different ADs which produce desensitization to norepinephrine and/or serotonin, the inhibitory response to iontophoretic GABA is unaltered (De Montigny and Aghajanian 1978; Siggins and Schultz 1979; Blier et al. 1984). In agreement with these results are the data showing that in vitro or ex vivo (after 5–10 mg kg^{-1} day^{-1} for 18 days) different ADs do not alter $GABA_A$ binding (Olsen et al. 1978). Only after a rather high dose of imipramine (32 mg kg^{-1} day^{-1} for 21 days) is there a decrease in $GABA_A$ binding (Suzdak and Gianutsos 1985). After repeated administration of different antidepressants benzodiazepine recognition sites are reported to be decreased in density (Suranyi-Cadotte et al. 1985), but a series of ten ECTs has no effect on this site (Bowdler et al. 1983). When ^3H-dihydropicrotoxin was used as the ligand for the $GABA_A$ receptor-linked chloride ion channel, 100 μM imipramine was inactive at this site (Olsen et al. 1978).

3.3 $GABA_B$ Receptors

3.3.1 Methods

Thus, different classes of ADs and ECT have very little in common with respect to presynaptic GABA neuron function, and there is little evidence for a shared mechanism at the $GABA_A$ receptor. In contrast, the $GABA_B$ receptor (Hill and Bowery 1981) seems to respond in a reproducible and predictable manner to clinically effective ADs and ECT. The methods used for this study have been published in detail (Pilc and Lloyd 1984; Lloyd et al. 1985). In brief, soluble compounds were administered s.c. via Alzet osmotic minipumps for 6–18 days, at which point the minipumps were removed. The animals were sacrificed 24–72 h later, after which the frontal cortex was removed and frozen. Membranes for $GABA_B$ binding were prepared within 48 h and the binding assays within 7 days thereafter. Membrane preparation and $GABA_B$ binding were performed essentially according to Hill and Bowery (1981). For single concentration studies, 10 n*M* ^{3}H-GABA was used in the presence of 40 μ*M* isoguvacine, with either 1 m*M* GABA or *dl*-baclofen to account for nonspecific binding (Lloyd 1986). For Scatchard analysis, 1–750 n*M* ^{3}H-GABA was used. Olfactory bulbectomies were performed as described by Broekkamp et al. (1980). These animals were sacrificed 14 days later; the frontal cortices were then removed and frozen, membranes prepared, and $GABA_B$ binding performed as described above. Detailed attention was paid to the integrity of the frontal cortex. In the case of any apparent damage the sample was rejected. The results of most of these studies have been published within the last few years (Lloyd and Pilc 1984; Lloyd et al. 1985, 1986; Lloyd and Pichat 1986).

3.3.2 Chronic Antidepressant Administration and $GABA_B$ Binding

Desipramine (5 mg kg^{-1} day^{-1} s.c. for 18 days) induced a reproducible increase in ^{3}H-$GABA_B$ (10 n*M*) binding to frontal cortex membranes. In 13 experiments performed between December 1982 and May 1985 this increase was always statistically significant ($P<0.05$–$P<0.01$) and ranged from a 20% to a 63% increase. The increase did not depend on the basal level which varied from 50 to 150 fmol/mg protein. This effect of desipramine was both time- and dose-dependent; 18 days of continuous infusion (5 mg kg^{-1} day^{-1}) produced a larger increase (62%) than a 6-day administration (39% increase). This particular study also demonstrated that the frontal cortex was more sensitive than the hippocampus; after 6 days of DMI there was no alteration in hippocampal $GABA_B$ binding. After 18 days of DMI infusion hippocampal $GABA_B$ binding was increased by 50%. Furthermore, a dose of 5 mg kg^{-1} day^{-1} DMI s.c. (for 18 days) was more effective ($P<0.01$) than 1.25 mg kg^{-1} day^{-1} (Lloyd et al. 1985).

This effect seemed to be a rather general phenomenon for the ADs tested (Table 4). Thus, antidepressant monoamine uptake inhibitors with varying degrees of specificity for dopamine, noradrenaline, or serotonin uptake mechanisms all produced an increase in ^{3}H-$GABA_B$ binding to rat frontal cortex membranes (for references dealing with biochemical specificity and clinical efficacy see Lloyd et al. 1985). Furthermore, the monoamine oxidase inhibitor pargyline evoked the same response. The exception to this was amphetamine, which did not significantly alter $GABA_B$ binding, although there was a trend towards an increase. This in itself is interesting, as amphetamine is currently considered not to be an antidepressant, but rather a psychostimulant (Mandel and Klerman 1978). If this is correct it implies that increased synaptic availability of monoamines per se is

Table 4. Effect of infusion or repeated administration of monoamine uptake inhibitors, an MAO inhibitor, GABA mimetics, electroshock, and diverse anti-depressants on $GABA_B$ binding in the rat frontal cortex

Compound ($mg\ kg^{-1}\ day^{-1}$)	Duration and route (No. of rats)	% Control	*P* value (*t* test)
A. *Uptake inhibitors*			
Nonspecific			
Amitriptyline (10)	18 days, s.c. (15)	154	<0.01
Amphetamine (2)	18 days, s.c. (10)	119	NS
Noradrenaline			
Desipramine (5)	18 days, s.c. (14)	151	<0.01
Maprotiline (10)	18 days, s.c. (9)	135	<0.001
Viloxazine (10)	18 days, s.c.	188	<0.001
Dopamine			
Nomifensine (5)	18 days, s.c. (10)	146	<0.01
Buproprion (5)	18 days, s.c. (10)	154	<0.01
Serotonin			
Citalopram (10)	18 days, s.c. (15)	172	<0.001
Fluoxetine (10)	6 days, i.p. (10)	183	<0.01
Zimelidine (10)	18 days, s.c. (10)	165	<0.01
B. *Monoamine oxidase inhibitor*			
Pargyline (20)	18 days, s.c. (5)	142	<0.05
C. *Electroshock*			
150 mA, 0.5 s/48 h	10 days (10)	177	<0.001
D. *GABA mimetics*			
Progabide (100)	18 days, i.p. (9)	127	<0.001
Fengabine (50)	6 days, i.p. (7)	159	<0.01
Sodium valproate (100)	18 days, i.p. (8)	120	<0.01
E. *Miscellaneous compounds*			
Trazodone (10)	18 days, s.c. (10)	155	<0.001
Iprindole (5)	18 days, s.c. (10)	129	<0.01
Mianserine (10)	18 days, s.c. (10)	133	<0.01
Idazoxan (5)	18 days, s.c. (10)	207	<0.001

Data from Lloyd et al. (1985) and Lloyd (unpublished).
The concentration of ^{3}H-GABA was 10 n*M* in the presence of 40 μ*M* isoguvacine.

insufficient to produce an increase in $^3H\text{-}GABA_B$ binding, and rather an effect related to the antidepressant properties is the important factor.

The increase in $GABA_B$ binding is not limited to ADs acting directly on monoaminergic synapses. The GABA mimetics progabide, fengabine, and valproate all increase $GABA_B$ binding to rat frontal cortex membranes (Table 4). These compounds have all shown clinical efficacy in affective disorders (Lloyd et al. 1983; Morselli et al. 1981, 1986; Musch 1986; Emrich et al. 1983, 1985), and thus these results are consistent with an AD–$GABA_B$ interaction. It should be noted that the signal is rather weak for two of these GABA mimetics, progabide and valproate. This may be due to an interplay (equilibrium) between $GABA_B$ receptor up-regulation related to the antidepressant aspect of the compound, and a tendency towards a subsensitivity often seen after long-term exposure of receptors to their agonists.

Other compounds with clinically demonstrated antidepressant effects, yet with little direct action on monoaminergic synapses (trazodone, iprindole, Table 4), or which block presynaptic alpha-2 adrenoceptors (mianserin, idazoxan) also up-regulate $GABA_B$ binding. As the clinical efficacy of idazoxan has yet to be substantiated, this may prove to be a false-positive.

3.3.3 Electroshock and $GABA_B$ Binding

An important observation is that a nonpharmacological antidepressant paradigm also increased $GABA_B$ binding to rat frontal cortex membranes. Thus, five electroshock treatments spaced over 10 days evoked an increase in $GABA_B$ binding of the same order as most ADs (Table 4). This indicates that the $GABA_B$ changes observed are not related simply to the prolonged presence of lipophilic compounds in brain membranes.

3.3.4 Kinetics of $GABA_B$ Binding to Frontal Cortex Membranes

Although the above changes are significant and highly consistent, the use of a single concentration of ligand (in this case 10 μM ^{3}H-GABA) does not provide an insight into the molecular mechanisms involved. Scatchard analysis of the $GABA_B$ binding to frontal cortex membranes from controls and rats treated with different ADs reveals that an increase in B_{max} is responsible for the changes following at least amitriptyline, the low dose of desipramine, viloxazine, citalopram, nomifensine, and pargyline (Table 5). However, the kinetics become more complex for the higher dose of imipramine and zimelidine as K_d changes occur (increased apparent affinity of the high-affinity site) together with the appearance of a lower affinity (130–140 nM) binding site and an increase in total binding (Table 5). It is at present impossible to say whether these lower affinity sites are

Table 5. Kinetic constants of $GABA_B$ binding to rat frontal cortex membranes after prolonged administration of antidepressant drugs or saline

Compound (mg kg^{-1} day^{-1} s.c.)	K_d (nM)	B_{max} (total) (% corresponding saline controls)
Saline	43.9	100
Amitriptyline (10)	42.3	163
Desipramine		
1.25	37.3	142
5.0	22.2; 144[a]	234
Viloxazine (10)	39.7	166
Citalopram (10)	37.9	152
Zimelidine (10)	22.0; 132[a]	332
Nomifensine (5)	28.3	116
Pargyline (20)	54.6	157

[a] Induction of low-affinity binding site observed.
Data from Lloyd et al. (1985).

being unmasked from a normally inaccessible state or whether new low-affinity recognition sites have been induced.

3.3.5 Nonantidepressant Drugs and $GABA_B$ Binding

This alteration in $GABA_B$ binding appears to be highly specific for ADs, as several other classes of psychotropic agents do not induce this phenomenon (Table 6). Compounds which activate the $GABA_A$ macromolecular complex are either inactive (diazepam) or decrease $GABA_B$ binding (phenobarbital, diphenylhydantoin). These latter results suggest that the $GABA_B$ receptor up-regulation by the antidepressant GABA mimetics (progabide, fengabine, valproate; see above), which also activate the $GABA_A$ receptor complex, is the net result of several competing effects.

Of the neuroleptics examined, haloperidol and chlorpromazine had no activity in this system. In contrast, reserpine resulted in a significant decrease in $GABA_B$ binding to rat frontal cortex membranes. Of these neuroleptics, only reserpine has been reported to induce depression in man (Johnson 1981; Goodwin et al. 1972; Whitlock and Evans 1978). The muscarinic agonist oxotremorine did not alter $GABA_B$ binding to rat frontal cortex membranes.

3.3.6 $GABA_B$ Receptors in Olfactory-Bulbectomized Rats

Potential alterations in $GABA_B$ synaptic activity in behavioral models of depression have yet to be investigated in detail. However, in the olfactory bulbectomy model $GABA_B$ binding is significantly decreased by more than 50% in the frontal cortex (70.0 fmol/mg protein vs 153.8 for sham-operated animals: $P < 0.001$) but not in the occipital cortex (27% decrease, NS), amygdala (36% increase, NS), hippocampus (103%: controls), or cerebellum (40% increase, NS). In a further experiment the B_{max} was found to be 40% lower in the frontal cortex

Table 6. $GABA_B$ binding to rat frontal cortex membranes: Effect of 18-day, s.c. infusion of nonantidepressant compounds

Compound	Dose ($mg\ kg^{-1}\ day^{-1}$)	$GABA_B$ binding (% control)	P vs saline (control)
$GABA_A$ complex interaction			
Diazepam	0.5	113	NS
Phenobarbital	40	71	<0.01
Diphenylhydantoin	30	67	<0.01
Neuroleptics			
Haloperidol	0.3	107	NS
Chlorpromazine	2	81	NS
Reserpine	1	70	<0.01
Cholinomimetic			
Oxotremorine	4	119	NS

Data from Lloyd et al. (1985) and Lloyd (unpublished)

of olfactory bulbectomized vs sham-operated animals, whereas the K_d's were similar (30–35 n*M*). Whether such changes parallel the behavior modifications seen in these animals is as yet unknown.

4 Discussion

Thus, a body of evidence exists supporting a deficit in GABAergic function in depression and a GABAergic mechanism of action of antidepressant drugs. Amongst the host of questions needing to be answered before such a hypothesis is established, two can presently be addressed: First, what brain region(s) may be involved; and second, whether the monoaminergic and GABAergic hypotheses of depression are mutually exclusive or represent different facets of a common mechanism.

The first question can only be partially answered at present; however, at least in rat models it appears that the frontal cortex is involved in the GABAergic mechanism of action of ADs. Thus, in the learned helplessness model, GABA injected into the frontal cortex prevents the learning deficits, as do ADs (Petty and Sherman 1982; Petty 1986). Furthermore, in the olfactory bulbectomy model $GABA_B$ receptors are decreased in the frontal cortex but not in other brain regions. As documented above, various ADs and electroshock increase $GABA_B$ binding in the frontal cortex, and at least for desipramine this region is more sensitive than the hippocampus. In the human, GABA synthesis (GAD activity) is decreased in the frontal cortex of depressed patients (Perry et al. 1977), and clinical observations relate EEG changes (Flor-Henry and Koles 1980) and pathology (Ross and Rusch 1981; Ruff and Russakoff 1980) of the frontal lobe to changes in mood (cf. Deutsch et al. 1979).

With regard to the second question, even with the limited results available it seems highly probable that the monoamine and GABA hypotheses can be integrated to form a more rational hypothesis of AD action. It is known that different ADs have varying actions on GABA synapses, in addition to the up-regulation of $GABA_B$ binding (see above). Furthermore, different GABA mimetics alter noradrenergic (increased activity) or serotonergic (decreased activity) neuron activity in different ways (Scatton et al. 1982; Zivkovic et al. 1986). However, none of these observations are consistent enough to fit into an overall hypothesis. In fact, the only two consistent observations (for all tested ADs and ECT) are the down-regulation of beta adrenergic binding (or the associated adenylate cyclase) (e.g., Enna et al. 1981; Sulser 1978; Vetulani et al. 1984) and the up-regulation of $GABA_B$ binding. These two phenomena are interrelated at several levels: (a) The integrity of 5-HT terminals is necessary for the down-regulation of beta adrenergic receptors (Kellar, this volume). From preliminary experiments (Scatton and Lloyd, unpublished) it appears that $GABA_B$ receptors are located on 5-HT terminals, as $GABA_B$ binding decreases after 5,7-dihydroxytryptamine administration; furthermore, baclofen alters 5-HT release from its terminals (Schlicker et al. 1984). (b) $GABA_B$ receptors also occur on adrenergic nerve terminals as baclofen alters cortical noradrenaline release (Hill and Bowery 1981; Langer et al. 1986) and $GABA_B$ sites are reduced by 6-OH dopmaine-induced lesions of noradrenergic neurons (Karbon et al. 1983). (c) A postsynaptic interaction between $GABA_B$ and beta adrenergic systems is also highly probable, as $GABA_B$ receptor stimulation (Hill 1985; Karbon et al. 1984) greatly potentiates the beta adrenergic receptor-linked adenylate cyclase activity.

Thus, the $GABA_B$ response and the beta adrenergic responses to repeated AD administration are probably different aspects of an integrated cellular response, linked to the eventual antidepressant action of the compounds.

References

Berrettini WH, Nurnberger JI, Hare T, Gershon ES, Post RM (1982) Plasma and CSF GABA in affective illness. Br J Psychiatry 14:483–487

Berrettini WH, Nurnberger JI, Hare TA, Gershon ES (1985) CSF and plasma GABA in bipolar patients. In: IVth World congress of biological psychiatry, 8–13 Sept. 1985, Philadelphia, Abstract 619.9

Blier P, De Montigny C, Tardiff D (1984) Effects of two antidepressant drugs mianserin and indalpine on the serotonergic system: Single cell studies in the rat. Psychopharmacology (Berlin) 84:242–249

Bowdler JM, Green AR, Minchin MCW, Nutt DJ (1983) Regional GABA concentration and ^3H-diazepam binding in rat brain following repeated electroconvulsive shock. J Neural Transm 56:3–12

Broekkamp CL, Garrigou D, Lloyd KG (1980) Serotonin-mimetic and antidepressant drugs on passive avoidance learning by olfactory bulbectomized rats. Pharmacol Biochem Behav 13:643–646

Coffman JA, Petty F (1986) Plasma GABA: a potential indicator of altered GABAergic function in psychiatric illness. In: Bartholini G, Lloyd KG, Morselli PL (eds) GABA and mood disorders. Raven, New York, pp 179–185

Delina-Stula A, Vassout A (1978) Influence of baclofen and GABA-mimetic agents on spontaneous and olfactory-bulb-ablation-induced muricidal behaviour in the rat. Arzneimittelforsch 28:1508–1509

De Montigny C, Aghajanian GK (1978) Tricyclic antidepressants: long term treatment increases responsivity of rat forebrain neurons to serotonin. Science 202:1303–1306

Depoortere H, Riou-Merle F (1986) Pharmaco-EEG profiles of progabide and fengabine compared with classical antidepressants. In: Bartholini G, Lloyd KG, Morselli PL (eds) GABA and mood disorders. Raven, New York, pp 97–99

Deutsch RD, Kling A, Steklis HD (1979) Influence of frontal lobe lesions on behavioural interactions in man. Res Commun Psych Psychiatr 4:415–431

Emrich HM, Altman H, Dose M, von Zerssen D (1983) Therapeutic effects of GABA-ergic drugs in affective disorders. Preliminary report. Pharmacol Biochem Behav 19:369–372

Emrich HM, Dose M, von Zerssen D (1985) The use of sodium valproate, carbamazepine and oxarbazepine in patients with affective disorders J Affective Disord 8:243–250

Enna SJ, Mann E, Kendall D, Stancel GM (1981) Effect of chronic antidepressant administration on brain neurotransmitter receptor binding. In: Enna SL, Kuhar M, Coyle J (eds) Antidepressants: neurochemical, behavioural and clinical perspectives. Raven, New York, pp 91–105

Flor-Henry P, Koles ZJ (1980) EEG studies in depression, mania and normals: Evidence for partial shifts of laterality in the affective psychoses. Adv Biol Psychiatry 4:21–43

Gerner RH, Fairbanks L (1985) Discriminate function of CSF neurochemistry among normals, depressed, schizophrenia, mania and anorexia subjects. IVth World congress of biological psychiatry, 8–13 Sept. 1985, Philadelphia, Abstract 500.1

Gerner RH, Hare TA (1981) CSF GABA in normal subjects and patients with depression, schizophrenia, mania and anorexia nervosa. Am J Psychiatry 138:1098–1101

Gerner RH, Fairbanks L, Andersen GM, Young JG, Scheinini M, Linnoila M, Hare TA, Shaywitz BA, Chen DJ (1984) CSF neurochemistry in depressed, mania and schizophrenia patients compared with that of normal controls. Am J Psychiatry 141:1533–1540

Gold BI, Bowers MB, Roth RH, Seeney DW (1980) GABA levels in CSF of patients with psychiatric disorders. Am J Psychiatry 137:362–364

Goodwin FK, Ebert MH, Bunney WE Jr (1977) Mental effects of reserpine in man: a review. In: Shader RI (ed) Psychiatric complications of medicinal drugs. Raven, New York, pp 73–101

Gottesfeld Z, Elliott KAC (1971) Factors that affect the binding and uptake of GABA by brain tissue. J Neurochem 18:683–690

Harris M, Hopkin JM, Neal MJ (1973) Effect of centrally acting drugs on the uptake of gamma-aminobutyric acid (GABA) by slices of rat cerebral cortex. Br J Pharmacol 47:229–239

Hill DR (1985) $GABA_B$ receptor modulation of adenylate cyclase activity in rat brain slices. Br J Pharmacol 84:249–257

Hill DR, Bowery NG (1981) ^{3}H-Baclofen and ^{3}H-GABA bind to bicuculline-insensitive $GABA_B$ sites in rat brain. Nature 290:149–152

Hollister LE (1978) Tricyclic antidepressants. N Engl J Med 299:1168–1172

Hrdina PD, Dubas TC, Riva E (1978) Brain distribution and pharmacokinetics of psychotropic drugs: Desipramine. In: Deniker P, Raduco-Thomas C, Villeneuve A (eds) Neuropsychopharmacology. Pergamon, New York, pp 841–848

Joffe RT, Post RM, Rubinow DR, Berrettini WH, Hare TA, Ballenger JC, Roy-Byrne PP (1986) Cerebrospinal fluid GABA in manic-depressive illness. In: Bartholini G, Lloyd KG, Morselli PL (eds) GABA and mood disorders. Raven, New York, pp 187–194

Johnson DAW (1981) Drug-induced psychiatric disorders. Drugs 22:57–69

Karbon EW, Duman R, Enna SJ (1983) Biochemical identification of $GABA_B$ binding sites: association with noradrenergic terminals in rat forebrain. Brain Res 274:393–396

Karbon EW, Duman RS, Enna SJ (1984) $GABA_B$ receptors and norepinephrine-stimulated cAMP production in rat brain cortex. Brain Res 306:327–332

Kasa K, Otsuki S, Yamamoto M, Sato M, Kuroda H, Ogawa N (1982) Cerebrospinal fluid gamma-aminobutyric acid and homovanillic acid in depressive disorders. Biol Psychiatry 17:877–883

Korf J, Venema K (1983) Desmethylimipramine enhances the release of endogenous GABA and other neurotransmitter amino acids from the rat thalamus. J Neurochem 40:946–950

Langer SZ, Arbilla S, Scatton B, Zivkovic B, Galzin AM, Lloyd KG, Bartholini G (1986) Progabide and SL 75102: interaction with GABA receptors and effects on neurotransmitter and receptor system. In: Bartholoni G, Bossi L, Lloyd KG, Morselli PL (eds) Epilepsy and GABA receptor agonists. Raven, New York, pp 81–90

Leonard BE (1984) The olfactory bulbectomized rat as a model of depression. Pol J Pharmacol Pharm 36:561–569

Lewis WC, Calden G, Thurston JR, Gelson WF (1957) Psychiatric and neurological reactions to cycloservine in the treatment of tuberculosis. Dis Chest 32:172–182

Lloyd KG (1986) GABA binding. In: Baker A, Boulton AA (eds) Neuromethods, vol 4. Humana, Clifton (in press)

Lloyd KG, Pichat P (1985) Decrease in $GABA_B$ binding in the frontal cortex of bulbectomized rats. Br J Pharmacol 87:36P

Lloyd KG, Pilc A (1984) Chronic antidepressants and $GABA_B$ binding sites. Neuroscience 10:117.5 (Abstract)

Lloyd KG, Bovier PH, Broekkamp CL, Worms P (1981) Reversal of the antiaversive and anticonvulsant actions of diazepam, but not progabide by a selective antagonist of benzodiazepine receptors. Eur J Pharmacol 75:77–78

Lloyd KG, Morselli PL, Depoortere H, Fournier V, Zivkovic B, Scatton B, Broekkamp CL, Worms P, Bartholini G (1983) The potential use of GABA agonists in psychiatric disorders: evidence from studies with progabide in animal models and clinical trials. Pharmacol Biochem Behav 18:957–966

Lloyd KG, Thuret F, Pilc A (1985) Upregulation of gamma-aminobutyric acid (GABA)"B" binding sites in rat frontal cortex: a common action of repeated administration of different classes of antidepressants and electroshock. J Pharmacol Exp Ther 235:191–199

Lloyd KG, Thuret F, Pilc A (1986) GABA and the mechanisms of action of antidepressant drugs. In: Bartholini G, Lloyd KG, Morselli PL (eds) GABA and mood disorders. Raven, New York, pp 33–42
Mandel MR, Klerman GL (1978) Clinical use of antidepressants, stimulants, tricyclics and monoamine oxidase inhibitors. In: Clark WG, Del Guidice J (eds) Principles of psychopharmacology, 2nd ed. Academic, New York, pp 537–551
Morselli PL, Henry JF, Macher JP, Bottin P, Huber JP, Van Landeghem VH (1981) Progabide and mood. In: Perris C, Struwe G, Jansson B (eds) Biological psychiatry. Elsevier, Amsterdam, pp 440–443
Morselli PL, Fournier V, Nacker JP, Orofiama B, Bottin P, Huber (1986) Therapeutic action of progabide in depressive illness: a controlled clinical trial. In: Bartholini G, Lloyd KG, Morselli PL (eds) GABA and mood disorders. Raven, New York, pp 118–125
Musch B (1986) The antidepressant activity of fengabide: a critical overview of the present results in open clinical studies. In: Bartholini G, Lloyd KG, Morselli PL (eds) GABA and mood disorders. Raven, New York, pp 171–177
Olsen RW, Ticku MK, Van Ness PC, Greenlee D (1978) Effects of drugs on gamma-aminobutyric acid receptors, uptake, release and synthesis in vitro. Brain Res 139:277–294
Patel GJ, Schatz RP, Constandinidis SM, Lal H (1975) Effect of desipramine and pargyline on brain gamma-aminobutyric acid. Biochem Pharmacol 24:57–60
Perry EK, Gibson PH, Blessed G, Perry RH, Tomlinson BE (1977) Neurotransmitter abnormalities in senile dementia. J Neurol Sci 34:247–265
Petty F (1986) GABA mechanisms in learned helplessness. In: Bartholini G, Lloyd KG, Morselli PL (eds) GABA and mood disorders. Raven, New York, pp 61–66
Petty F, Schlesser MA (1981) Plasma GABA in affective illness. J Affective Disord 3:339–343
Petty F, Sherman AD (1982) Plasma GABA: a blood test for bipolar affective disorder trait? Res Commun Psychol Psychiatr Behav 7:431–440
Petty F, Sherman AD (1984) Chronic antidepressants and GABA "B" receptors: a GABA hypothesis of antidepressant drugs action. Life Sci 35:2149–2154
Post RM, Balenger JC, Hare TA, Goodwin FK, Lake CR, Jimerson DC, Bunney WE (1980) Cerebrospinal fluid GABA in normals and patients with affective disorders. Brain Res Bull 5[Suppl 2]:755–759
Rampello L, Patti F, Condorelli DF, Reggio A, Prato A, Canonico PL, Nicoletti F (1982) Effects of some typical and atypical antidepressants on GAD activity in various brain regions. Encephale 8:89–94
Ross ED, Rusch AJ (1981) Diagnosis and neuroanatomical correlates of depression in brain-damaged patients. Arch Gen Psychiatry 38:1344–1354
Ruff RL, Russakoff LM (1980) Catatonia with frontal lobe atrophy. J Neurol Neurosurg Psychiatry 43:185–187
Ruiz RC (1964) D-Cycloserine in the treatment of pulmonary tuberculosis resistant to the standard drugs. Dis Chest 45:181–186
Sanger DJ, Joly D, Depoortere H, Zivkovic B, Lloyd KG (1986) Behavioural profile of progabide in tests for anxiolytics and antidepressant drugs. In: Bartholini G, Lloyd KG, Morselli PL (eds) GABA and mood disorders. Raven, New York, pp 77–84
Scatton B, Zivkovic B, Dedek J, Lloyd KG, Constantinidis J, Tissot R, Bartholini G (1982) γ-Aminobutyric acid (GABA) receptor stimulation. III. Effect of progabide (SL 76002) on norepinephrine, dopamine and 5-hydroxytryptamine turnover in rat brain areas. J Pharmacol Exp Ther 220:678–687
Schlicker E, Classen K, Gothert M (1984) $GABA_B$ receptor-mediated inhibition of serotonin release in the rat brain. Naunyn Schmiedebergs Arch Pharmacol 326:99–105
Sherman AD, Petty F (1982) Additivity of neurochemical changes in learned helplessness and imipramine. Behav Neural Biol 35:344–353
Sherman AD, Sacquitne JL, Petty F (1982) Specificity of the learned helplessness model of depression. Pharmacol Biochem Behav 16:449–454
Siggins GR, Schultz JE (1979) Chronic treatment with lithium or desipramine alters discharge frequency and norepinephrine responsiveness of cerebellar Purkinje cells. Proc Natl Acad Sci USA 76:5987–5991

Snodgrass SR, Heddley-Whyte ET, Lorenzo AV (1973) GABA transport by nerve ending fractions of cat brain. J Neurochem 20:771–782

Sulser F (1978) Functional aspects of the norepinephrine receptor coupled adenylate cyclase system in the limbic forebrain and its modification by drugs which precipitate or alleviate depression: molecular approaches to an understanding of affective disorders. Pharmacopsychiatria 11:43–52

Suranyi-Cadott BE, Dam TV, Quirion R (1985) Antidepressant-anxiolytic interaction: decreased density of benzodiazepine receptors in rat brain following chronic administration of antidepressants. Eur J Pharmacol 106:673–675

Suzdak PD, Gianutsos G (1985) Parallel changes in the sensitivity of gamma-aminobutyric acid and noradrenergic receptors following chronic administration of antidepressant and GABAergic drugs. Neuropharmacology 24:217–222

Tunnicliff G (1976) Centrally acting drugs and the formation of brain gamma-aminobutyric acid. Gen Pharmacol 7:259–262

Vetulani J, Antiewicz-Michaluk L, Rokorz-Pelc A, Pilc A (1984) Alpha up-beta down adrenergic regulation: a possible mechanism of antidepressant treatments. Pol J Pharmacol Pharm 36:231–248

Walker WC, Murdoch JM (1957) Cycloserine in the treatment of pulmonary tuberculosis. Tubercle 38:297–302

Whitlock FA, Evans LEJ (1978) Drugs and depression. Drugs 15:53–71

Willner P (1984) The ability of antidepressant drugs to desensitize beta-receptors is inversely correlated with their clinical potency. J Affective Disord 7:53–58

Winek CL (1976) Tabulation of therapeutic toxic and lethal concentrations of drugs and chemicals in blood. Clin Chem 22:832–836

Zivkovic B, Lloyd KG, Scatton B, Sanger DJ, Depoortere H, Dedek J, Arbilla S, Langer SZ, Bartholini G (1986) The pharmacological and neurochemical spectrum of fengabine, a new antidepressant agent. In: Bartholini G, Lloyd KG, Morselli PL (eds) GABA and mood disorders. Raven, New York, pp 85–95

Antidepressant Monoamine Oxidase Inhibitors Enhance Serotonin but not Norepinephrine Neurotransmission

P. Blier and C. de Montigny

1 Introduction

Monoamine oxidase inhibitors (MAOIs) were the first effective drugs in the treatment of major depression (Klein et al. 1980). Given their inhibiting action on the catabolism of monoaminergic neurotransmitters, they constitute unique tools for investigating the neurobiological basis of the antidepressant response.

The MAOIs used clinically, mainly phenelzine and tranylcypromine, are nonselective inhibitors, as they block the action of both the A and the B forms of monoamine oxidase (MAO). In vivo, serotonin (5-HT) and norepinephrine (NE) are metabolized by the A form of MAO, whereas dopamine is inactivated by both forms (Hall et al. 1969; Yang and Neff 1974). The therapeutic efficacy of nonselective MAOIs is currently attributed to their effect on MAO-A, since clorgyline and moclobemide, which selectively inhibit this isoenzyme, are clearly effective in the treatment of endogenous depression (Cassachia et al. 1984; Murphy et al. 1981; Stefanis et al. 1984), whereas the efficacy of MAO-B inhibitors is in question (Man et al. 1984; Murphy et al. 1981). Hence, both the 5-HT and the NE systems appear to be likely candidates for mediating the antidepressant effect of MAOIs. However, several biochemical (Savage et al. 1979; Sulser 1983), behavioral (Lucki and Fraser 1982), and electrophysiological (Olpe and Schellenburg 1980, 1981) studies have shown that in certain brain regions postsynaptic neurons become subsensitive to 5-HT and NE following long-term treatment with MAOIs. Therefore, the question as to whether the net efficacy of 5-HT and NE neurotransmission is modified by MAOI administration has remained unanswered. In other words, it is not known whether the gain expected from an increased availability of 5-HT and NE is cancelled out by an adaptation of the target neurons.

In order to address this question, we developed an electrophysiological model to evaluate the net change in 5-HT and NE neurotransmission produced by MAOIs. This model is presented schematically in Fig. 1. The first parameter assessed is the firing activity of the presynaptic neurons. This step is essential, since the amount of 5-HT and NE released from terminals in postsynaptic areas is impulse-flow dependent (Aghajanian 1978). The sensitivity of any autoreceptors, which contributes to the regulation of the firing rate of these neurons (Aghajanian 1978), can also be evaluated by the microiontophoretic ejections of agonists di-

Centre de Recherche en Sciences Neurologiques, Faculté de Medecine, Université de Montreal, C. P. 6128, Succursale A, Montreal, Quebec, Canada, H3C 3J7.

Clinical Pharmacology in Psychiatry
Editors: Dahl, Gram, Paul, Potter
(Psychopharmacology Series 3)

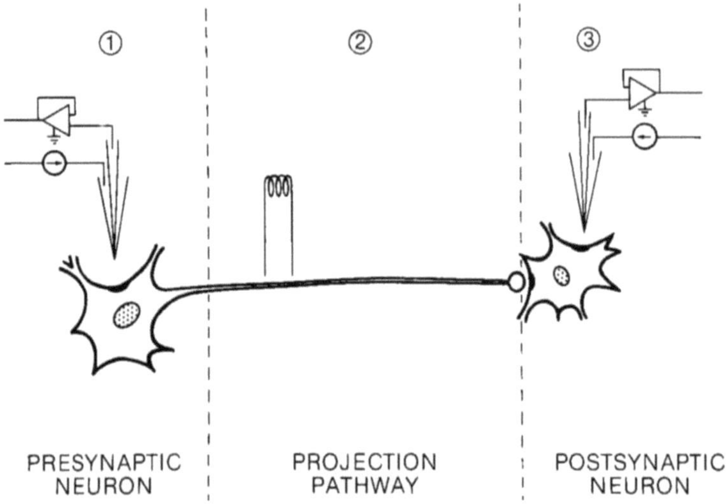

Fig. 1. Electrophysiological paradigm used to assess the effect of MAOIs on 5-HT and NE neurotransmission. *1*, Firing activity of the presynaptic neuron and sensitivity of the autoreceptor (assessed by either microiontophoresis or systemic administration of agonists); *2*, effect of the electrical stimulation of the ascending pathway on the firing activity of the postsynaptic neuron; *3*, responsiveness of the postsynaptic neuron to microiontophoretic applications of 5-HT and NE

rectly onto the recorded neuron or by injecting selective agonists of these receptors i.v. The second step consists in measuring the effect of the electrical stimulation of the ascending pathway on the firing activity of postsynaptic neurons. This provides a direct estimate of the global efficacy of synaptic transmission, which can be modulated by both presynaptic (e.g., availability of the neurotransmitter) and postsynaptic factors (e.g., sensitivity of postsynaptic receptors). The third step permits the determination of the sensitivity of the postsynaptic moiety to the neurotransmitter studied, using microiontophoresis.

2 Effects of MAOIs on Presynaptic Neurons

Rats were treated with clorgyline (1 mg kg^{-1} day^{-1} s.c.), a selective inhibitor of MAO-A (Johnston 1968), deprenyl (0.1 or 0.25 mg kg^{-1} day^{-1} s.c.), a selective inhibitor of MAO-B (Knoll 1976), or with phenelzine (2.5 mg kg^{-1} day^{-1} i.p.), a nonselective MAOI, for 2, 7, or 21 days. All experiments were carried out 24 h after the last dose. Dorsal raphe 5-HT neurons showed a drastic reduction of their firing rate after 2 days of treatment with phenelzine or clorgyline, a partial recovery after 7 days, and a complete restoration after 21 days of treatment (Fig. 2). This recovery of firing activity, in the presence of a sustained increase in the brain levels of 5-HT (Blier et al. 1986) can be attributed to a desensitization of the somatic 5-HT autoreceptor, since LSD is less effective in reducing the firing of 5-HT neurons after a 21-day treatment with either phenelzine or clorgyline. These data on 5-HT neurons stand in sharp contrast to those obtained in NE neurons. With

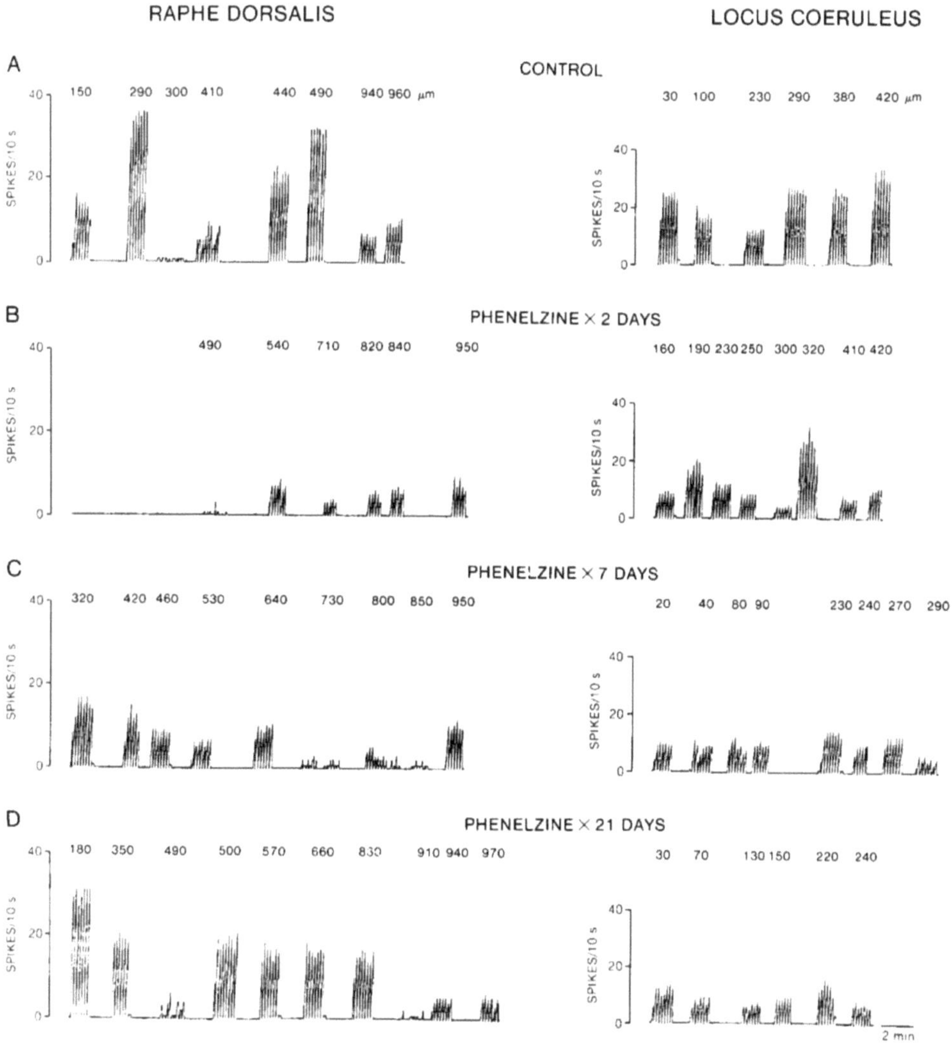

Fig. 2 a–d. Integrated firing rate histograms of 5-HT and NE neurons obtained during single electrode descents in the dorsal raphe and locus ceruleus in control rats and in rats treated with phenelzine (2.5 mg kg^{-1} day^{-1} i.p.) for 2, 7, or 21 days. Recordings were obtained 24 h after the last dose. The depth of recording for each neuron is indicated in micrometers from the floor of the Sylvius aqueduct for the raphe and from the floor of the fourth ventricle for the locus. Time base applies to all traces

both phenelzine and clorgyline, the firing rate of locus ceruleus NE neurons was decreased by more than 50% after 2 days of treatment and showed no recovery after 7 or 21 days of treatment (Fig. 2). Consistent with this finding, the responsiveness of their α_2-autoreceptors to clonidine remained unchanged. In keeping with its lack of effect on MAO-A, deprenyl failed to alter firing of 5-HT and NE neurons, or the sensitivity of their autoreceptors, as measured by iontophoresis of LSD or clonidine, respectively.

Hence, these results suggest a fundamental difference between the properties of 5-HT and NE neurons: 5-HT, but not NE neurons, have the capacity to adapt to an increased availability of their neurotransmitters. 5-HT neurons possess a plasticity that NE neurons appear to lack. The differential adaptability of these two neuronal populations might prove crucial in unravelling the neurobiological modifications responsible for the antidepressant activity of MAOIs.

3 Sensitivity of Postsynaptic Neurons to Exogenous 5-HT and NE

Microiontophoretic experiments were carried out to determine the sensitivity of postsynaptic neurons to 5-HT and NE in control rats and in rats treated for 21 days with the same three MAOIs. The responsiveness of hippocampal pyrami-

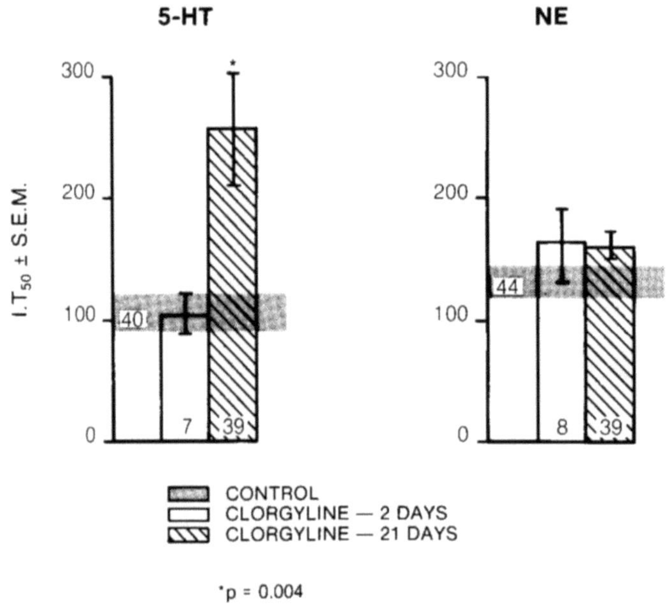

Fig. 3. Histograms representing the responsiveness of postsynaptic hippocampal pyramidal neurons, expressed as mean IT_{50} values ($\pm$sem) for 5-HT and NE in rats treated for 2 or 21 days with clorgyline (1 mg kg^{-1} day^{-1} i.p.). The IT_{50} value (I in nA x T50 in s) represents a charge required to obtain a 50% decrease in the firing rate of the neuron recorded. The number of units tested is given at the bottom of each *column* and within the *shaded areas* representing the range obtained in the controls. The responsiveness to either 5-HT or NE was not modified by the 21-day treatment with phenelzine or deprenyl (data not shown)

dal neurons to microiontophoretically-applied NE was not altered by any of the treatments. As for the responsiveness to 5-HT, it was decreased in the clorgyline group (Fig. 3), but not in the phenelzine or deprenyl groups. To ascertain that the subsensitivity to 5-HT following the long-term clorgyline treatment was a chronic adaptive effect, we assessed the sensitivity of the pyramidal neurons following a 2-day treatment. This short-term treatment failed to modify the responsiveness of hippocampal pyramidal neurons to 5-HT (Fig. 3). The difference between the effects of the long-term phenelzine and clorgyline regimens might stem from the more rapid MAO-A inhibition produced by clorgyline (Blier et al. 1986), which could result in a longer exposure of postsynaptic neurons to increased 5-HT. A similar desensitization of postsynaptic neurons to 5-HT has already been observed by Olpe and Schellenburg (1980) in the rostral and cingulate cortices following clorgyline administration.

4 Assessment of the Efficacy of Synaptic Transmission

In light of the decreased sensitivity to 5-HT of postsynaptic neurons in clorgyline-treated rats, it was important to assess whether impulses over the ascending 5-HT pathway produce a greater (or a smaller) effect on target neurons. The effects of stimulating the 5-HT and the NE pathways were assessed on the same neurons on which the microiontophoretic applications were carried out.

The effectiveness of the electrical stimulation of the dorsal NE bundle was not modified by any of the treatments. This may appear paradoxical, since NE brain levels were nearly doubled in rats treated with phenelzine or clorgyline (Blier et al. 1986). The lack of effect of MAOIs might be due to an increased activation of the α_2-autoreceptors located on NE terminals controlling the amount of NE released per impulse (Langer 1981). This possibility is all the more likely insofar as these receptors might fail to desensitize, as is the case for their somatic congeners (Sect. 2).

The electrical activation of the ascending 5-HT pathway produced a greater suppression of the firing of hippocampal pyramidal neurons in phenelzine- and clorgyline-treated rats, and its effectiveness was unchanged in deprenyl-treated rats. Given the decreased responsiveness of these same neurons to microiontophoretically applied 5-HT in the clorgyline-treated rats, the increased effectiveness of the stimulation indicates that the enhancing effect of clorgyline on the efficacy of 5-HT neurons themselves overcomes the attenuation of responsiveness of the target neurons. These results underscore the necessity of assessing overall synaptic transmission before a conclusion can be reached regarding a change in the net efficacy of neurotransmission.

5 Conclusion

From these results, it appears that adaptive changes in the NE system cannot account for the delayed antidepressant effect of MAOIs, since acute and chronic drug administration had the same effect; the net effect was a decreased NE neuro-

Table 1. Effects of long-term administration of MAOI on the 5-HT and NE systems[a]

Treatment	Firing rate of the presynaptic neuron		Sensitivity of the postsynaptic neuron[c]		Net effect on neurotransmission[d]	
	5-HT	NE	5-HT	NE	5-HT	NE
Phenelzine	Normal[b]	↓	0	0	↑	↓
Clorgyline	Normal[b]	↓	↓	0	↑	↓
Deprenyl	0	0	0	0	0	0

↑, increased; ↓, decreased; 0, no change.
[a] Rats were treated daily for 21 days (doses are given in the text).
[b] The firing rate was markedly decreased at the beginning of the treatment, but progressively recovered due to a desensitization of the somatic 5-HT autoreceptor.
[c] Assessed by microiontophoresis.
[d] Determined from the firing activity of the presynaptic neuron and the effect of stimulating the ascending pathways on postsynaptic neurons.

transmission resulting from an unchanged synaptic transmission in the presence of a decreased firing rate (Table 1). The 5-HT system, on the other hand, appears to be a good candidate for mediating the delayed therapeutic effect of MAOIs; during the first few days of treatment, 5-HT neurotransmission cannot be substantially increased even in the presence of elevated neuronal 5-HT, since the presynaptic neurons are firing at a much diminished rate. As the treatment continues, however, firing rate returns to normal in the continued presence of increased levels of 5-HT, thus producing a net increase in 5-HT neurotransmission (Table 1).

The conclusion reached from these electrophysiological data, that the 5-HT system might be involved in mediating the antidepressant effect of MAOI drugs, is in keeping with several lines of clinical evidence. First, Price al. (1985) have shown that 5-HT transmission is increased following treatment with an MAOI. Since the 5-HT system is known to exert a stimulatory effect on the secretion of prolactin (Dannies 1980), they measured the prolactin response to an i.v. injection of L-tryptophan, a precursor of 5-HT, in depressed patients before and following tranylcypromine treatment. The prolactin response to L-tryptophan was enhanced by tranylcypromine, indicating that at least along some pathways, 5-HT neurotransmission may be increased. Secondly, that such an increase in 5-HT transmission is relevant to the antidepressive efficacy of MAOIs was shown earlier by studying the effect of para-chlorophenylalanine, a 5-HT synthesis inhibitor, in depressed patients who had recovered on being treated with tranylcypromine (Shopsin et al. 1976). A rapid return of the depressive syndrome was induced by the addition of the synthesis inhibitor, and remission was reinstated upon discontinuation of this agent. The last source of clinical evidence involves the addition to an MAOI regimen of substances that augment the efficacy of the 5-HT system. Two strategies have been used: First, the combination of an MAOI and L-tryptophan, and secondly, the addition to an MAOI of lithium, which enhances serotonergic neurotransmission (Blier and de Montigny 1985a). L-Tryptophan potentiated the antidepressant effect of MAOIs (Ayuso Guttirez and Lopez-Ibor

1971; Coppen et al. 1963; Glassman and Platman 1969; Pare 1963), and the addition of lithium to an MAOI regimen was reported to be effective in MAOI-resistant patients (Louie and Meltzer 1984; Nelson and Byck 1982).

In conclusion, the electrophysiological studies reviewed here show that MAOIs increase 5-HT neurotransmission with a time-course that is congruent with their therapeutic effect. In addition, there is strong clinical evidence to support a role of the 5-HT system in mediating the antidepressant response to MAOI administration. Clinical investigations with an MAOI selective for 5-HT neurons, such as amiflamine (Ask et al. 1984; Blier et al. 1985), could provide additional information on the links the 5-HT system has with other chemospecific neuronal systems in mediating the antidepressant response.

References

Aghajanian GK (1978) Feedback regulation of central monoaminergic neurons: evidence from single-cell recording studies. In: Youdim MBH, Lovenberg W, Sharman DF, Lagnado JR (eds) Essays in neurochemistry and neuropharmacology, vol 3. Wiley, New York, p 1

Ask AL, Fagervall I, Kelder D, Nygren R, Ross SB (1984) Effects of acute and repeated administration of amiflamine on monoamine oxidase inhibition in the rat. Biochem Pharmacol 33:2839–2847

Ayuso Guttirez JL, Lopez-Ibor AJJ (1971) Tryptophan and a MAOI (nialamide) in the treatment of depression. A double-blind study. Int Pharmacopsychiatry 7:92–97

Blier P, de Montigny C (1985a) Short-term lithium administration enhances serotonergic neurotransmission: electrophysiological evidence in the rat CNS. Eur J Pharmacol 113:69–77

Blier P, de Montigny C (1985b) Serotonergic but not noradrenergic neurons in rat CNS adapt to long-term treatment with monoamine oxidase inhibitors. Neuroscience 16:949–955

Blier P, de Montigny C, Azzaro AJ (1985) Selective effect of amiflamine, a reversible monoamine oxidase inhibitor, on serotonergic neurotransmission. Soc Neuroci 11:60.1 (Abstract)

Blier P, de Montigny C, Azzaro AJ (1986) Modification of serotonergic and noradrenergic neurotransmission by repeated administration of monoamine oxidase inhibitors: electrophysiological studies in the rat CNS. J Pharmacol Exp Ther 237:987–994

Cassachia M, Carolei A, Barba C, Rossi A (1984) Moclobemide (Ro-11-1163) versus placebo: a double-blind study in depressive patients. In: Tipton KF, Dostert P, Strolin Benedetti M (eds) Monoamine oxidase and disease. Academic, New York, p 607

Coppen A, Shaw DM, Farrell JP (1963) Potentiation of the antidepressive effects of a monoamine oxidase inhibitor by tryptophan. Lancet 1:79–81

Dannies PS (1980) Prolactin. Trends Pharmacol Sci 1:206–208

Glassman A, Platman SR (1969) Potentiation of a monoamine oxidase inhibitor by tryptophan. J Psychiatry Res 7:83–88

Hall DWR, Logan BW, Parsons GH (1969) Further studies on the inhibition of monoamine oxidase by M and B 9302 (Clorgyline). Biochem Pharmacol 18:1447–1454

Johnston JP (1968) Some observations upon a new inhibitor of monoamine oxidase in brain tissue. Biochem Pharmacol 17:1285–1297

Klein DF, Gittelman R, Quitkin F, Rifkin A (1980) Diagnosis and treatment of psychiatric disorders: adults and children. Williams and Wilkins, Baltimore

Knoll J (1976) Analysis of the pharmacological effects of selective monoamine oxidase inhibitors. In: Wolstenholme GEW, Knight J (eds) Monoamine oxidase and its inhibition. Elsevier, Amsterdam, p 135

Langer SZ (1981) Presynaptic regulation of the release of catecholamines. Pharmacol Rev 32:337–360

Louie AK, Meltzer HY (1984) Lithium potentiation of antidepressant treatments. J Clin Psychopharmacol 4:316–320

Lucki I, Frazer A (1982) Prevention of the serotonin syndrome by repeated administration of monoamine oxidase inhibitors but not tricyclic antidepressants. Psychopharmacology (Berlin) 77:205–211

Mann JJ, Fox Aarrons S, Frances A, Bernstein W, Brown RD (1984) Studies of selective and reversible monoamine oxidase inhibitors. J Clin Psychiatry 45:62–66

Murphy DL, Lipper S, Pickar D, Jimerson D, Cohen RM, Garrick NA, Alterman IS, Campbell IC (1981) Selective inhibition of monoamine oxidase type A: clinical antidepressant effects and metabolic changes in man. In: Youdim MBH, Paykel ES (eds) Monoamine oxidase inhibitors – The state of the art. Wiley, New York, P 189

Nelson JC, Byck R (1982) Rapid response to lithium in phenelzine non-responders. Br J Psychiatry 141:85–86

Olpe HR, Schellenburg A (1980) Reduced sensitivity of cortical neurons to noradrenaline after chronic treatments with antidepressant drugs. Eur J Pharmacol 63:7–13

Olpe HR, Schellenburg A (1981) The sensitivity of cortical neurons to serotonin: effect of chronic treatment with antidepressant serotonin uptake inhibitors and mono-amine oxidase blocking drugs. J Neural Transm 51:233–244

Pare CMB (1963) Potentiation of monoamine oxidase inhibitors by tryptophan. Lancet 2:527–528

Price LH, Charney DS, Heninger GR (1985) Effects of tranylcypromine treatment on neuroendocrine, behavioral, and autonomic responses to tryptophan in depressed patients. Life Sci 37:809–818

Savage DD, Frazer A, Mendels J (1979) Differential effects of monoamine oxidase inhibitors and serotonin reuptake inhibitors on ^{3}H-serotonin receptor binding in rat brain. Eur J Pharmacol 58:87–98

Shopsin B, Friedman E, Gershon S (1976) Parachlorophenylalanine reversal of tranylcypromine effects in depressed patients. Arch Gen Psychiatry 33:811–819

Stefanis CN, Alevizos B, Papadimitriou GN (1984) Controlled clinical study of moclobemide (Ro 11-1163), a new MAO inhibitor, and desipramine in depressive patients. In: Tipton KF, Dostert P, Strolin Benedetti M (eds) Monoamine oxidase and disease. Academic, New York, p 377

Sulser F (1983) Deamplification of noradrenergic signal transfer by antidepressants: a unified catecholamine-serotonin hypothesis of affective disorders. Psychopharmacol Bull 19:300–304

Yang HYT, Neff NH (1974) The monoamine oxidase of the brain: selective inhibition with drugs and the consequences for the metabolism of the biogenic amines. J Pharmacol Exp Ther 189:733–740

Selective Amine Oxidase Inhibitors: Basic to Clinical Studies and Back

D. L. Murphy[1], T. Sunderland[1], N. A. Garrick[1], C. S. Aulakh[1], and R. M. Cohen[2]

1 Introduction

The monoamine oxidase (MAO)-inhibiting antidepressants, which have been in general clinical use in various parts of the world for the past 25 years, are all nonselective agents. They have marked effects on the metabolism of over 15 different monoamines, including major brain neurotransmitters (norepinephrine, dopamine, and serotonin) and on that of many other amines, which may act as co-transmitters, false transmitters, amine-releasing agents, or neuromodulators (e.g., tryptamine, tyramine, octopamine, and phenylethylamine).

Recently, knowledge concerning new drugs with selective MAO-inhibiting actions has expanded rapidly. Part of this development has been spurred by the delineation of at least three different amine oxidases: MAO type A, MAO type B, and a clorgyline-resistant, semicarbazide-sensitive, benzylamine oxidase (Singer et al. 1979; Buffoni 1983; Tipton et al. 1984; Kuhn et al. 1986).

Drugs are now available with very highly selective inhibitory activity against either MAO-A or MAO-B. A series of amine substrates are clearly differentially affected in vitro and in vivo by these selective inhibitors. For example, serotonin and norepinephrine metabolism are considerably altered by MAO-A inhibitors, while phenylethylamine, phenylethanolamine, and benzylamine metabolism are more markedly affected by inhibitors of MAO-B. It should be noted that selectivity is a function of drug concentration, and agents which are very selective at low concentrations become nonselective at high concentrations. Some of these agents also exhibit tissue selectivity, affecting MAO in brain and some specific cell groups or tissues to a greater extent than MAO in, for example, liver. Selective MAO inhibitors also differ in their physiological consequences for blood pressure and sleep, as well as in their therapeutic efficacy as antidepressants.

2 Different Classes of Selective Amine Oxidase Inhibitors

Clorgyline, pargyline, and deprenyl (Fig. 1), three 2-propinylamine inhibitors, have been the most studied irreversible selective inhibitors of MAO-A or MAO-B. The acetylenic ($C \equiv N$) substituent that they possess interacts with a pentapep-

[1] Section on Clinical Neuropharmacology, Laboratory of Clinical Science, National Institute of Mental Health, NIH Clinical Center, 10-3D41 Bethesda, MD 20892, USA.
[2] Section on Clinical Brain Imaging, Laboratory of Cerebral Metabolism, National Institute of Mental Health, NIH Clinical Center, 10-4N 317 Bethesda, MD 20892, USA.

Clinical Pharmacology in Psychiatry
Editors: Dahl, Gram, Paul, Potter
(Psychopharmacology Series 3)

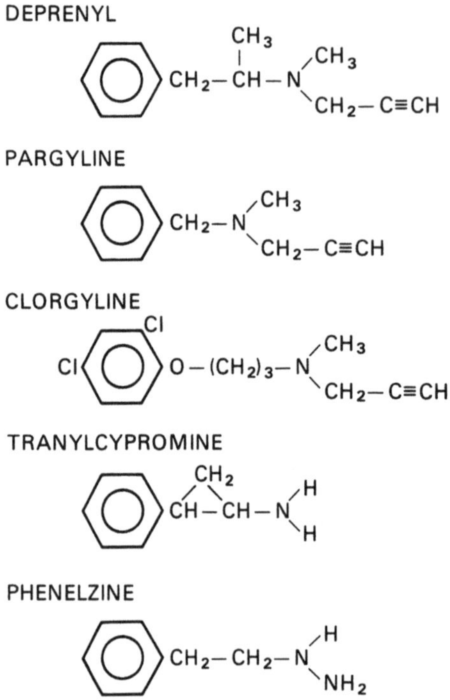

Fig. 1. Structures of three selective acetylenic MAO inhibitors (deprenyl, pargyline and clorgyline) and two nonselective MAO inhibitors

tide-FAD segment of the active site of both MAO-A and MAO-B to inactivate the enzyme irreversibly. It is of note that while all three drugs are structurally similar to phenylethylamine, including the nonselective hydrazine inhibitor phenelzine and the cyclopropylamine inhibitor tranylcypromine (Fig. 1), clorgyline is distinguished by a longer side chain, with an oxygen atom linking the side chain to the phenyl ring, and chloro substituents on the phenyl ring. Clorgyline, while among the first of the selective MAO-inhibitors recognized (Johnston 1968; Hall et al. 1969), remains the most highly selective irreversible inhibitor yet identified (Table 1). L-Deprenyl, which was shown by Knoll et al. (1965) to possess what are now recognized as MAO-B selective inhibiting actions, manifests lesser selectivity. An N-substituted cyclopropylamine with highly selective, irreversible MAO-A-inhibiting properties, Lilly 51641, was also identified during the same period by Fuller (1968). Lilly 51641, like clorgyline, differs from a series of MAO-B selective congeners in possessing a longer side chain containing oxygen, and an *o*-chloro substituent on its phenyl ring (Murphy et al. 1978).

Much of what is known about the physiological consequences of selective inhibition of MAO-A or MAO-B has resulted from studies with the acetylenic or *N*-cyclopropylamine irreversible inhibitors (Murphy 1978). In the last few years, however, in vitro and in vivo animal studies and, in a few cases, clinical investigations have been initiated to investigate several new classes of reversible inhibitors of MAO-A or MAO-B (Bieck et al. 1983; Ask et al. 1984, 1985; Da Prada et al. 1984; Strolin Benedetti and Dostert 1985; Tipton et al. 1984). A comparison of the selectivity and potency of these newer agents with those properties of the

Table 1. MAO inhibitors: Relative selectivity and potency

	Selectivity ratio	Potency (IC_{50}[a] or K_i, n*M*)
MAO-A-selective (A:B) inhibitors		
Irreversible		
Clorgyline	4000	0.5
LY 51641	1990	2
Reversible		
Brofaremine (CGP 11305 A)	3000	10
Moclobemide (RO 11-1163)	1000	1000
Amiflamine	525	400
(+)Amphetamine	38	20000
Toloxatone	24	1800
Cimoxatone (MD 780515)	20	4
MAO-B-selective (B:A) inhibitors		
Irreversible		
(−)Deprenyl	107	26
Pargyline	32	20
LY 54761	10	1600
Reversible		
RO 16-6491	250	50
MDL 72145	100	2500
MD 240926	6	300
Imipramine	7	40
Other irreversible inhibitors (A:B)		
Phenelzine	2	1000
Tranylcypromine	4	2000

[a] IC_{50}, inhibitor concentration that produces 50% inhibition of enzyme activity.

irreversible selective inhibitors determined in rodent or human brain in vitro is presented in Table 1. As these data were compiled from several sources with different assay procedures, tissue preparations, and other experimental procedures, this information can only be considered a rough approximation for orienting purposes (Tipton et al. 1984; Murphy et al. 1979; Ask et al. 1984; Kettler et al. 1985; McDonald et al. 1985). The selectivity ratios for the different inhibitors in Table 1 have generally been derived from a comparison of the deamination of the MAO substrate serotonin with that of either phenylethylamine or benzylamine as MAO-B substrates. The concentrations producing 50% inhibition of the enzyme activity (IC_{50}), or in the case of the reversible inhibitors, The K_i's, were generally derived using tyramine or a similarly nonselective substrate. Of particular note are two instances of structurally similar compounds which exemplify MAO-A selectivity (moclobemide and cimoxatone) while their respective congeners (RO 16-6491 and MD 240926) possess MAO-B selective properties.

3 Tissue Localization of the MAO-A or MAO-B Enzyme Forms as a Factor in Inhibitory Selectivity In Vivo

Most mammalian tissues contain both MAO-A and MAO-B, and hence the effects of MAO inhibition in vivo often correspond to the in vitro relationships summarized in Table 1. Two major exceptions exist, however. The most obvious are exemplified in the tissues listed in Table 2, which contain essentially only MAO-A or MAO-B and hence are only affected by one inhibitor type when it is used in MAO-selective doses. The pineal gland is an interesting organ in this respect, as pinealocyte cells, which synthesize, store, and release serotonin and melatonin, contain only MAO-B, while the presynaptic sympathetic neurons which innervate these cells and synthesize and store norepinephrine contain only MAO-A (Goridis and Neff 1971). Human platelets, which also possess specialized transport and storage processes for serotonin, also contain only MAO-B (Donnelly and Murphy 1977), as do serotonin-rich areas in rodent and primate brain (Levitt et al. 1982; Westlund et al. 1985). In contrast, norepinephrine-synthesizing cell bodies in the locus ceruleus in the brain and in sympathetic nerve endings in the periphery contain predominantly if not exclusively MAO-A, as do rodent (but not primate) dopamine nerve endings in brain (Demarest et al. 1980; Garrick and Murphy 1980). Thus, although serotonin and norepinephrine are the two substrates which behave as highly selective substrates for MAO-A in vitro, the different localization of MAO-A versus MAO-B in neurons and other cells which utilize these monoamines suggests the possibility of different functional roles for the two enzymes in these tissues.

Similar questions regarding evolutionary development, differentiation for specialized functions, and dedifferentiation as part of tumorigenesis are raised by the presence of MAO-A alone in placental trophoblasts and in many tumor tissues such as neuroblastoma and glioma cells (Donnelly et al. 1976; Murphy, Donnelly and Richelson 1976; Cawthorn and Breakefield 1983) and in the occurrence of MAO-B alone in adrenal medullary chromaffin cells, but MAO-A in the PC-12 tumor cell line derived from adrenal medullary cells (Youdim et al. 1984).

Table 2. Localization of monoamine oxidase subtypes

	MAO-A	MAO-B
Periphery	Sympathetic nerve endings Placental trophoblasts	Platelets Adrenal medullary chromaffin cells
Brain	Locus ceruleus Striatal dopamine nerve endings (rodents)	Astrocytes Pinealocytes Serotonin-rich areas
Others	Neuroblastoma C6 glial cells PC-12 adrenal medullary cells Most hepatoma cell lines	

4 Other Factors Affecting In Vivo-Selective Actions of MAO Inhibitors

As with other drugs, some MAO inhibitors require metabolic transformation in vivo to become potent inhibitors. The prototype hydrazine inhibitor, iproniazid, is in fact inactive in vitro. Some selective MAO inhibitors possess metabolites which differ in potency and duration of action, e.g., cimoxatone's metabolite MD 770222 (Garrick et al. 1985 a). Metabolites of other selective MAO inhibitors may have different MAO selectivity or pharmacological actions. Deprenyl, for example, is metabolized to amphetamine and methamphetamine, which are weak, reversible MAO-A inhibitors and also possess direct stimulant properties (Knoll 1978). Amiflamine has been suggested to have greater MAO-inhibitory effects in vivo on serotonergic than catecholaminergic neurons, in part because it is more readily transported by the serotonin membrane uptake pump (Ask et al. 1985), although the ultimate functional significance of this property is controversial (Garrick et al. 1985 b). Several MAO-inhibitor precursors have been synthesized in attempts to obtain agents which act only in the central nervous system; for example, MD 72394 requires decarboxylation to become effective and, if given together with a peripheral decarboxylase inhibitor, may be converted in the brain but not in the periphery to active inhibitors (Palfreyman et al. 1984).

Interestingly, clorgyline given chronically to rodents produces substantially more inhibition in brain than in liver, partly because the half-life of MAO-A in liver is 3.5 days, as against more than 12 days in brain; deprenyl demonstrates similar, although smaller, tissue-selective differences following administration (Felner and Waldmeier 1979; Cohen et al. 1982 b). The selectivity of deprenyl is dependent only partly on its affinity for the MAO-B site; its selectivity is enhanced by a greater rate of formation of the irreversible adduct with MAO-B than MAO-A (Fowler et al. 1982). Fuller (1978) and Strolin Benedetti and Dostert (1985) have presented theoretical outlines of these and other approaches to developing new MAO inhibitors with tissue and substrate selectivity and other desirable properties in vivo.

5 Physiologic Consequences of Selective MAO Inhibitor Administration to Rodents, Nonhuman Primates and Humans

Yang and Neff (1974) were among the first to demonstrate that the substrate-selective actions of clorgyline observed in vitro could result in greater changes in serotonin and norepinephrine concentrations in rodent brain; in contrast, deprenyl preferentially altered phenylethylamine metabolism. Although this selectivity can be lost with chronic administration of the drugs at high doses, careful titration of drug dosage over time has now been shown in rodents, nonhuman primates, and humans to lead to highly selective alterations in metabolism during clorgyline administration (Felner and Waldmeier 1979; Waldmeier et al. 1981; Cohen et al. 1982 b; Garrick et al. 1984; Murphy et al. 1979, 1981).

As noted above, additional factors besides direct drug-enzyme interactions account for the monoamine metabolism changes which occur in vivo, and in some

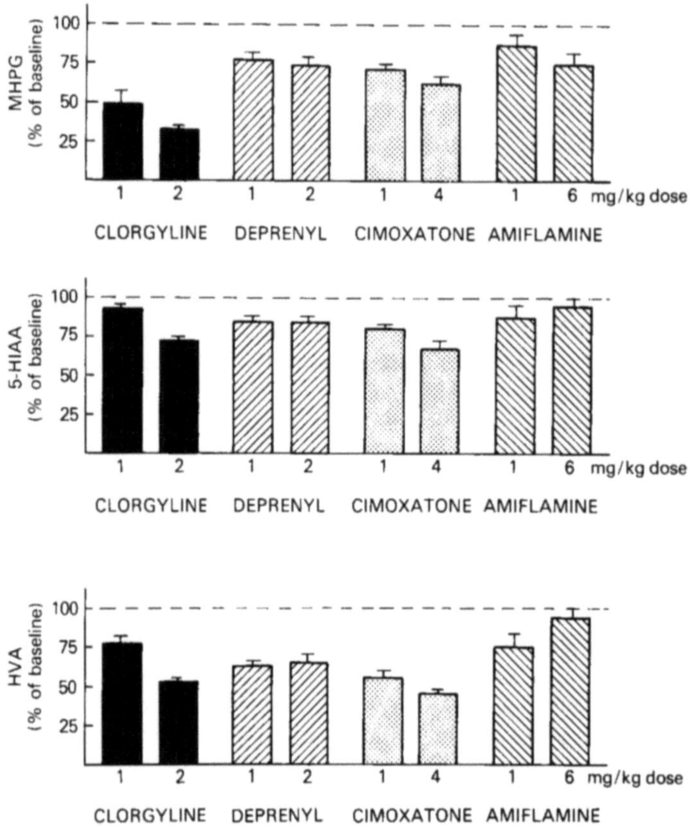

Fig. 2. Reductions in rhesus monkey CSF amine metabolites following acute MAO inhibitor administration

cases greater selectivity may be found in specific brain areas or tissues, and after longer term rather than single-dose administration. An example of this complexity is presented in Fig. 2, which illustrates the changes in the major metabolites of norepinephrine (3-methoxy, 4-hydroxyphenylglycol, MHPG), serotonin (5-hydroxyindoleacetic acid, 5-HIAA), and dopamine (homovanillic acid, HVA) after single doses of four selective MAO inhibitors given to rhesus monkeys (Garrick et al. 1984, 1985 a, 1985 b). Of all the drugs, clorgyline produced the most marked reductions in MHPG, but these changes did not approach the 85%–90% reductions in MHPG observed with considerably smaller doses of clorgyline (0.25–0.5 mg/kg) given chronically to rhesus monkeys (Garrick et al. 1984). Reductions in 5-HIAA after clorgyline were considerably smaller than those in MHPG, despite the in vitro data obtained in rhesus monkey brain, indicating that serotonin rather than norepinephrine was the substrate most selectively deaminated by MAO-A according to comparisons of the relative inhibitory activities of clorgyline versus deprenyl (Garrick and Murphy 1982). Amiflamine and cimoxatone, two reversible MAO-A inhibitors, which were given in doses chosen to approximate those under study in human antidepressant efficacy trials, did not yield

MHPG reductions comparable to those found with clorgyline (Fig. 2). Amiflamine also did not show evidence of the selectivity towards greater inhibition of serotonin deamination found in vitro in rodents (Fig. 2; see also Ask et al. 1984, 1985).

Human cerebrospinal fluid (CSF) data obtained during therapeutic trials with clorgyline, pargyline, and two different doses of deprenyl revealed strong evidence that sustained, low-dose administration of these drugs was capable of maintaining quite selective actions on monoamine metabolites. As illustrated in Fig. 3, low doses (10 mg/day) of deprenyl (which inhibited platelet MAO-B activity in these patients >95%) produced only 10%–15% reductions in MHPG and 5-HIAA, and 20% reductions in HVA, while MAO-A-selective doses of clorgyline yielded 90% reductions in MHPG, 50% reductions in 5-HIAA, and 25% reductions in HVA. High, nonselective doses of pargyline reduced all three metabolites (Major et al. 1979; Sunderland et al. 1985). Additional evidence from studies of urinary, plasma, and CSF amines and amine metabolites and of platelet

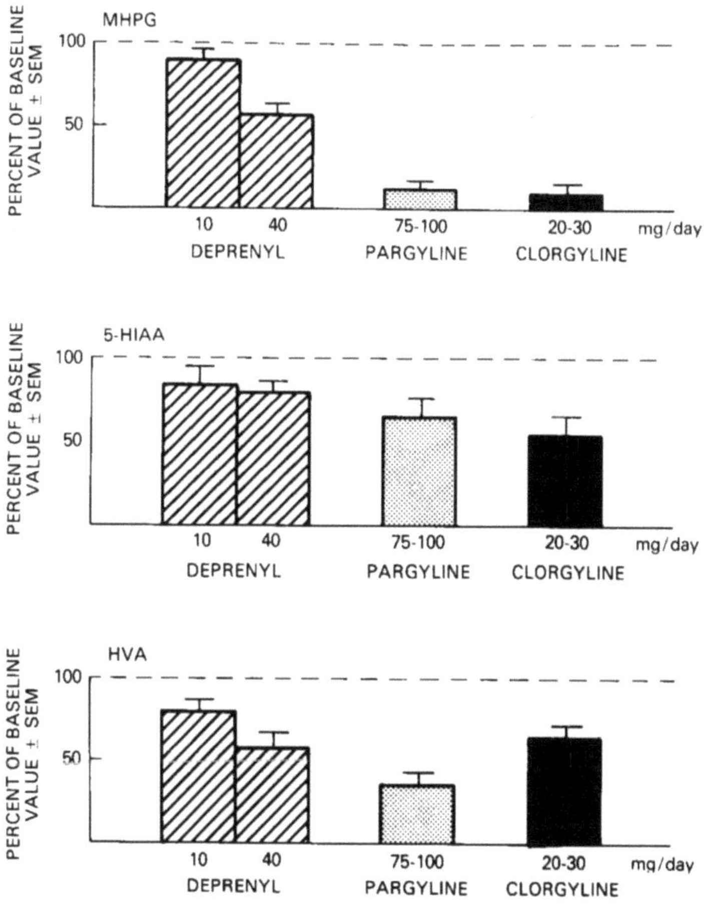

Fig. 3. Human CSF amine metabolites following chronic MAO inhibitor administration

MAO-B activity summarized in Table 3 provides more comprehensive data on the selectivity achievable with these drugs in humans (Murphy et al. 1979, 1981; Linnoila et al. 1982; Sunderland et al. 1985).

These data on monoamine metabolism changes with selective inhibitors have direct functional and clinical implications. We have recently reviewed elsewhere the evidence that clorgyline given chronically in low doses produces α- and β-adrenoceptor changes, as well as serotonin receptor changes and other alterations in serotonin metabolism, which are accompanied by behavioral, cardiovascular, sleep, and neurohormonal changes in animals and humans (Murphy et al. 1984; Cohen et al. 1982a, c, 1983; Roy et al. 1986; Siever et al. 1981; Campbell et al. 1985; Murphy et al. 1986; Aulakh et al. 1983a, b). These changes include altered brain self-stimulation responses, food intake, locomotion, blood pressure, rapid eye movement sleep, and plasma and CSF melatonin changes, and are consistent with expected selective changes in MAO activity. In contrast, minimal or no changes have been observed in these measures during chronic low-dose deprenyl administration.

Similarly, there is substantial evidence from studies examining antidepressant efficacy in random-assignment, double-blind studies suggesting that MAO-A inhibitors are more therapeutically effective than MAO-B inhibitors (Table 4). In recent experiments, we have been able to confirm that the metabolic changes observed in catecholamine metabolism and the physiologic changes attributable to

Table 3. Indices of MAO-B and MAO-A inhibition in man

	Clorgyline (30 mg)	Pargyline		Deprenyl (10 mg)
		(30 mg)	(90 mg)	
Indices of MAO-B inhibition				
Platelet MAO-B activity inhibition	22%	99%	99%	99%
Urinary phenylethylamine increase	Unchanged	–	100 ×	24 ×
Indices of MAO-A inhibition				
Plasma MHPG reduction	86%	65%	–	17%
Urinary MHPG excretion reduction	85%	58%	82%	–
CSF MHPG reduction	91%	–	89%	9%
CSF 5-HIAA reduction	45%	–	34%	14%

Table 4. Antidepressant effects of selective MAO inhibitors: Double-blind, randomized trials

Selective MAO-A inhibitors		
Clorgyline	> Amitriptyline	(Herd 1969)
(3/3 studies positive)	= Imipramine	(Wheatley 1970)
	> Pargyline	(Lipper et al. 1979)
Meclobemide	> Placebo	(Casachia et al. 1984)
(3/3 studies positive)	= Clomipramine	(Larsen et al. 1984)
	= Desipramine	(Stefanis et al. 1984)
Selective MAO-B inhibitors		
Deprenyl	= Placebo	(Mendis et al. 1981)
(1/2 studies positive)	> Placebo	(Mendlewicz and Youdim 1983)

these found with selective MAO inhibitors are in fact attributable to differences in the relative magnitude of MAO-A versus MAO-B inhibition, by comparing the effects of low (10 mg/day), moderate (30 mg/day), and high (60 mg/day) doses of deprenyl (Sunderland et al. 1985). With the higher deprenyl doses, plasma MHPG becomes progressively reduced and orthostatic hypotension and enhanced tyramine pressor sensitivity become more prominent, approaching the magnitude of changes found with clorgyline and with nonselective MAO inhibitors such as tranylcypromine.

It will be important to continue to seek selective metabolic and physiologic actions of the irreversible and the newly available reversible inhibitors of MAO-A and MAO-B to identify possible therapeutic advantages in treating depression and other disorders which may accompany selective monoamine system changes. Similarly, the possibilities provided by these selectively acting drugs to explore the importance of different monoamine systems in the mechanisms of action and side effects of psychotropic durgs, and in psychiatric and other medical disorders, continue to be important areas for further investigation.

Acknowledgments. We thank our many scientific coworkers for assistance in studies accomplished at NIMH and cited in the reference list. We also thank Audrey Reid for editorial assistance and Gloria Goldsmith, Nancy Glaros, and Dottie Drake for assistance with the manuscript preparation.

References

Ask AL, Fagervall I, Jonze M, Kelder D, Nygren R, Ross SB (1984) Effects of acute and repeated administration of amiflamine on monoamine oxidase inhibition in the rat. Biochem Pharmacol 33:2839–2847

Ask AL, Fagervall I, Florvall L, Ross SB, Ytterborn S (1985) Inhibition of monoamine oxidase in 5-hydroxytryptaminergic neurones by substituted *p*-aminophenylalkylamines. Br J Pharmacol 85:683–690

Aulakh CS, Cohen RM, Pradhan SN, Murphy DL (1983a) Self-stimulation responses are altered following long-term but not short-term treatment with clorgyline. Brain Res 270:383–386

Aulakh CS, Cohen RM, McLellan C, Murphy DL (1983b) Correlation of changes in α_2-adrenoceptor number and locomotor responses to clonidine following clorgyline discontinuation. Br J Pharmacol 80:10–12

Bieck P, Antonin KH, Jedrychowski M (1983) Monoamine oxidase inhibition in healthy volunteers by CGP 11305 A, a new specific inhibitor of MAO-A. Mod Probl Pharmacopsychiatry 19:53–62

Buffoni F (1983) Biochemical pharmacology of amine oxidases. Trends Pharmacol Sci 4:313–315

Campbell IC, Gallager DW, Hamburg MA, Tallman JF, Murphy DL (1985) Electrophysiological and receptor studies in rat brain: effects of clorgyline. Eur J Pharmacol 111:355–364

Casacchia M, Carolei A, Barba C, Rossi A (1984) Moclobemide (Ro 11-1163) versus placebo: a double-blind study in depressive patients. In: Tipton KF, Dostert P, Strolin Benedetti M (eds) Monoamine oxidase and disease. Prospects for therapy with reversible inhibitors. Academic, London, pp 607–608

Cawthon RM, Breakefield XO (1983) Differences in the structures of monoamine oxidases A and B in rat clonal cell lines. Biochem Pharmacol 32:441–448

Cohen RM, Campbell IC, Yamaguchi I, Pickar D, Kopin IJ, Murphy DL (1982a) Cardiovascular changes in response to selective monoamine oxidase inhibition in the rat. Eur J Pharmacol 80:155–160

Cohen RM, Ebstein RP, Daly JW, Murphy DL (1982b) Chronic effects of a monoamine oxidase-inhibiting antidepressant: decreases in functional alpha-adrenergic autoreceptors precede the decrease in norepinephrine-stimulated cyclic adenosine 3′:5′-monophosphate systems in rat brain. J Neurosci 2:1588–1595

Cohen RM, Pickar D, Garnett D, Lipper S, Gillin JC, Murphy DL (1982c) REM sleep suppression induced by selective monoamine oxidase inhibitors. Psychopharmacology (Berlin) 78:137–140

Cohen RM, Aulakh CS, Murphy DL (1983) Long-term clorgyline treatment antagonizes the eating and motor function responses to *m*-chlorophenylpiperazine. Eur J Pharmacol 94:175–179

Da Prada M, Kettler R, Burkard WP, Haefely WE (1984) Moclobemide, an antidepressant with short-lasting MAO-A inhibition: brain catecholamines and tyramine pressor effects in rats. In: Tipton KF, Dostert P, Strolin Benedetti M (eds) Monoamine oxidase and disease. Prospects for therapy with reversible inhibitors. Academic, London, pp 137–154

Demarest KT, Smith DJ, Azzaro AJ (1980) The presence of the type A form of monoamine oxidase within nigrostriatal dopamine-containing neurons. J Pharmacol Exp Ther 215:461–468

Donnelly CH, Murphy DL (1977) Substrate and inhibitior-related characteristics of human platelet monoamine oxidase. Biochem Pharmacol 26:853–858

Donnelly DH, Richelson E, Murphy DL (1976) Properties of monoamine oxidase in mouse neuroblastoma NIE-115 cells. Biochem Pharmacol 27:959–963

Felner AE, Waldmeier PC (1979) Cumulative effects of irreversible MAO inhibitors in vivo. Biochem Pharmacol 28:995–1002

Fowler CJ, Mantle TJ, Tipton KF (1982) The nature of the inhibition of rat liver monoamine oxidase types A and B by the acetylenic inhibitors clorgyline, *l*-deprenyl and pargyline. Biochem Pharmacol 31:3555–3561

Fuller RW (1968) Influence of substrate in the inhibition of rat liver and brain monoamine oxidase. Arch Int Pharmacodyn Ther 174:32–37

Fuller RW (1978) Selectivity among monoamine oxidase inhibitors and its possible importance for development of antidepressant drugs. Prog Neuropsychopharmacol Biol Psychiatry 2:303–311

Garrick NA, Murphy DL (1980) Species differences in the deamination of dopamine and other substrates for monoamine oxidase in brain. Psychopharmacology (Berlin) 72:27–33

Garrick NA, Murphy DL (1982) Monoamine oxidase type A: differences in selectivity towards levo-norepinephrine compared to serotonin. Biochem Pharmacol 31:4061–4066

Garrick Na, Scheinin M, Chang WH, Linnoila M, Murphy DL (1984) Differential effects of clorgyline on catecholamine and indoleamine metabolites in the cerebrospinal fluid of rhesus monkeys. Biochem Pharmacol 33:1423–1427

Garrick NA, Seppala T, Linnoila M, Murphy DL (1985a) Rhesus monkey cerebrospinal fluid amine metabolite changes following treatment with the reversible monoamine oxidase type-A inhibitor cimoxatone. Psychopharmacology (Berlin) 86:265–269

Garrick NA, Seppala T, Linnoila M, Murphy DL (1985b) The effects of amiflamine on cerebrospinal fluid amine metabolites in the rhesus monkey. Eur J Pharmacol 110:1–9

Goridis C, Neff NH (1971) Evidence for a specific monoamine oxidase associated with sympathetic nerves. Neuropharmacology 10:557–564

Hall DWR, Logan BW, Parsons GH (1969) Further studies on the inhibition of monoamine oxidase by M+B 9302 (clorgyline): I. Substrate specificity in various mammalian species. Biochem Pharmacol 18:1447–1454

Herd JA (1969) A new antidepressant – M and B 9302. A pilot study and double-blind controlled trial. Clin Trials 6:219–225

Johnston JP (1968) Some observations upon a new inhibitor of monoamine oxidase in brain tissue. Biochem Pharmacol 17:1285–1297

Kettler R, Keller HH, Bonetti EP, Wyss PC, Da Prada M (1985) Ro 16-6491: a new highly selective and reversible MAO-B inhibitor. J Neurochem 44:S94

Knoll J (1978) The possible mechanisms of action of (−)deprenyl in Parkinson's disease. J Neural Transm 43:117–198

Knoll J, Ecseri Z, Kelemen K, Nievel J, Knoll B (1965) Phenylisopropylmethylpropinylamine (E-250), a new spectrum psychic energizer. Arch Int Pharmacodyn Ther 155:154–164
Kuhn DM, Murphy DL, Youdim MBH (1986) Physiological and clinical aspects of monoamine oxidase. In: Mondori B (ed) Monoamine oxidases. CRC Publications Press, New York (in press)
Larsen JK, Mikkelsen PL, Holm P (1984) Moclobemide (Ro 11-1163) in the treatment of major depressive disorder. A randomized clinical trial. In: Tipton KF, Dostert P, Strolin Benedetti M (eds) Monoamine oxidase and disease. Prospects for therapy with reversible inhibitors. Academic, London, p 609
Levitt P, Pintar JE, Breakefield XO (1982) Immunocytochemical demonstration of monoamine oxidase B in brain astrocytes and serotonergic neurons. Proc Natl Acad Sci USA 79:6385–6389
Linnoila M, Karoum F, Potter WZ (1982) Effect of low-dose clorgyline on 24-h urinary monoamine excretion in patients with rapidly cycling bipolar affective disorder. Arch Gen Psychiatry 39:513–516
Lipper S, Murphy DL, Slater S, Buchsbaum MS (1979) Comparative behavioral effects of clorgyline and pargyline in man: a preliminary evaluation. Psychopharmacology (Berlin) 62:123–128
Major LF, Murphy DL, Lipper S, Gordon E (1979) Effects of clorgyline and pargyline on deaminated metabolites of norepinephrine, dopamine and serotonin in human cerebrospinal fluid. J Neurochem 32:229–231
McDonald IA, Lacoste JM, Bey P, Paltreyman MG, Zreika M (1985) Enzyme-activated irreversible inhibitors of monoamine oxidase phenylallylamine structure-activity relationships. J Med Chem 28:186–193
Mendelewicz J, Youdim MBH (1983) L-Deprenyl, a selective monoamine oxidase type-B inhibitor, in the treatment of depression: a double-blind evaluation. Br J Psychiatry 142:508–511
Mendis N, Pare CMB, Sandler M, Glover V, Stern M (1981) Is the failure of L-deprenyl, a selective monoamine oxidase B inhibitor, to alleviate depression related to freedom from the cheese effect. Psychopharmacology (Berlin) 73:87–90
Murphy DL (1978) Substrate-selective monoamine oxidases: inhibitor, tissue, species and functional differences. Biochem Pharmacol 27:1889–1893
Murphy DL, Donelly CH, Richelson E, Fuller RW (1978) *N*-Substituted cyclopropylamines as inhibitors of MAO A and B forms. Biochem Pharmacol 27:1767–1769
Murphy DL, Donnelly CH, Richelson E (1976) Substrate and inhibitor-related characteristics of monoamine oxidase in C6 rat glial cells. J Neurochem 26:1231–1235
Murphy DL, Lipper S, Campbell IC, Major LF, Slater SL, Buchsbaum MS (1979) Comparative studies of MAO-A and MAO-B inhibitors in man. In: Singer TP, von Korff RW, Murphy DL (eds) Monoamine oxidase: structure, function and altered functions. Academic, New York, pp 457–475
Murphy DL, Pickar D, Jimerson D, Cohen RM, Garrick NA, Karoum F, Wyatt RJ (1981) Biochemical indices of the effects of selective MAO inhibitors (clorgyline, pargyline and deprenyl) in man. In: Usdin E, Dahl SG, Gram LF, Lingjaerde O (eds) Clinical pharmacology in psychiatry: Neuroleptic and antidepressant research. Macmillan, London, pp 307–316
Murphy DL, Garrick NA, Aulakh CS, Cohen RM (1984) New contributions from basic science to understanding the effects of monoamine oxidase inhibiting antidepressants. J Clin Psychiatry 45:37–43
Murphy DL, Tamarkin L, Sunderland T, Garrick NA, Cohen RM (1986) Human plasma melatonin is elevated during treatment with the monoamine oxidase inhibitors clorgyline and tranylcypromine but not deprenyl. Psychiatry Res 17:119–127
Palfreyman MG, McDonald I, Zreika M, Fozard JR (1984) The prodrug approach to brain selective MAO inhibition. In: Tipton KF, Dostert P, Strolin Benedetti M (eds) Monoamine oxidase and disease. Prospects for therapy with reversible inhibitors. Academic, London, pp 561–562
Roy BF, Murphy DL, Lipper S, Siever L, Alterman IS, Jimerson D, Lake CR, Cohen RM (1986) Cardiovascular effects of the selective monoamine oxidase-inhibiting antidepressant clorgyline: correlations with clinical responses and changes in catecholamine metabolism. J Clin Psychopharmacol (in press)

Siever LJ, Uhde TW, Murphy DL (1981) Possible sensitization of alpha$_2$-adrenergic receptors by chronic monoamine oxidase inhibitor treatment in psychiatric patients. Psychiatry Res 6:293–302
Singer TP, von Korff RW, Murphy DL (eds) (1979) Monoamine oxidase: structure, function and altered functions. Academic, New York
Stefanis CN, Alevizos B, Papadimitriou GN (1984) Controlled clinical study of moclobemide (Ro 11-1163), a new MAO inhibitor, and desipramine in depressive patients. In: Tipton KF, Dostert P, Strolin Benedetti M (eds) Monoamine oxidase and disease. Prospects for therapy with reversible inhibitors. Academic, London, pp 377–392
Strolin Benedetti M, Dostert P (1985) Stereochemical aspects of MAO interactions: reversible and selective inhibitors of monoamine oxidase. Trends Pharmacol Sci 6:249–251
Sunderland T, Mueller EA, Cohen RM, Jimerson DC, Pickar D, Murphy DL (1985) Tyramine pressor sensitivity changes during deprenyl treatment. Psychopharmacology (Berlin) 86:432–437
Tipton KF, Dostert P, Strolin Benedetti M (eds) (1984) Monoamine oxidase and disease: prospects for therapy with reversible inhibitors. Academic, London
Waldmeier PC, Felner AE, Maitre L (1981) Long-term effects of selective MAO inhibitors on MAO activity and amine metabolism. In: Youdim MBH, Paykel ES (eds) Monoamine oxidase inhibitors. The state of the art. Wiley, New York, pp 87–102
Westlund KN, Denney RM, Kochersperger LM, Rose RM, Abell CW (1985) Distinct monoamine oxidase A and B populations in primate brain. Science 230:181–183
Wheatley D (1970) Comparative trial of a new monoamine oxidase inhibitor in depression. Br J Psychiatry 117:547
Yang HYT, Neff NH (1974) The monoamine oxidases of brain: selective inhibition with drugs and the consequences for the metabolism of the biogenic amines. J Pharmacol Exp Ther 733–740
Youdim MBH, Banerjee DK, Pollard HB (1984) Isolated chromaffin cells from adrenal medulla contain primarily monoamine oxidase B. Science 224:619–621

Therapeutic Effect of Selective 5HT Reuptake Inhibitors in Comparison with Tricyclic Antidepressants

P. KRAGH-SØRENSEN[1], P. LE FÈVRE HONORÉ[3], and L. F. GRAM[2]

1 Introduction

A recent count suggests that there are more than a hundred compounds at various stages of development as possible new antidepressants. These include "pure" norepinephrine and serotonin reuptake inhibitors. Most of these compounds, however, have not reached the stage of clinical research at which it would be wise, from a clinical point of view, to discuss their efficacy or draw conclusions on toxicity and unwanted side effects. This is especially evident for the pure norepinephrine reuptake blockers.

Therefore, this review will only focus on the data concerning compounds having a selective effect in blocking serotonin reuptake. The review is tentative rather than conclusive, because of difficulties in evaluating the various clinical studies published up to now. In this connection, the assessment of the efficacy of new potentially antidepressant compounds is currently of particular concern, and stringent trial methodology is required to ensure that effective antidepressants are not overlooked or that ineffective compounds are not accepted as antidepressants.

2 Clinical Expectations of New Antidepressants

Clinicians and their patients have the right to expect that any new antidepressant introduced onto the market will be at least as effective as antidepressants already available. The overall efficacy of existing tricyclic antidepressants (TCAs) leaves room for much improvement. At least 20%–25% of all patients respond poorly. The antidepressant effect is slow and gradual, and complete response is achieved after 3–6 weeks. The newer antidepressants introduced in recent years usually have about the same final efficacy as the TCAs, but do not appear to have a faster onset of action.

In the development of new antidepressants, the search for compounds less toxic than the TCAs is given high priority. The dangerous overdose toxicity is a major problem with TCAs, and the risk of cardiovascular toxicity at therapeutic doses is of concern in the treatment of the elderly and of patients with heart dis-

[1] Department of Psychiatry and
[2] Department of Clinical Pharmacology, Odense University Hospital, DK-5000 Odense C, Denmark
[3] Research Division, Danish Ferrosan Group, DK-2860 Søborg, Denmark.

Clinical Pharmacology in Psychiatry
Editors: Dahl, Gram, Paul, Potter
(Psychopharmacology Series 3)

ease. The development of orthostatic hypotensive reactions in about 50% of elderly patients is a particularly troublesome problem (Gram et al. 1984; Christensen et al. 1985). The marked anticholinergic action of the TCAs causes many of the distressing side effects often found to be intolerable to patients, thus compromising compliance with treatment (Kragh-Sørensen 1985).

Results from experimental pharmacology and phase II and III studies suggest that the new selective serotonin reuptake blockers are less toxic than TCAs (e.g., Wernicke 1985). The effects on the cholinergic, histaminergic, and adrenergic receptors that are typical of TCAs but considered not essential for the therapeutic effect have been avoided, so that the corresponding adverse reactions have also been eliminated. The assumption (Carlsson 1982) that serotonin is particularly involved in mood regulation has led to the development of a series of compounds resulting in selective blockade of the reuptake of serotonin.

3 Methodological Issues in the Clinical Evaluation of New Antidepressants

Therapeutic efficacy of new antidepressants can only be assessed when stringent trial methodology is applied (Table 1). We have focused on four of the new selective inhibitors of 5-HT reuptake, citalopram, femoxetine, fluoxetine, and fluvoxamine. Pharmacodynamically these compounds are rather similar (Hyttel 1984), but they show some differences in pharmacokinetics (Table 2). Clinical studies published recently with these drugs are placebo-controlled studies (only fluoxetine and fluvoxamine), multicenter or single-center studies comparing the new drugs with TCAs or placebo/TCAs. Not surprisingly, most reports state that the new compounds are superior to placebo and equal to TCAs. But is this enough to desribe the new compounds as antidepressants? Many of the studies reviewed highlight several methodological issues that ought to be considered before such a conclusion can be drawn (Table 1).

Table 1. Methodological issues in evaluation of therapeutic effectiveness of new antidepressants

1. Diagnostic criteria
2. Assessment of severity of depression (inclusion)
3. Operational response criteria
4. Patient status (inpatients)
5. "Adequate" sample size (> 50 patients in each group)
6. Control groups:
   A. Placebo
   B. Reference drug (TCAs)
   C. Placebo + reference drug (TCAs)
7. Initial placebo washout
8. Adequate length of trial (4–6 weeks)
9. Dosage (fixed/flexible)
10. Plasma concentration monitoring (including active metabolites)

Table 2. Elimination half-life and protein binding of citalopram, femoxetine, fluoxetine, fluvoxamine, and their active metabolites

Drug	Half-life (h)	Protein binding (%)	Ratio drug/ active meta- bolite in plasma	Ref.[b]
Citalopram	33	50		
Norcitalopram	–	–	2/1	[1]
Fluoxetine	60	94		
Norfluoxetine	200	–	–[a]	[2]
Femoxetine	20	90–95		
Norfemoxetine	20	90–95	1	[3]
Fluvoxamine	15	77	–	[4]

[a] Data not available from C_{SS} measurement.
[b] [1] Kragh-Sørensen et al. (1981); [2] Lemberger et al. (1985); [3] Lund et al. (1979); [4] Claasen (1983).

3.1 Diagnostic Criteria

For diagnostic classification DSM III (1980) has often been used, but this system gives rather vague criteria for the classification of depressive illness and does not define endogenous depression precisely enough to identify patients in whom the antidepressants can be expected to have a clear therapeutic effect. A combination of DSM III and other diagnostic classification systems, e.g., diagnostic rating scales such as the Newcastle Inventory I and II (Carney et al. 1965; Gurney 1971; Gurney et al. 1972), is recommended (World Health Organization 1984).

3.2 Assessment and Response Criteria

The measures used to assess the severity of depression must be valid, sensitive, and reliable (Bech 1981), and only patients with sufficiently severe illness should be included.

The frequently reported changes in group average rating score are not a suitable means of answering the clinicians' question: How many patients achieved a complete response? A relevant criterion of response should be defined in the protocol. A final rating scale score indicating full recovery [e.g., 17-item Hamilton depression rating scale $\leqq 7$ points (Bech 1981)] and/or a global clinical assessment that the patient has experienced marked (or even moderate) improvement is preferable. Percentage changes, which were often used in the studies reviewed, do not answer the question of whether or not the patient has recovered (Hamilton 1982).

3.3 Patient Status

Therapeutic efficacy should initially be established in a sample of depressed patients most likely to respond to antidepressants. This can best be done under inpatient conditions (American Psychiatric Association 1985). An inpatient study provides better control of variables such as compliance, concurrent medication, and diagnostic accuracy. It is evident from the outpatient studies (e.g., Cohn and Wilcox 1985) that a marked proportion of outpatients treated with TCAs stop their medication because of intolerable side effects, while this is not the case in inpatient studies. This raises several statistical problems and makes any conclusion on the efficacy and side effects profile difficult. Outpatient studies should preferably be done late in phase III, when the therapeutic effect has been established in inpatient studies (World Health Organization 1984).

3.4 Sample Size and Control Groups

What clinicians wish to know is whether the efficacy of the new compound is comparable to that of TCAs. There is thus a need for both placebo- and TCA-controlled studies. The function of placebo-controlled studies is to exclude clearly inferior drugs, whereas the documentation of superiority to placebo always has to be followed by comparative studies with established antidepressants. The latter requires larger patient samples, with due consideration for sample size in relation to the minimal difference considered important to detect variance in outcome: type I and type II error probability (Prien and Levine 1984). To achieve a sufficient sample size multicenter studies are often required, but this usually increases the variability at all levels. Application of a similar protocol and adequate intra- and interrater reliability studies may help to even out on the variances between centers in multicenter studies (DUAG 1986). This methodology does not seem to have been applied consistently in all the multicenter studies reviewed (Guelfi et al. 1983; Stark and Hardison 1985).

3.5 Initial Placebo Washout – Length of Trial

An initial placebo treatment period allows early placebo responders to be identified and excluded. The trial period most likely to demonstrate a difference between treatments is usually at least 4–6 weeks. The vast majority of the studies reviewed included a placebo washout period and lasted 4 weeks or more.

3.6 Dosage and Plasma Concentration Monitoring

Both standard reference drug and experimental drug should be administered in optimum doses. For reference drug the recommended daily doses should be used, but ideally dosage should be based on drug level monitoring (Gram et al. 1981). The appropriate dosage of the new compound should be established in initial dose-finding studies.

Most of the standard TCAs have elimination half-lives of 17–30 h, and steady state levels are reached within a week. Fluoxetine, and sometimes the active metabolite norfluoxetine, have very long half-lives (Table 2), and steady state levels are thus not achieved until after 2–3 weeks, of administration. Plasma concentration measurements should be included in the trial design to control for drug compliance, especially in outpatient studies (Johnson 1974), and to establish possible concentration-effect relationships (Kragh-Sørensen 1985).

4 Clinical Studies with 5HT Reuptake Inhibitors with Especial Reference to Femoxetine vs TCAs

Many trials fail to demonstrate significant differences in therapeutic effect because they usually include only 40–50 patients in total, which would only allow detection of vast differences. A larger number of patients can be obtained by combining several small studies carried out with similar methodology and with the results recorded in a way permitting pooling. In a number of femoxetine studies the design, patient samples, assessment measures and analyses of data followed the same principles and were available from the published papers and internal reports (data on file, held by the Ferrosan Group).

Eight randomized, double blind studies were included in the analyses. Control therapy (amitriptyline, desipramine, or imipramine), number of patients, patient status, dosage and diagnostic criteria are shown in Table 3. With a few minor exceptions, the design, diagnostic classification systems, patient status and control therapy were identical. The Hamilton Depression Scale (HDS) (Hamilton 1967) was administered after a placebo drug-free washout period, and after 2, 4, and 6 weeks of active treatment. An HDS score $\geqq 17$ was required for inclusion.

The sum scores on HDS [total and six-item subscale (HDSS); Bech et al. 1975] and the four factors according to Cleary and Guy (1977) were used as primary variables for evaluating clinical response. Nonparametric tests were used (Fisher's exact test, Mann-Whitney U test, Kruskal-Wallis, and Friedman analysis of variance). The 95% confidence limits have been calculated for intertreatment differences in the median reduction on HDS from baseline to week 6. The significance level was 0.05 (two-tailed).

Table 3. Patient status, diagnostic classification, no. of patients, dosage, and control therapy in femoxetine studies reviewed

Study[a]	Treatment setting	Diagnosis/ classification	No. of patients allocated		Dosage Fem[d]	(mg)[c] Ref.[d]
			Fem	Ref		
[1]	Inpatients	MRC-criteria	10	10	600	150 AT
[2]	Inpatients	ICD (8)	21	17	600	150 AT
[3]	Outpatients	ICD/Newcastle II	20	22	600	150 (DMI)
[4]	Inpatients	ICD (8)/Newcastle II	44	42	9 mg/kg	2.2 mg/kg AT
[5]	Inpatients	ICD/Newcastle II	21	21	600	150 (DMI)
[6]	Inpatients	ICD/Newcastle II	20	25	600	150 AT
[7]	Outpatients	RDC[b]	39	36	600	150 AT
[8]	Inpatients	ICD-RDC/ Newcastle II	25	27	600	150 IP

[a] [1] Ghose et al. (1977); [2] Bøjholm et al. (1979); [3] Dahl et al. (1982); [4] Reebye et al. (1982); [5] Ahlberg et al. (1982); [6] Tamminen et al. (1982); [7] Skrumsager and Jeppesen (1986); [8] Suominen et al. (1986).

[b] Retrospectively.

[c] Standard dosage flexible according to therapeutic effect and tolerance.

[d] Ref, reference compound; AT, amitriptyline; DMI, desipramine; IP, imipramine; Fem, Femoxetine

5 Results

Of the 400 randomly allocated patients, 36 receiving femoxetine and 34 receiving control therapy were dropouts. Side effects, especially anticholinergic, dominated in the reference group (TCAs), whereas lack of effect or deterioration was more frequent in the femoxetine group. However, the differences were not statistically significant.

Analyses of clinical response profile, and therapeutic effect were based only on patients completing the 6-week study period. The pretrial distribution according to various patient characteristics showed no significant differences. The severity of the depression was reduced significantly in both groups, as seen from the reduction in mean score on the total HDS and the HDSS. The cumulated response during treatment, based on categorical response criteria, showed a tendency toward a higher proportion of patients with complete response (HDS $\leqq 7$)/ partial response (HDS: 8–15) in the reference group in weeks 2 and 4, whereas there was only a minor differences after 6 weeks. In all studies combined, the 95% confidence limits for the difference between femoxetine and reference drug ranged from −2.15–0.24 for the HDS and from −1.23–0.19 for the HDSS (Fig. 1). This suggests a more pronounced reduction in the reference group, although the difference does not reach the level of statistical significance.

The 95% confidence limits for the difference in individual studies using the HDS included zero in all studies except one (Ahlberg et al. 1982). Thus, one of the eight studies indicates a significant difference in favor of the reference treatment (AT). When the HDSS was used the confidence limits included zero in all

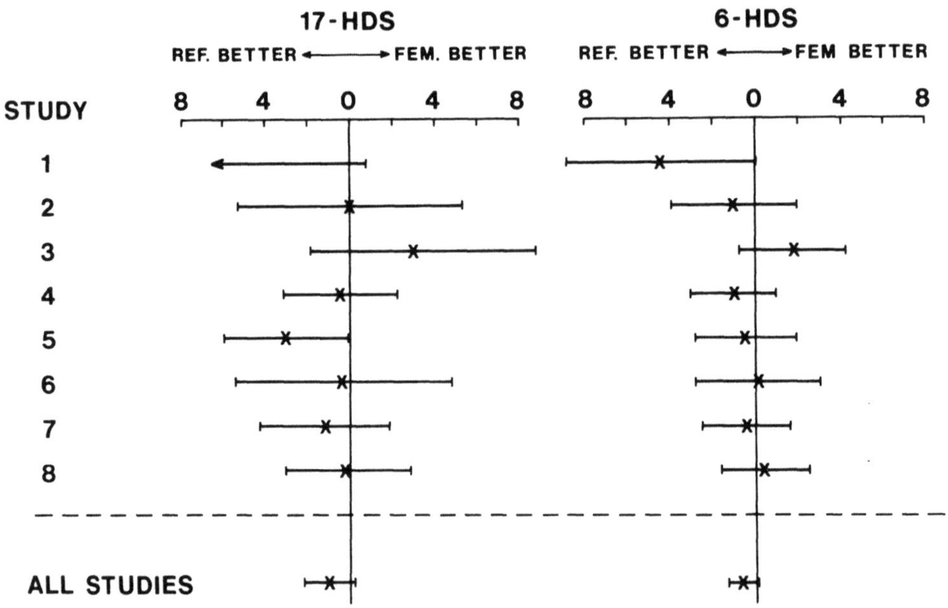

Fig. 1. 95% confidence limits for the difference between femoxetine and reference in median reduction of total HDS and HDSS (6-HDS) from baseline to week 6

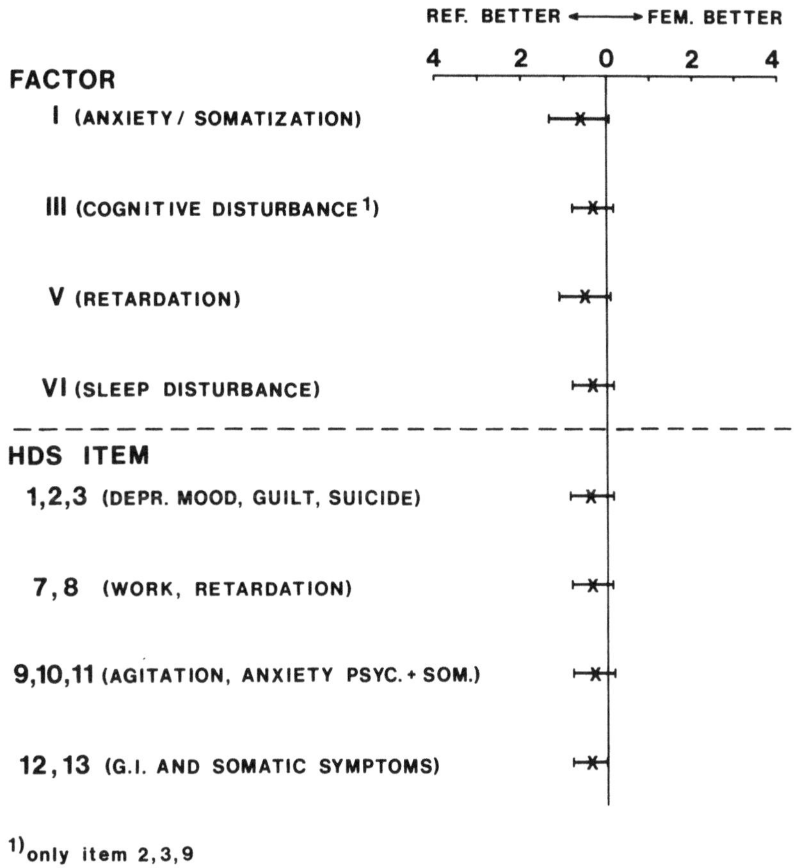

Fig. 2. 95% confidence limits for the difference between femoxetine and reference in median reduction of HDS factors from baseline to week 6

studies. Also, the centers of the intervals were close to zero in seven of the studies.

For the various subgroups of HDS items (Fig. 2) the 95% confidence intervals all included zero, with weak tendencies in favor of the reference treatment. Taking all studies together, the 95% confidence limits for the HDS total the HDSS and the factors are small and show that the true difference between femoxetine and reference treatment in terms of median reduction is 1–2 points on the HDS total scale.

6 Discussion

The overall results derived from the pooled data from these eight studies comparing femoxetine and TCAs were that in efficacy femoxetine and the standard reference drugs (AT, DMI, IP) were clinically comparable. However, there was a tendency towards a moderate difference in favor of the reference compounds. The time-course showed a higher proportion of responders in the reference drug group at weeks 2 and 4, but no difference at week 6.

Pooling data from studies with different protocols or no coordination should be viewed with caution even if the same treatments and outcome measures are used. Even minor deviations in design or conduct may introduce enough variability to offset the advantages of combining the data. However, we found that in this case the deviations were small, and we could not identify specific factors accounting for the overall results.

In a recent Danish multicenter study (DUAG 1986) in which most of the critical points described above concerning trial methodology were dealt with, the clinical effect of citalopram, a selective 5HT reuptake inhibitor, was evaluated in comparison with clomipramine. In all, 102 patients were included in the analyses of therapeutic efficacy. After 5 weeks' treatment a complete response according to HDS (both endogenous and nonendogenous depression) was seen in about 60% of the patients treated with clomipramine and in about 30% of the patients treated with citalopram. The corresponding values for 6 weeks treatment in the pooled femoxetine studies were 60% and 49% for TCAs and femoxetine, respectively.

The problems with trial design, homogeneity of patients, sample size, patient status, response criteria, etc., as exemplified in the fluoxetine and fluvoxamine studies (Guelfi et al. 1983; Dick and Ferrebo 1983; De Wilde et al. 1983; Itil et al. 1983; Feighner and Cohn 1985; Cohn and Wilcox 1985; Chouinard 1985; Stark and Hardison 1985), is probably not the only reason why many authors in recent years have questioned the clinical efficacy of many new antidepressants (e.g., Zis and Goodwin 1979; Hollister 1981; Kragh-Sørensen et al. 1983). It may be that these new compounds, including the specific serotonin blockers, have a different and sometimes more limited spectrum of effects, and their therapeutic effect may be weaker than that of the TCAs. Other questions are which patients will benefit from treatment with these drugs, and whether the efficacy varies from drug to drug in this group. It has been postulated that different receptor systems may be affected in different types of depression. Drugs acting selectively on 5-HT reuptake or norepinephrine reuptake, for example, may thus have optimal therapeutic effects in subgroups of patients. As yet, studies addressing this hypothesis have not produced convincing evidence of the selectivity of clinical antidepressant effect. It may be postulated that the selectivity of action results in a weaker antidepressant effect and that the otpimum antidepressant effect is obtained with compounds active on both serotonin and norepinephrine reuptake and possibly on other receptor systems (Gram et al., this volume).

References

Ahlberg B, Palm O, le Fèvre Honoré P (1982) Femoxetine in the treatment of patients with depressive illness. A randomized comparison with amitriptyline. Nord Psychiatr Tidsskr 36:329–333

American Psychiatric Association (1980) Task force on nomenclature and statistics. Diagnostic and statistical manual of mental disorders. American Psychiatric Association, Washington, DC

American Psychiatric Association (1985) Tricyclic antidepressants – blood level measurements and clinical outcome: an APA task force report. Am J Psychiatry 142:155–162
Bech P (1981) Rating scales for affective disorders: their validity and consistency. Acta Psychiatr Scand [Suppl 295]64:1–101
Bech P, Gram LF, Dein E, Jacobsen O, Vitger J, Bolwig TG (1975) Quantitative rating of depressive states. Acta Psychiatr Scand 51:161–170
Bech P, Allerup P, Gram LF, Reisby N, Rosenberg P, Jacobsen O, Nagy A (1981) The Hamilton depression scale, evaluation of objectivity using logistic models. Acta Psychiatr Scand 63:290–299
Bøjholm, S, Børup C, Kvist J, Petersen IM, le Fèvre Honoré (1979) A double-blind study of femoxetine and amitriptyline in patients with endogenous depression. Nord Psychiatr Tidsskr 33:455–460
Carlsson A (1982) Recent observations on new potential and established antidepressant drugs. Pharmacopsychiatria 15:116–120
Carney MWP, Roth M, Garside RF (1965) The diagnosis of depressive syndromes and prediction of ECT response. Br J Psychiatry 111:659–674
Chouinard G (1985) A double-blind controlled clinical trial of fluexitine and amitriptyline in the treatment of outpatients with major depressive disorder. J Clin Psychiatry 46:32–37
Christensen P, Thomsen HY, Pedersen OL, Thayssen P, Oxhøj H, Kragh-Sørensen P, Gram LF (1985) Cardiovascular effects of amitriptyline in the treatment of elderly depressed patients. Psychopharmacology (Berlin) 87:212–215
Claassen V (1983) Review of the animal pharmacology and pharmacokinetics of fluvoxamine. Br J Clin Pharmacol 15:349–355
Cleary P, Guy W (1977) Factor analysis of the Hamilton depression scale. Drugs Exp Clin Res 1(1–2):115–120
Cohn JB, Wilcox C (1985) A comparison of fluoxetine, imipramine and placebo in patients with major depressive disorder. J Clin Psychiatry 46:26–31
Dahl LE, Lundin L, le Fèvre Honoré P, Dencker SJ (1982) Antidepressant effect of femoxetine and desipramine and relationship to the concentration of amine metabolites in cerebrospinal fluid. Acta Psychiatr Scand 66:9–17
Danish University Antidepressant Group (DUAG) (1986) Citalopram: clinical effect profile in comparison with clomipramine. A controlled multicenter study. Psychopharmacology (Berlin) 90:131–138
De Wilde JE, Mertens C, Wakelin JS (1983) Clinical trials of fluvoxamine vs chlorimipramine with single and three times daily dosing. Br J Clin Pharmacol 15:427–431
Dick P, Ferrero E (1983) A double-blind comparative study of the clinical efficacy of fluvoxamine and chlorimipramine. Br J Clin Pharmacol 15:419–425
Feighner JP, Cohn JB (1985) Double-blind comparative trials of fluoxetine and doxepin in geriatric patients with major depressive disorder. J Clin Psychiatry 46:20–25
Ghose K, Gupta R, Coppen A, Lund J (1977) Antidepressant evaluation and the pharmacological actions of FG 4963 in depressive patients. Eur J Pharmacol 42:31–37
Gram LF, Bech P, Reisby N, Jørgensen OS (1981) Methodology in studies on plasma level/effect relationship of tricyclic antidepressants. In: Usdin E (ed) Clinical pharmacology in psychiatry. Elsevier/North-Holland, New York, pp 155–179
Gram LF, Kragh-Sørensen P, Kristensen CB, Møller M, Pedersen OL, Thayssen P (1984) Plasma level monitoring of antidepressants: theoretical basis and clinical application. In: Usdin E, Åsberg M, Bertilsson L, Sjöqvist F (eds) Frontiers in biochemical and pharmacological research in depression (Nobel Conference 1982). Raven, New York, pp 399–411
Guelfi JD, Dreyfus JF, Pichot P (1983) A double-blind controlled clinical trial comparing fluvoxamine with imipramine. Br J Clin Pharmacol 15:411–417
Gurney C (1971) Diagnostic scales for affective disorders. Proceedings of the 5th world conference of Psychiatry, 28 Nov. to 4 Dec. 1971, Mexico City, p 330
Gurney C, Roth M, Garside RB, Kerr TA, Schapira K (1972) Studies in the classification of affective disorders. The relationship between anxiety states and depressive illnesses: II. Br J Psychiatry 121:162–166
Hamilton M (1967) Development of a rating scale for primary depressive illness. Br J Soc Clin Psychol 6:278–296

Hamilton M (1982) The effect of treatment on the melancholias (depressions). Br J Psychiatry 140:223–230
Hollister LE (1981) "Second generation" antidepressant drugs. Psychosomatics 22:872–879
Hyttel J (1984) Experimental pharmacology of selective 5-HT reuptake inhibitors: differences and similarities. Clin Neuropharmacol 7 [Suppl 1]:866–867
Itil TM, Shrivastava RK, Mukherjee S, Coleman BS, Michael ST (1983) A double-blind placebo-controlled study of fluvoxamine and imipramine in out-patients with primary depression. Br J Clin Pharmacol 15:433–438
Johnson DAW (1974) A study of the use of antidepressant medication in general practice. Br J Psychiatry 125:186–192
Kragh-Sørensen P (1985) Monitoring plasma concentration of nortriptyline. Dan Med Bull 32(1):29–53
Kragh-Sørensen P, Overø KF, Pedersen OL, Jensen K, Parnas W (1981) The kinetics of citalopram: single and multiple dose studies in man. Acta Pharmacol Toxicol 48:53–60
Kragh-Sørensen P, Christensen P; Gram LF, Kristensen CB, Muller M, Pederone OL, Thayssen P (1983) Phase-4 studies in psychopharmacology – new antidepressant drugs. In: Gram LF, Uschin E, Dahl SG, Kragh-Sørensen P, Sjöqvist F, Morselli PL (eds) Clinical pharmacology in psychiatry. Bridging the experimental-therapeutic gap. Macmillan, London, pp 114–126
Lemberger L, Bergstrom RF, Wolen RL, Nagy AF, Greg GE, Aronoff GR (1985) Fluoxetine: clinical pharmacology and physiologic disposition. J Clin Psychiatry 46:14–19
Lund J, Christensen JA, Bechgaard E, Molander L, Larsson H (1979) Pharmacokinetics of femoxetine in man. Acta Pharmacol Toxicol 44:177–184
Prien RF, Levine J (1984) Research and methodological issues for evaluating the therapeutic effectiveness of antidepressant drugs. Psychopharmacol Bull 20(2):250–257
Quitkin FM, Rabkin JG, Ross D, McGrath PJ (1984) Duration of antidepressant drug treatment. Arch Gen Psychiatry 41:238–245
Reebye PN, Yiptong C, Samsoon J, Schulsinger F, Fabricius J (1982) A controlled double-blind study of femoxetine and amitriptyline in patients with endogenous depression. Pharmacopsychiatria 15:164–169
Skrumsager BK, Jeppesen K (1986) Femoxetine and amitriptyline in general practice: a randomized double-blind group comparison. Pharmacopsychiatria (in press)
Stark P, Hardison CD (1985) A review of multicenter controlled studies of fluoxetine vs imipramine and placebo in outpatients with major depressive order. J Clin Psychiatry 46:53–58
Suominen J, Tamminen T, Elosuo R, Manniche P (1986) Femoxetine vs. imipramine. A randomized, double-blind study (in press)
Tamminen T, Salminen JK, Skrumsager BK (1982) A double-blind controlled trial of the selective serotonin uptake inhibitor femoxetine and amitriptyline in depression. Nord Psychiatr Tidsskr 36:335–339
Wernicke JF (1985) The side effect profile and safety of fluoxetine. J Clin Psychiatry 46:59–67
World Health Organization (1984) Guidelines for the clinical investigation of antidepressant drugs. European drug guideline series 3. Regional Office for Europe, Copenhagen
Zis AP, Goodwin FK (1979) Novel antidepressants and the biogenic amine hypothesis of depression. The case for iprindole and mianserin. Arch Gen Psychiatry 36:1097–1107

Accidental Antidepressants: Search for Specific Action

M. V. RUDORFER[1], M. LINNOILA[2], and W. Z. POTTER[1]

1 Introduction

Serendipity has been invoked to explain a number of discoveries in psychopharmacology. These have included the pharmacoconvulsive therapies in the 1930s (which originated in the idea of using transfused blood from schizophrenics to treat epileptics), and the "uricosuric agent" lithium, studied in the 1940s for the treatment of gout. Today electroconvulsive therapy and lithium carbonate are standard treatments for affective disorders. Of the primary antidepressant medications developed in the 1950s, monoamine oxidase inhibitors evolved from the clinical observation of euphoric reactions of tuberculosis patients to iproniazid; the prototype tricyclic antidepressant, imipramine, was synthesized in the search for a better neuroleptic. So, the classic antidepressants were the truly accidental ones.

2 Current "Accidental" Antidepressants

The last 30 years have witnessed the development of a host of clinically effective compounds. While some are novel, few are truly accidental, since they were active in animal screening models developed using the original antidepressants. The biochemical actions of some such drugs active in animal tests were superficially different from those of the traditional agents. For instance, iprindole, the "first of the second-generation antidepressants" (Maxwell 1983) is a very weak reuptake inhibitor for either norepinephrine (NE) or serotonin (5-HT), and until recently it was thought not to produce significant effects on the noradrenergic system. Similarly, as an even less potent reuptake inhibitor, the tetracyclic mianserin caused a stir in the field (Zis and Goodwin 1979) until its action of blocking presynaptic alpha-2 receptors was appreciated. Another new compound of uncertain biochemical action and equally uncertain antidepressant potency (Shopsin et al. 1981) is trazodone, a relatively selective but poor inhibitor of 5-HT reuptake, which offers the unique clinical combination of sedation without anticholinergic effects (Rudorfer et al. 1984c); its active metabolites are under study. The closest recent candidate for a truly accidental antidepressant has emerged from the ad-

[1] Section on Clinical Pharmacology, Laboratory of Clinical Science, National Institute of Mental Health, Building 10, Room 2D46, Bethesda, MD 20892, USA.
[2] Laboratory of Clinical Studies, National Institute on Alcohol Abuse and Alcoholism, Bethesda, MD 20892, USA.

Clinical Pharmacology in Psychiatry
Editors: Dahl, Gram, Paul, Potter
(Psychopharmacology Series 3)

dition of a nitrogen-containing ring to the basic benzodiazepine structure; this produced the triazolobenzodiazepine alprazolam with apparent antidepressant properties at high doses. This drug does not block monoamine reuptake but has just been reported to enhance coupling between adrenergic receptors and adenylate cyclase in a platelet model (Mooney et al. 1985), which permits one to conceive of it as "belonging" to the monoamine-active system of antidepressant agents.

More clearly premeditated was the synthesis of a new generation of transmitter reuptake blockers designed chemically to be more selective than the original series and to have fewer adverse side effects (Rudorfer et al. 1984c). Thus, maprotiline and +oxaprotiline are selective NE reuptake inhibitors, with zimelidine, citalopram, fluvoxamine, and several others showing equal selectivity of effect on the serotonergic system. Moreover, involvement of the dopamine (DA) system is also new. Nomifensine blocks DA as well as NE reuptake, and bupropion (to be discussed in detail below) acutely inhibits only DA reuptake in vitro. In addition to blocking the reuptake of NE, amoxapine and its 7-hydroxymetabolite exhibit the neuroleptic-like action of dopamine receptor blockade. Among the monoamine oxidase (MAO) inhibitors, there has also been a major advance in the direction of increased biochemical specificity, most notably in the form of clorgyline, a highly potent antidepressant and anticycling agent (Potter et al. 1982), which inhibits only the A type of MAO (Johnston 1968).

3 Common Biochemical Effects of Antidepressant Drugs

Given the myriad acute biochemical effects of drugs sharing a common clinical effect, are there shared mechanisms of action? The search for a universal antidepressant mechanism of action has led to a number of discoveries focusing on the role of the noradrenergic system and the interactions among neurotransmitter systems.

An integrated measure of the state of the noradrenergic system is the "whole-body turnover" of this transmitter, representing its daily synthesis, output, and degradation. This can be approximated by summating the concentration of NE and its three major metabolites, normetanephrine, 3-methoxy-4-hydroxyphenylglycol (MHPG), and vanillylmandelic acid (VMA) in 24-h urine collections. We have found consistent reductions in this indicator of NE turnover compared with pretreatment values in depressed patients treated with antidepressant agents for 4 weeks, regardless of clinical outcome. The six treatments for which this effect and the extent of relative fall from baseline have been demonstrated in patients and/or volunteers are desipramine (−40%), zimelidine (−22%), lithium (−38%), clorgyline (−60%), electroconvulsive therapy (−19%), and, most recently, bupropion (−18%) (Linnoila et al. 1982a, b, 1983a; Rudorfer et al. 1984a; Golden et al. 1986a). Preliminary unpublished data from our laboratory show decreases in NE turnover in patients treated with alprazolam or citalopram.

We also find that the major metabolites of both NE and 5-HT are reduced in cerebrospinal fluid following the three drug treatments for which we have data, desipramine, zimelidine and clorgyline, suggesting that the turnovers of both 5-

HT and NE are reduced in the central nervous system (Potter et al. 1985). The few preliminary reports of antidepressant effects on a potential indicator of central NE turnover, i.e., plasma free MHPG, also reveal reductions (Charney et al. 1981 b; Zavadil et al. 1984; Charney and Heninger 1985).

A number of preclinical studies in recent years have converged on the postsynaptic beta receptor as subject to change under the influence of a variety of antidepressant agents. Antidepressants administered chronically (2–4 weeks), but not acutely (consistent with the clinical time course) decrease postsynaptic beta receptor-stimulated cyclic AMP formation and/or number of beta receptors in either the frontal cortex or the hypothalamus of rats (Vetulani et al. 1976; Banerjee et al. 1977; Wolfe et al. 1978) and generally tend to decrease 5-HT_2 binding sites (Peroutka and Snyder 1980), except with electroconvulsive stimulation, where the density of 5-HT_2-binding sites is increased (Stockmeier and Kellar 1986; for reviews see Charney et al. 1981 a; Sugrue 1983).

These binding studies have proven useful in the evaluation of novel antidepressants. Alprazolam down-regulates rat cortical beta receptors only at high doses (Pandey and Davis 1983), as does the hydroxymetabolite (but not parent compound) of bupropion (Ferris and Beaman 1983; Cooper et al. 1984; also see below). Mianserin also fails to alter rat adrenoceptors (Choudhury and O'Donnell 1985). We are currently pursuing studies of beta receptors on lymphocytes and neutrophils of human subjects treated with antidepressants, in an effort to extend these findings to the clinical setting. The previously mentioned preliminary finding of Mooney et al. (1985) on functional up-regulation (increased capacity) of adrenergic receptors on platelets following alprazolam suggests the value of this approach.

We have suggested, on the basis of our clinical studies, that these antidepressant-induced alterations of output or receptor response can be best understood as reflections of increased efficiency of the noradrenergic system (Linnoila et al. 1982a; Ross et al. 1983, 1985; Rudorfer et al. 1984a, b, 1985a) – in other words, in the face of less NE, necessary functions deficient in the depressed state are restored. On the basis of a review of the previous literature, mostly in animals, Stone (1983) advanced the notion that antidepressants increase the efficiency of the noradrenergic system. As is made clear in discussions in his paper, however, efficiency is not precisely enough defined to be tested in humans. We use the term "increased efficiency" to describe a condition documented by actual data recorded in humans. Our findings on noradrenergic efficiency are derived from ongoing studies of plasma NE response to a standardized orthostatic challenge (Rudorfer et al. 1985 b) administered before and after treatment. To date, three treatments have been evaluated in both healthy volunteers and depressed patients: desipramine, zimelidine, and lithium, whereas two others (clorgyline and ECT) have been studied only in patients. Supine NE and the absolute and/or the relative increase of NE on changing from a lying to a standing position have been altered after each treatment except for lithium in volunteers (Ross et al. 1983, 1985; Rudorfer et al. 1984a, b, 1985a; Golden et al. 1986a; unpublished data). These plasma findings along with the results for the urinary measure of whole-body NE turnover and basic indices of cardiovascular function are summarized in Table 1. As can be seen, despite drug treatments reducing total NE turnover,

Table 1. Antidepressant effects on the noradrenergic system in depressed patients and healthy volunteers

Drug	Type of subject	Whole-body NE output	Plasma				Heart rate	Supine MAP	Hydroxy-melatonin output
			MHPG	Supine NE	Δ NE on standing	Fractional NE Δ on standing			
Desipramine	Volunteers		↓	↑	↑↑	↑	↑↑	↑	
Tricyclic antidepressants	Patients	↓↓	↓	↑	↑	0	↑	0	0–↑
Zimelidine	Volunteers	↓	(↓)[a]	0	↑	↑	0	0	?
	Patients	(↓)	?	(↑)	(↑)	0	0	0	?
Lithium	Volunteers	0	0	0	0	0	0	0	?
	Patients	↓↓	?	?	?	?	0	0	?
Clorgyline	Patients	↓↓	↓↓	↓	0	↑	0	0	0–↑
Bupropion	Patients	↓	?	0	0	0	0	↑	?
ECT	Patients	↓	(↓)	↓	↓	↓	0	0	?

Data from Linnoila et al. (1982a, b, 1983a), Ross et al. (1983, 1985), Veith et al. (1983), Rudorfer et al. (1984a, b, 1985a), Golden et al. (1984, 1986a).
[a] Symbols in parentheses represent trends of $P<0.10$ by two-tailed tests. ?, no data available; 0, no change; ↓ or ↓↓/↑ or ↑↑, moderate or pronounced decrease/increase, respectively.

cardiovascular function is maintained and either supine NE or the absolute or fractional NE rise on standing is increased. After ECT, not only is total turnover reduced, but NE release on standing is reduced without associated orthostatic hypotension. In other words, a lower rate of NE turnover is functionally accomplishing as much or more – the NE system is more efficient than before treatment.

Two details in Table 1 require comment. The failure of lithium to have an effect in volunteers on *any* of the parameters (Rudorfer et al. 1985), despite a clear-cut effect in patients (Linnoila et al. 1983 a), can most probably be interpreted as the absence of any effect of lithium on a healthy NE system. The data on ECT should be taken as preliminary (Rudorfer et al. 1984 b); a more extended study is under way.

Another possible index of beta adrenergic function is the release of the pineal hormone melatonin, assessed in an integrated manner by the 24-h output of urinary hydroxymelatonin. Thus far we have recorded urinary hydroxymelatonin measures only after desipramine and MAOIs, including clorgyline. In contradistinction to results in rodents with melatonin (Heydorn et al. 1982), hydroxymelatonin output was *increased* after desipramine and the MAOIs under conditions which decreased whole-body NE turnover (Golden et al. 1984) (Table 1). Moreover, there appeared to be a positive relationship between 5-HIAA in the CSF and hydroxymelatonin output (Golden et al. 1984), reminding us that "hormone" output is usually not controlled by any single neurotransmitter. We are currently evaluating the effects of several other treatments on hydroxymelatonin output.

4 Interactions Among Neurotransmitter Systems

The development of antidepressant drugs with relatively selective acute biochemical actions in vitro seemed to provide tools for factoring out the contribution of various transmitter systems in the pathophysiology of hypothesized chemically distinct subtypes of depressive illness (Rudorfer et al. 1984 c). A growing body of data, however, challenges such an assumption in the living organism. For example, some investigators report 90% response rates to NE reuptake inhibitors (DMI and nortriptyline) when dose and/or plasma concentrations are adjusted (Kragh-Sørensen et al. 1976; Stewart et al. 1980); this argues against a subpopulation needing a more "serotonergic" antidepressant. Against expectations, the antidepressant efficacy of clomipramine is related more closely to concentrations of its potent NE reuptake inhibiting metabolite than to the serotonergic parent drug (Träskman et al. 1979).

As already noted, in the long term nearly all antidepressant treatments, regardless of in vitro properties, reduce the number and functioning of both noradrenergic beta receptors and 5-HT_2 receptors. Furthermore, animal studies demonstrate interactions between the noradrenergic and serotonergic systems. Several preclinical studies have shown that in order for antidepressants to affect noradrenergic receptors the serotonergic system must be intact (Brunello et al. 1982; Janowsky et al. 1982) and that serotonergic functions are modified by noradrenergic input (Cowen et al. 1982; Hallberg et al. 1982; Jones 1980).

In the clinical setting, we have documented a progressive reduction in NE turnover in healthy volunteers during a week of administration of the 5-HT reuptake inhibitor zimelidine (Rudorfer et al. 1984a). Furthermore, we have identified common biochemical effects in the cerebrospinal fluid (CSF) of the disparate antidepressants DMI, zimelidine, and clorgyline, which have very different pharmacological profiles. All three drugs significantly reduced CSF MHPG (by 20%–72%: clorgyline > DMI > zimelidine) and 5-HIAA concentrations (by 26% –39%: zimelidine ≧ DMI ≧ clorgyline); only clorgyline was associated with a decrement in the primary dopamine metabolite, homovanillic acid (HVA) (Potter et al. 1985). The latter finding was surprising given the in vitro data suggesting 5-HT as the substrate with the highest affinity and dopamine as that with the lowest affinity for MAO type A. Thus, it may be impossible in vivo to chronically alter one transmitter system without affecting others which are anatomically and functionally linked.

Another aspect of neurotransmitter interaction suggested by these CSF metabolite levels concerns the relationship between the serotonergic and dopaminergic systems. While electrophysiological studies have suggested an inhibitory input of 5-HT on dopamine transmission, pharmacological interventions in animals have shown the reverse. In an effort to address this issue in patient data, Ågren et al. (1986) collated CSF 5-HIAA and HVA concentrations from 175 medication-free depressed patients in Sweden and the United States. The 0.7 to > 0.8 correlations between these metabolites – not significantly different among six depressive subtypes – replicate other reports in the literature. A structural analysis as well as a nonlinear regression analysis suggest a unidirectional correlation, with 5-HIAA influencing HVA and not vice versa.

This patient material was supplemented by animal data. Healthy dogs not subjected to pharmacological manipulation were sacrificed and neurotransmitter substances were measured in 20–50 micropunched brain areas. Positive correlations between 5-HT and dopamine and between 5-HIAA and HVA were observed in all nuclei except for the basal ganglia (Ågren et al. 1986). Together, these human and animal data suggest a widespread serotonergic influence on dopamine *turnover* in brain, presumably of a facilitatory nature. This is not to suggest, however, that turnover and *function* directly covary. In fact, they may go in opposite directions. The implication for novel antidepressants is that with the possible exception of dopaminergic effects (reduced turnover) of the anticycling drugs lithium and clorgyline (Linnoila et al. 1983b; Potter et al. 1985) initial selectivity in drug action coalesces into a common, shared biochemical effect during the course of treatment.

5 Example of Biochemical Study of a Novel Antidepressant: Bupropion

The search for a specific action of new antidepressants can be illustrated by our experience with the novel antidepressant bupropion. Although characterized preclinically as a weak dopamine reuptake inhibitor without appreciable effects on

NE uptake, in a double blind clinical study bupropion reduced whole-body NE turnover without altering plasma NE levels at rest and following orthostatic challenge (Golden et al. 1986a; Table 1). The decline in NE turnover did not appear to be a consequence of NE reuptake inhibition by bupropion or one of its active metabolites (see below). The ratio of urinary normetanephrine to MHPG+VMA, an index of extraneuronal vs intraneuronal metabolic processing of NE, did not increase, as is seen following NE reuptake blockade by DMI (Linnoila et al. 1982a). This finding supports the hypothesis, developed above, that reduction in total NE production is a final common pathway for antidepressant treatments and perhaps a necessary, though not sufficient, condition for a therapeutic antidepressant effect.

There was a trend toward reductions in CSF MHPG and HVA concentrations following bupropion treatment, with no effect on CSF 5-HIAA. This lack of significant effects on CSF monoamine metabolite concentrations was surprising, in light of our earlier results with other drugs (see above) and bupropion's effects on the dopamine sytem in vitro. However, a dopaminergic effect of the drug did emerge in plasma HVA data. Six responders to bupropion (300–500 mg/day) showed no change in plasma HVA concentrations (41.7 vs 42.1 pmol/ml). In contrast were four nonresponders to the medication, three of whom became clearly psychotic while taking the drug. This subgroup had nonsignificantly higher plasma HVA levels at baseline while medication-free (52.1 pmol/ml), which rose 36% to a mean of 70.9 pmol/ml, which is in the range recorded in unmedicated schizophrenic patients and reported by Pickar et al. (1984).

In attempts to understand the actions of antidepressants, old and new, the role of active metabolites has achieved increasing importance over the past decade. In the case of bupropion, at steady state the three major metabolites predominated (up to 40-fold) over the parent drug in both plasma and CSF. Plasma concentrations of each metabolite (but not bupropion itself) correlated with the respective CSF concentrations. Moreover, higher plasma metabolite concentrations were associated with poor clinical outcome. This was most striking with hydroxybupropion: plasma levels of this metabolite exceeded 1250 ng/ml in all five nonresponders (including one patient for whom no biochemical studies were performed) and were lower than 1200 ng/ml in all seven responders studied. Interestingly, plasma hydroxybupropion concentrations correlated ($r=0.72$, $P<0.05$) with post-treatment plasma HVA levels (Golden et al. 1986b). Thus, high levels of bupropion metabolites may be associated with poor clinical outcome due to toxic effects on the central nervous system dopaminergic systems. Alternatively, a curvilinear dose-response relationship may exist for bupropion metabolites. An important implication of these findings is the inadequacy of animal models to predict these kinetic variables. These bupropion metabolites have very short half-lives in the rat (Schroeder 1983), whereas in humans we observed elimination half-lives of 27–50 h (Golden et al. 1986b), about 2–3 times in excess of that of the parent compound.

In conclusion, the development of new antidepressants has moved on from the accidental discovery of therapeutic agents to planned, measured, incremental improvements to or imitations of existing compounds. What has proven surprising is that preclinical information about drug metabolism and actions has often been inadequate to predict medication effects in humans. The complexity of normal and abnormal physiology and nervous system function in humans necessitates that actual studies in volunteers and patients be continued to define the unique and common properties of antidepressant treatments and "accidentally" discover new ones.

References

Ågren H, Mefford IN, Rudorfer MV, Linnoila M, Potter WZ (1986) Interacting neurotransmitter systems. A non-experimental approach to the 5HIAA-HVA correlation in human CSF. J Psychiatr Res (in press)

Banerjee SP, Kung LR, Riggi SJ, Chanda SK (1977) Development of beta-adrenergic receptor subsensitivity by antidepressants. Nature 268:455–456

Brunello N, Barbaccia ML, Chuang DM, Costa E (1982) Down regulation of beta-adrenergic receptors following injections of desmethylimipramine. Permissive role of serotonergic axons. Neuropharmacology 21:1145–1149

Charney DS, Heninger GR (1985) Noradrenergic function and the mechanism of action of anti-anxiety treatment. I. The effect of long-term alprazolam treatment. Arch Gen Psychiatry 42:458–467

Charney DS, Menkes DB, Heninger GR (1981 a) Receptor sensitivity and the mechanism of action of antidepressant treatment – implications for the etiology and therapy of depression. Arch Gen Psychiatry 38:1160–1180

Charney DS, Heninger GR, Sternberg DE, Redmond DE, Leckman JF, Maas JW, Roth RH (1981 b) Presynaptic adrenergic receptor sensitivity in depression: The effect of chronic desipramine treatment. Arch Gen Psychiatry 38:1334–1340

Choudhury L, O'Donnell JM (1985) Effects of chronic administration of amitriptyline or mianserin on rat cardiac and central adrenoceptors. Br J Pharmacol 85:635–638

Cooper TB, Perumal AS, Suckow RF, Glassman A (1984) Bupropion: possible role of major metabolites in mode of action. Clin Pharmacol Ther 37:187

Cowen PJ, Grahame-Smith DG, Green AR, Heal DJ (1982) Beta-adrenoceptor agonists enhance 5-hydroxytryptamine-mediated behavioral responses. Br J Pharmacol 76:265–270

Ferris RM, Beaman OJ (1983) Bupropion: a new antidepressant drug, the mechanism of action of which is not associated with down-regulation of post-synaptic B-adrenergic, serotonergic (5HT-2), alpha-adrenergic, imipramine and dopamine receptors in brain. Neuropharmacology 22:1257–1262

Golden RN, Markey SP, Potter WZ (1984) A new marker for noradrenergic function in man (Abstract) New Research Section, Annual Meeting of the American Psychiatric Association, 5–11 May 1984, Los Angeles

Golden RN, Rudorfer MV, Sherer MA, Linnoila M, Potter WZ (1986 a) Bupropion: biochemical effects and clinical response in depressed patients. Arch Gen Psychiatry (in press)

Golden RN, De Vane CL, Laizure SC, Rudorfer MV, Sherer MA, Potter WZ (1986b) Bupropion: the role of metabolites in clinical outcome. Arch Gen Psychiatry (in press)

Hallberg H, Almgren O, Svensson TH (1982) Reduced brain serotonergic activity after repeated treatment with beta adrenoceptor antagonists. Psychopharmacology (Berlin) 76:114–117

Heydorn WE, Brunswick DJ, Frazer A (1982) Effect of treatment of rats with antidepressants on melatonin concentrations in the pineal gland and serum. J Pharmacol Exp Ther 222:534–543

Janowsky A, Okada F, Manier DH, Applegate CD, Sulser F, Steranka LR (1982) Role of serotonergic input in the regulation of the beta-adrenergic receptor coupled adenylate cyclase system. Science 218:900–901

Johnston JP (1968) Some observations upon a new inhibitor of monoamine oxidase in brain tissue. Biochem Pharmacol 17:1285–1297

Jones RSG (1980) Enhancement of 5-hydroxytryptamine-induced behavioral effects following chronic administration of antidepressant drugs. Psychopharmacology (Berlin) 69:307–311

Kragh-Sørensen P, Eggert Hansen C, Baastrup PC, Hvidberg EF (1976) Self-inhibiting action of nortriptyline's antidepressive effect at high plasma levels. Psychopharmacology (Berlin) 45:305–312

Linnoila M, Karoum F, Calil HM, Kopin IJ, Potter WZ (1982 a) Alteration of norepinephrine metabolism with desipramine and zimelidine in depressed patients. Arch Gen Psychiatry 39:1025–1028

Linnoila M, Karoum F, Potter WZ (1982 b) Effect of low-dose clorgyline on 24-h urinary monoamine excretion in patients with rapidly cycling bipolar affective disorder. Arch Gen Psychiatry 39:513–516

Linnoila M, Karoum F, Rosenthal N, Potter WZ (1983 a) Electroconvulsive treatment and lithium carbonate: their effects on norepinephrine metabolism in patients with primary, major depression. Arch Gen Psychiatry 40:677–680

Linnoila M, Karoum F, Potter WZ (1983 b) Effects of antidepressant treatments on dopamine turnover in depressed patients. Arch Gen Psychiatry 40:1015–1017

Maas JW, Koslow S, Katz MM, Bowden CL, Gibbons RL, Stokes PE, Robins E, Davis JM (1984) Pretreatment neurotransmitter metabolite levels and response to tricyclic antidepressants. Am J Psychiatry 141:1159–1171

Maxwell RA (1983) Second generation antidepressants: the pharmacological and clinical significance of selected examples. Drug Dev Res 3:203–211

Mooney JJ, Schatzberg AF, Cole JO, Kizuka PP, Schildkraut JJ (1985) Enhanced signal transduction by adenylate cyclase in platelet membranes of patients showing antidepressant responses to alprazolam: Preliminary data. J Psychiatr Res 19:65–75

Pandey GN, Davis JM (1983) Treatment with antidepressants and down regulation of beta-adrenergic receptors. Drug Dev Res 3:393–406

Peroutka SJ, Snyder SH (1980) Long-term antidepressant treatment decreases spiroperidol-labeled serotonin receptor binding. Science 210:88–90

Pickar D, Labarca R, Linnoila M, Roy A, Hommer D, Everett D, Paul SM (1984) Neuroleptic-induced decrease in plasma homovanillic acid and antipsychotic activity in schizophrenic patients. Science 225:954–957

Potter WZ, Murphy DL, Wehr TA, Linnoila M, Goodwin FK (1982) Clorgyline: a new treatment for refractory rapid cycling patients. Arch Gen Psychiatry 39:505–510

Potter WZ, Scheinin M, Golden RN, Rudorfer MV, Cowdry RW, Calil HM, Ross RJ, Linnoila M (1985) Selective antidepressants and cerebrospinal fluid: lack of specificity on norepinephrine and serotonin metabolites. Arch Gen Psychiatry 42:1171–1177

Ross RJ, Zavadil AP III, Calil HM, Linnoila M, Kitanaka I, Blombery P, Kopin IJ, Potter WZ (1983) Effects of desmethylimipramine on plasma norepinephrine, pulse, and blood pressure. Clin Pharmacol Ther 33:429–437

Ross RJ, Scheinin M, Lesieur P, Rudorfer MV, Hauger RL, Siever LJ, Linnoila M, Potter WZ (1985) The effect of clorgyline on noradrenergic function. Psychopharmacology (Berlin) 85:227–230

Rudorfer MV, Scheinin M, Karoum F, Ross RJ, Potter WZ, Linnoila M (1984 a) Reduction of norepinephrine turnover by serotonergic drug in man. Biol Psychiatry 19:179–193

Rudorfer MV, Golden RN, Linnoila M, Potter WZ (1984 b) ECT dampens norepinephrine system reactivity in depressed patients. Presented at annual meeting of the Society of Biological Psychiatry, 2–6 May, Los Angeles

Rudorfer MV, Golden RN, Potter WZ (1984 c) Second generation antidepressants. Psychiatr Clin North Am 7:519–534

Rudorfer MV, Karoum F, Ross RJ, Potter WZ, Linnoila M (1985 a) Differences in lithium effects in depressed and healthy subjects. Clin Pharmacol Ther 37:66–71

Rudorfer MV, Ross RJ, Linnoila M, Sherer MA, Potter WZ (1985 b) Exaggerated orthostatic responsivity of plasma norepinephrine in depression. Arch Gen Psychiatry 42:1186–1192

Schroeder DH (1983) Metabolism and kinetics of bupropion. J Clin Psychiatry 44(Sec 2):79–81

Shopsin B, Cassano GB, Conti L (1981) An overview of new "second generation" antidepressant compounds: research and treatment implications. In: Enna SJ, Molick J, Richelson E (eds) Antidepressants: neurochemical, behavioral and clinical perspectives. Raven, New York, pp 219–251

Stewart JW, Quitkin F, Fyer A, Klein DF (1980) Efficacy of desmethylimipramine in endogenomorphically depressed patients. Psychopharmacol Bull 16:52–54

Stockmeier CA, Kellar KJ (1986) In vivo regulation of the serotonin-2 receptor in rat brain. Life Sci 38:117–127

Stone EA (1983) Problems with current catecholamine hypotheses of antidepressant agents: speculation toward a new hypothesis. Behav Brain Sci 6:535–547; "Open Peer Commentary," ibid, 548–577

Sugrue MF (1983) Chronic antidepressant therapy and associated changes in central monoaminergic receptor functioning. Pharmacol Ther 21:1–33

Träskman L, Åsberg M, Bertilsson L, Cronhold B, Mellström B, Neckers LM, Sjöqvist F, Thoren P, Tybring G (1979) Plasma levels of chlorimipramine and its demethyl metabolite during treatment of depression. Clin Pharmacol Ther 26:600–610

Veith RC, Raskind MA, Barnes RF, Gumbrecht G, Ritchie JL, Halter JB (1983) Tricyclic antidepressants and supine, standing, and exercise plasma norepinephrine levels. Clin Pharmacol Ther 33:763–769

Vetulani J, Stawarz RJ, Dingell JW, Sulser F (1976) A possible common mechanism of action of antidepressant treatments. Reduction in the sensitivity of the noradrenergic cyclic AMP generating system in the rat limbic forebrain. Naunyn-Schmiedebergs Arch Pharmacol 239:109–114

Wolfe BB, Harden TK, Sporn JR, Molinoff PB (1978) Presynaptic modulation of beta-adrenergic receptors in rat cerebral cortex after treatment with antidepressants. J Pharmacol Exp Ther 207:446–457

Zavadil AP, Ross RJ, Calil HM, Linnoila M, Blombery P, Jimerson DC, Kopin IJ, Potter WZ (1984) The effect of desmethylimipramine on the metabolism of norepinephrine. Life Sci 35:1061–1068

Zis AP, Goodwin FK (1979) Novel antidepressants and the biogenic amine hypothesis of depression: the case for iprindole and mianserin. Arch Gen Psychiatry 36:1097–1107

Antidepressants and EEG Sleep: Search for Specificity

D. J Kupfer, J. A. Shipley, J. M. Perel, B. Pollock,
P. A. Coble, and D. G. Spiker

1 EEG Sleep in Depression

The measurement of electroencephalographic (EEG) sleep parameters in depressed patients provides opportunities both to understand the characteristic features of EEG sleep in depression and to examine the interaction of antidepressants, EEG sleep, and disease. On the basis of studies completed to date, we can state that the EEG sleep profile in such patients improves the diagnostic classification of affective states, offers an objective set of indicators in assessing the severity of illness, and provides an aid to the choice and length of treatment. Indeed, since the effects of antidepressant agents on sleep are immediate and pronounced, studies of these drug-induced effects on sleep may also represent a rational method for drug classification. However, despite the fact that sleep investigations represent an attractive laboratory aid in understanding the possible relationship between central nervous system functioning and affective disorders, relatively few studies with antidepressants have been undertaken. Even fewer studies have been designed to test a specific set of hypotheses.

2 Sleep Patterns in Antidepressant Drug Treatment

Over a period of several years we have been interested in finding out whether various constellations of sleep pattern changes in depressed patients are altered by different antidepressants and whether these changes correlate with or predict clinical response. For example, examinations of the early or acute effects of amitriptyline on EEG sleep patterns suggest that specific EEG sleep changes are predictive of amitriptyline response (Kupfer et al. 1981). While it appears that even predrug EEG sleep characteristics may separate clinical responders from nonresponders, the analysis of sleep changes during the early period of drug administration increases the precision with which treatment response for amitriptyline can be predicted. To expand these findings and ascertain the extent to which it is possible to generalize from such a predictive strategy, in addition to amitriptyline, we have been using two secondary amine tricyclic antidepressants, nortriptyline and desipramine, and also a bicyclic antidepressant (zimelidine), which appears to act specifically on serotonin reuptake blockade. We have been investigating whether the

Department of Psychiatry, University of Pittsburgh School of Medicine, Western Psychiatric Institute and Clinic, 3811 O'Hara Street, Pittsburgh, PA 15213, USA.

Clinical Pharmacology in Psychiatry
Editors: Dahl, Gram, Paul, Potter
(Psychopharmacology Series 3)

degree of immediate REM suppression predicts clinical response, regardless of which antidepressant is administered, and, if there are different effects, whether these changes can be categorized by the "class" of antidepressants, e.g., type of reuptake blocker.

As a first step we assessed the effects of nortriptyline on the EEG sleep of 20 inpatients with major depressive syndrome. While 25 mg nortriptyline had an immediate effect on REM sleep variables, sleep continuity measures were influenced relatively little. Subsequent administration of 75 and 100 mg nortriptyline produced continued REM sleep suppression over several weeks. In essence, nortriptyline altered EEG sleep in a pattern similar to that brought about by amitriptyline. REM latency and REM sleep time were consistently reduced by drug administration, whereas REM activity was only transiently decreased, as with amitriptyline (Kupfer et al. 1982 a).

Preliminary results with zimelidine (ZIM) have demonstrated immediate suppression of rapid eye movement (REM), marked by prolongation of REM latency and decrease in REM as a percentage of total sleep, unassociated with significant sleep continuity alterations. The REM sleep suppression persisted throughout the 4½-week drug protocol without major sleep continuity changes. For example, when the effects of amitriptyline or zimelidine on the EEG sleep of hospitalized depressed patients were compared in a double blind protocol, zimelidine did not affect sleep continuity; after 3 weeks of zimelidine treatment patients tended to have somewhat longer sleep latency, more awakening, and lighter NREM (non-REM) sleep than before drug treatment. Zimelidine did, however, induce a rapid and persistent alteration in sleep architecture and selected REM measures. Thus, REM sleep, which was suppressed over the first two nights of zimelidine administration, showed maximal suppression after 1 week, but by 3 weeks some tolerance for selected REM measures was noted. While zimelidine had none of the sedative qualities (increased sleep maintenance and sleep continuity) of amitriptyline, both drugs were equivalent in their REM-suppressant effects (Shipley et al. 1984).

We also recently documented the effects of desipramine (DMI) on EEG sleep in this group of depressed patients. Compared with placebo, patients receiving DMI showed somewhat worsened sleep continuity, particularly after 1 week of administration. On the other hand, REM measures showed a rapid suppression of REM sleep, followed by partial tolerance of this effect with continued administration of DMI for 3 weeks (Shipley et al. 1985).

All four antidepressant drugs (AMI, NT, DMI, and ZIM) in our most recent set of studies showed pronounced effects on the sleep patterns of depressed patients. The results indicate major similarities with respect to REM sleep and differences with respect to arousals and the sedative qualities of the compounds. The drugs also differed in their effects on sleep continuity and sleep architecture. Only amitriptyline was associated with consistently improved sleep continuity. In contrast, the patients treated with nortriptyline or desipramine showed no improvement in sleep maintenance, while patients treated with zimelidine showed poorer sleep continuity and a lightening of NREM sleep with continued administration. The effects of these drugs on REM sleep were more uniform, with all four drugs being associated with rapid and sustained suppression of several measures of

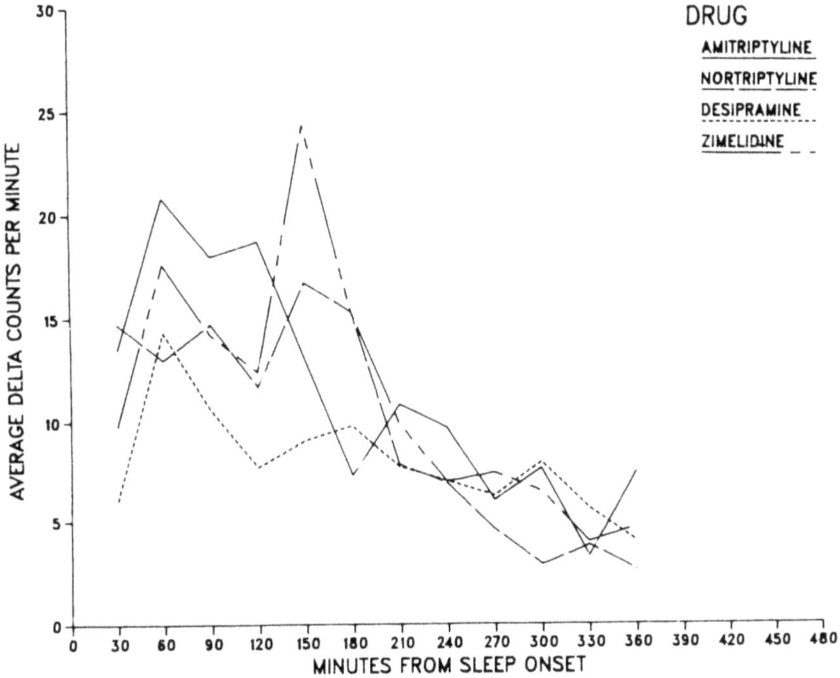

Fig. 1. Average delta counts at baseline

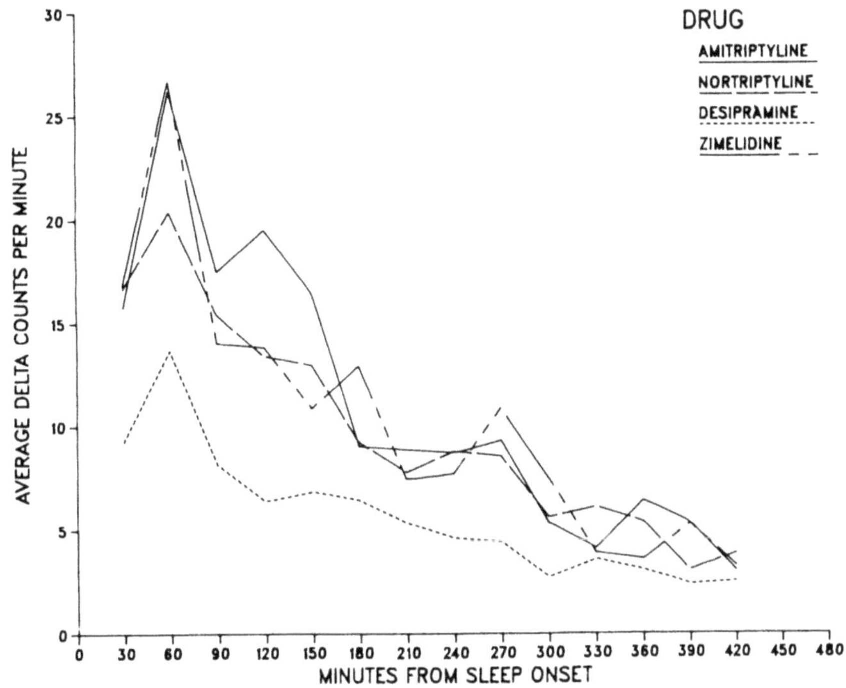

Fig. 2. Average delta counts after 2 days of antidepressant medication

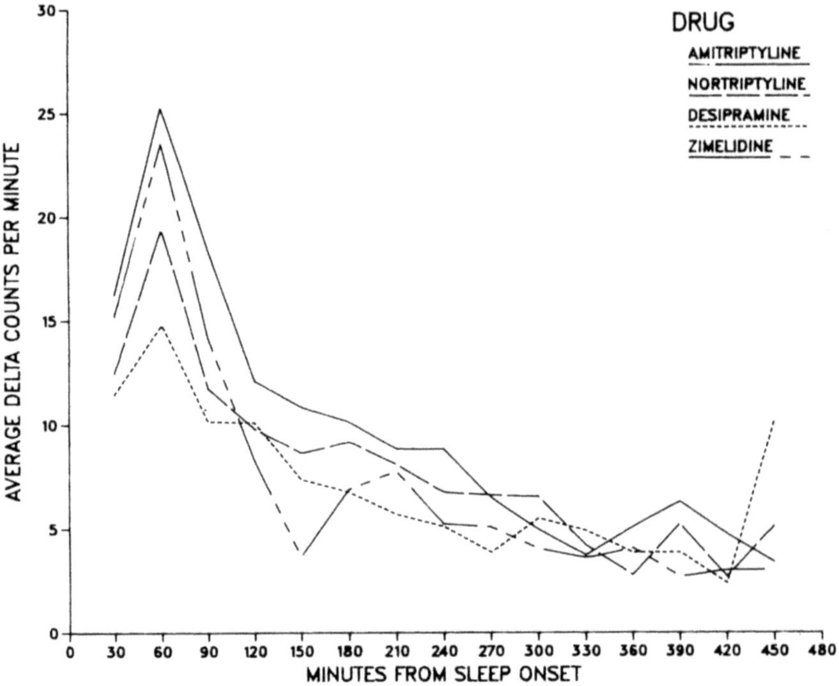

Fig. 3. Average delta counts after 1 week of antidepressant medication

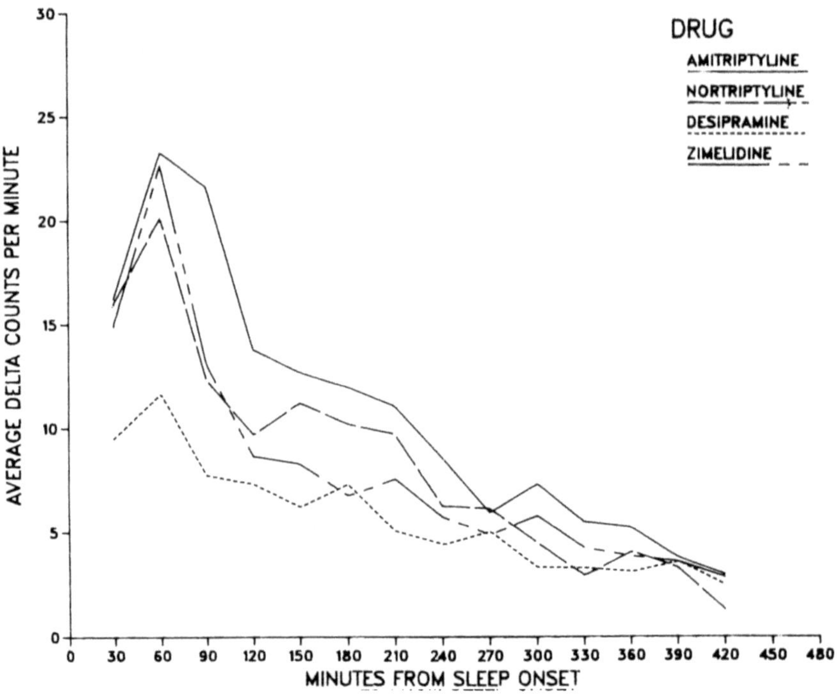

Fig. 4. Average delta counts after 3 weeks of antidepressant medication

REM sleep. On the other hand, ZIM and DMI showed a different sedative effect than AMI and NT, as reflected in the number of arousals and awake time, even after 3 weeks of drug administration.

Automated scoring techniques have been applied to delineate both REM and delta sleep measures in patients treated with amitriptyline, resulting in a fine-grained analysis of individual REM and NREM periods. In the first study of depressed patients, the average REM count for an individual REM period gradually decreased in the second half of the REM period, and this differentiated patients who subsequently did not respond well to amitriptyline (Kupfer et al. 1982b). This type of investigation has been extended to a study of the distribution of slow-wave sleep (SWS) before and during antidepressant drug treatment for the four antidepressants used in the overall design. We have tested one basic prediction derived from Borbély's (1982) two-process model of sleep regulation: If the S process (sleep propensity or ability) is indeed deficient in depression, then one would predict increased slow-wave sleep following successful treatment with antidepressants, as shown in either total delta counts or average delta counts per minute of sleep. One would also predict that clinical responders might show a greater change than nonresponders in these measures of SWS.

Aided by automated analysis, we recently examined 43 depressed patients, who were then treated randomly with one of these four antidepressants (amitriptyline $n=11$, nortriptyline $n=9$, desipramine $n=12$, and zimelidine $n=11$). The immediate effect of all four antidepressants within two nights of drug administration was to increase the average delta wave count in the first NREM period (concurrent with prolongation of REM latency, i.e., the first NREM period), especially within the first 60–90 min of sleep. In other words, a very early consolidation of delta sleep occurred in depressed patients (within 48 h of drug administration) (Fig. 1 and 2). As drug administration continued, increased consolidation and a more prominent peak in average delta counts was found early in the night, along with a steeper linear decay in average delta count across consecutive NREM periods during the night after 4 weeks of drug treatment, than at baseline (Fig. 3 and 4). Average delta counts were reduced significantly as treatment progressed, while total delta counts did not change as a function of drug administration due to the increased time spent asleep.

3 Possible Mechanisms

These results suggest that a simple linear increase in the average delta count may not be a function of the antidepressive sleep effect. It is likely that antidepressant drugs may affect the SWS patterning differently than sleep deprivation. Further analysis, involving the time-course of the slope decay in SWS during various periods of antidepressant administration compared with baseline studies, is necessary to test the applicability of the two-process model of sleep regulation for integrating therapeutic/biological measurements in depression.

To date, we have found no evidence for dramatic changes in average delta sleep production during the first 4 weeks in a treatment trial for acute depression, although the temporal distribution of slow-wave activity was altered in the direction of normal, with greater SWS intensity in the first NREM period. These findings must be tempered with two caveats: First, these automated examinations have focused only on the 0.5–2.0 Hz band of delta sleep. Ongoing investigations of the 2.0–3.0 Hz band are now being undertaken to ascertain whether this bandwidth will demonstrate a parallel set of findings. Second, it has been repeatedly suggested that a 4-week clinical trial is not necessarily associated with complete clinical remission, and that perhaps certain biological alterations may not recover for at least 3–6 months after treatment has been initiated. Only an examination of patients treated for longer periods of time and followed into complete remission can address this question.

To discriminate among potential neurochemical influences on EEG sleep, it is important to separate effects related to sedation (sleep continuity effects) from those related to REM sleep. Our data support the notion that the sedative effects of antidepressants seem to be related to anticholinergic, antihistaminic, or serotonergic effects, with a prime emphasis on anticholinergic effects. The action of amitriptyline, in contrast to that of zimelidine or desipramine, illustrates this point. It is appealing to assume that the REM sleep abnormalities seen in depression are associated with decreased norepinephrine and increased acetylcholine. Therefore, the administration of drugs that either increase norepinephrine or decrease available acetylcholine would alter this balance. It is also possible that drugs that operate on only one neurotransmitter system may have as much of an effect as those that affect both systems.

Other clinical investigations support these conclusions. In particular, our own studies of recurrent depressives treated with imipramine on a long-term basis report findings that parallel our findings with desipramine. Patients receiving imipramine tended to show a pronounced and sustained decrease in REM sleep without signs of significant sedative effects (Kupfer et al., unpublished observations, 1985).

In general, our clinical findings are also analogous to the available animal data. Reyes et al. (1983) studied zimelidine-treated rats and found pronounced REM suppression. More recently, Ursin has investigated the acute effect of zimelidine on the sleep of cats and rats. In both species, REM sleep decreased significantly (Ursin et al. 1984). However, since zimelidine appeared to increase to proportion of delta sleep over baseline, changes with specific serotonergic reuptake blockers will await further verification.

However, the present overall findings are difficult to explain on the basis of current hypotheses in relation to sleep and depression, especially those theories that advocate a major role for cholinergic mechanisms. We have continued our interest in potential differences with those compounds that act more specifically on serotonin reuptake. At present, we are planning to address this question with rigorous pharmacokinetic control by systematic studies of both fluvoxamine, a monocyclic antidepressant drug with highly selective serotonergic enhancing activity, and i.v.-infused clomipramine, a clinical tricyclic antidepressant with serotonergic activity. The principal metabolite of clomipramine (CMI) is the *N*-desmethyl compound (DCMI) which, because of its much longer half-life, is found in much greater steady-state plasma concentrations than the parent drug, i.e., DCMI : CMI ratios usually range from 3 : 1–5 : 1 after oral administration. CMI is a potent serotonergic (5-HT) reuptake blocker, whereas DCMI is mostly noradrenergic (NA); both compounds also act on other neurotransmitter systems. Intravenous CMI infusions minimize the hepatic presystemic clearance effects by reducing *N*-demethylation, as evidenced by DCMI : CMI ratios of less than one.

Recent pilot studies with i.v. clomipramine and fluvoxamine demonstrate a rapid REM suppression and an association of sleep continuity changes which actually appear to be somewhat dichotomous. While the patient reports a "better" night's sleep, clear objective evidence of greater sleep disruption is present. Studies are currently under way to examine whether the rapidity of REM suppression, especially with i.v. clomipramine, is correlated with a more rapid clinical response. It is expected that these strategies offer an opportunity to examine the specificity of the EEG sleep effect, which in turn may have important ramifications for understanding the specificity for drug mechanisms, as well as the specificity of clinical response.

References

Borbély AA (1982) A two-process model of sleep regulation. Hum Neurobiol 1:195–204

Kupfer DJ, Spiker DG, Coble PA, Neil JF, Ulrich RF, Shaw DH (1981) Sleep and treatment prediction in endogenous depression. Am J Psychiatry 138:429–434

Kupfer DJ, Spiker DG, Rossi A, Coble PA, Shaw DH, Ulrich RF (1982a) Nortriptyline and EEG sleep in depressed patients. Biol Psychiatry 18:535–546

Kupfer DJ, Shaw DH, Ulrich R, Coble PA, Spiker DG (1982b) Application of automated REM analysis in depression. Arch Gen Psychiatry 39:569–573

Reyes R, Hill SY, Kupfer DJ (1983) Effects of aute doses of zimelidine on REM sleep in rats. Psychopharmacology (Berlin) 80:214–216

Shipley JE, Kupfer DJ, Sewitch DE, Coble PA, McEachran AB, Grochocinski VJ (1984) Differential effects of amitriptyline and zimelidine on EEG sleep of depressed patients. Clin Pharmacol Ther 2:251–259

Shipley JE, Kupfer DJ, Griffin SJ, Dealy RS, Coble PA, McEachran AB, Grochocinski VJ, Ulrich R, Perel JM (1985) Comparison of effects of desipramine and amitriptyline on EEG sleep of depressed patients. Psychopharmacology (Berlin) 85:14–22

Ursin R, Sommerfelt L, Hauge E (1984) Similar effects on REM sleep but differential effect on slow-wave sleep of two selective 5-HT uptake inhibitors. Proceedings of the 7th European sleep conference, Munich, 3–7 Sept. 1984, pp 311

Possible Teratogenic Effects of Imipramine in the Rat

C. L. DeVane[1,3] and J. W. Simpkins[2,3]

1 Introduction

Tricyclic antidepressants are sometimes used during pregnancy (Crombie et al. 1972; Scanlon 1969). In reviews of studies which examine the teratogenic potential of antidepressants in humans it is frequently concluded that these drugs are relatively safe for use in pregnant patients (Calabrese and Gulledge 1985; Csernansky and Hollister 1984). While ethical and experimental restraints prohibit a thorough assessment of the results of prenatal drug exposure in humans, animal experiments have indicated that physiologic, biochemical, and behavioral effects may result from in utero drug exposure. Collectively, our pharmacokinetic and dynamic studies indicate that third trimester administration of imipramine (IMI) to rats in doses that do not cause dysmorphic effects in the fetus results in substiantial fetal drug and metabolite exposure, enhances infant mortality, and has teratogenic effects persisting into adulthood on neuronal systems which regulate growth and reproductive function. These data imply that maternal ingestion of imipramine may result in subclinical teratogenic effects, which may not be evident, if at all, until offspring have matured past adolescence.

2 Paradigm for Fetal Drug Exposure and Teratogenicity

Female Sprague-Dawley rats whose pregnancies were accurately timed were each given a single i.p. drug injection of 30 mg/kg, a dose for many psychoactive drugs which does not result in obvious malformations in animal offspring. At timed intervals six animals were sacrificed and various tissues retained for drug analysis.

Another group of rats was allowed to complete gestation following drug administration during the third trimester of pregnancy. For each experimental group there was a parallel control group in which the animals received injections of drug vehicle. The following parameters were monitored: (a) gestation length; (b) maternal weight during the injection period; (c) number of offspring per liter; (d) birth weights; (e) infant mortality rate; (f) growth rate; and (g) for female offspring, the age and body weight at vaginal opening. Beginning at 5 weeks of age, indirect systolic blood pressure was determined weekly for male progeny by the tail cuff method.

Departments of [1]Pharmacy Practice, [2]Psychiatry, and [3]Pharmacodynamics, University of Florida, Gainesville, FL 32610, USA.

Clinical Pharmacology in Psychiatry
Editors: Dahl, Gram, Paul, Potter
(Psychopharmacology Series 3)

The responsiveness of the heart to beta adrenergic stimulation was determined by constructing dose-response curves for the chronotropic response to 1-isoproterenol. Contractility and adrenergic responsiveness were measured in vitro in rings of aortic smooth muscle obtained from the male offspring (Simpkins et al. 1985).

Female offspring of drug-exposed mother rats were monitored for the pattern of estrous cycles by obtaining daily vaginal lavages for 16 consecutive days. To determine the effects of prenatal exposure to psychoactive drugs on the regulation of luteinizing hormone (LH) secretion, groups of the female progeny from treatment and control groups were bilaterally ovariectomized, and 14 days later these rats received single injections of estradiol benzoate (EB) followed by an injection 2 days later of progesterone. Serum LH concentrations were determined from samples obtained 2 weeks after ovariectomy, 2 days after EB treatment, and 6.5 h after progesterone treatment.

Finally, the effects of maternal drug exposure on hypothalamic catecholamine metabolism were determined in groups of female offspring. Subgroups of animals were treated with alpha methylparatyrosine and were sacrificed 45 or 90 min later. The tissue concentrations of dopamine (DA), norepinephrine (NE), and the dopamine metabolite, 3,4-dihydroxyphenylacetic acid (DOPAC) were determined in the medial basal hypothalamus (MBH) and the preoptic area of the anterior hypothalamus (POA-AH). These two regions mediate the stimulatory and inhibitory feedback effects of gonadal sterioids on LH secretion. Turnover rates for each catecholamine were determined by the non-steady-state method of Brodie et al. (1966).

3 Imipramine Pharmacokinetics in Pregnant Rats and Their Fetuses

Tissues obtained from pregnant rats treated acutely with IMI revealed that IMI and its metabolites 2-hydroxy-imipramine and desipramine (DMI) rapidly and extensively appeared in the fetus (DeVane and Simpkins 1985). The concentrations of DMI quickly exceeded those of IMI in all tissues and persisted longer. Comparison of the areas under the drug concentration-time curves (AUC) indicated that the fetal liver and fetal brain were exposed to concentrations of IMI and its metabolites that were 10–17 times those in the maternal plasma. In addition, the AUC for DMI in whole fetus and fetal brain was, respectively, 5.46 and 5.35 times the AUC of IMI in these tissues. This demonstrates that the major drug to which the fetal brain was exposed following maternally administered IMI was DMI.

4 Imipramine Effects on Developmental Parameters

Maternal exposure to imipramine clearly enhanced infant mortality, reduced birth weight, appeared to cause a persistent retardation of growth in progeny of both sexes, and delayed the onset of female sexual maturation as reflected by the age at vaginal opening (Table 1).

Table 1. Birth and developmental parameters of progeny of rats treated with imipramine during pregnancy

Parameter	Maternal treatment	
	Saline	Imipramine
Length of pregnancy (days)	21.9±0.14	22.2±0.2
Young per litter (no.)	9.0±0.4	9.1±1.0
Mean birth weight (g)	6.9±0.06	5.5±0.06 c
Live mass delivered (g/litter)	62.0±2.7	52.5±1.9 a
Infant mortality (deaths/total # of young)	0/108	9/91 d
Age at vaginal opening (days)	36.4±0.3	37.7±0.3 b
Weight at vaginal opening (g)	129 ±2	123 ±2

[a] $P<0.025$
[b] $P<0.005$
[c] $P<0.001$ versus saline group, Student's *t*-test
[d] $P<0.005$ versus saline group according to χ^2 analysis

5 Imipramine Effects on Reproductive Parameters

Maternal exposure to IMI adversely affected reproductive function in surviving female progeny. While in control progeny 75% had normal 4- to 5-day estrous cycles, only 23% of IMI-exposed female progeny showed normal estrous cycles at 3–4 months of age. These observations indicate that prenatal IMI exposure can adversely affect the ability of the hypothalamo-hypophysial-ovarian axis to cyclically alter their secretory activity and hence to regulate phasic changes in ovarian

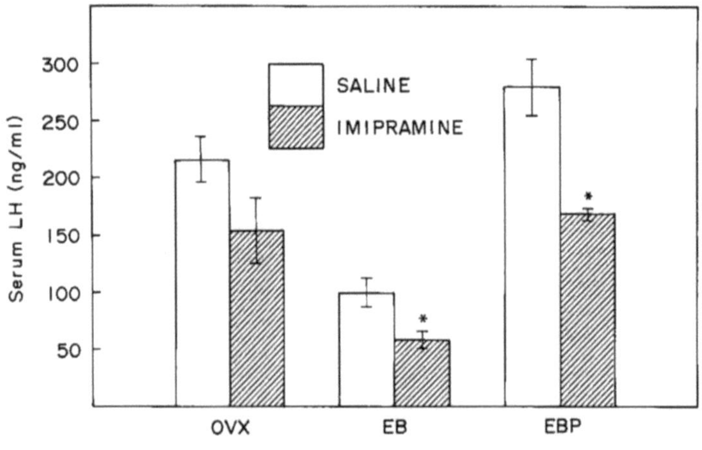

Fig. 1. Effects of ovariectomy and gonodal steroid treatment on serum LH concentration in female progeny from rats treated with saline or imipramine during pregnancy. OVX = 14 days after ovariectomy; EB = 2 days after estradiol benzoate (7.5 µg/rat) treatment; EBP = 6.5 h after progesterone treatment of estradiol benzoate-primed rats. Each group consisted of six to seven rats. *P < 0.025 versus saline group exposed to the same steroid treatment

follicular development and hormone secretion. Consistent with this hypothesis is the observation that IMI-exposed female progeny differ significantly in their LH-secretory responses to gonadal steroids. Imipramine-exposed progeny were significantly more responsive to the negative feedback effects of estradiol on LH release (Simpkins and Geagan 1985; Fig. 1).

6 Imipramine Effects on Catecholamine Concentrations and Turnover

Associated with the effects of prenatal IMI exposure on development and reproductive function were significant alterations in the concentrations and turnover rate of dopmaine in the hypothalamus (Table 2; Simpkins and Geagan 1985). In the POA-AH, DA concentrations were increased by 21% and DA turnover was enhanced by 65%. Associated with this increased activity of POA-AH neurons was a 34% increase in levels of DOPAC, the major acid metabolite of DA. Similarly, in the MBH, DA concentrations were increased by 15%, DA turnover by 24%, and levels of DOPAC by 14%. This persistent enhancement in the activity of dopaminergic neurons in the two brain regions which regulate body temperature, food and water intake behavior, sexual behavior, reproductive cycles, and anterior pituitary hormone secretion indicates that prenatal IMI exposure, through these aminergic neurons, could adversely affect a variety of physiological processes in progeny.

Table 2. Effects of maternal imipramine exposure on concentrations and turnover rate of norephinephrine and dopamine in the preoptic area-anterior hypothalamus and medial basal hypothalamus of female progeny

Brain region	Prenatal treatment	Amine	Initial concentration (ng/mg protein)	Rate constant of amine loss	Turnover rate (ng/mg protein per h.)
POA-AH	Saline	NE	12.3 ±0.8	0.200±0.123	2.46±1.48
	IMI	NE	12.2 ±0.8	0.240±0.054	2.93±0.66
POA-AH	Saline	DA	2.2 ±0.08	0.589±0.102	1.29±0.22
	IMI	DA	2.8 ±0.23[b]	0.761±0.098[a]	2.13±0.27[b]
POA-AH	Saline	DOPAC	0.41±0.01	–	–
	IMI	DOPAC	0.55±0.03[c]	–	–
MBH	Saline	NE	13.8 ±0.9	0.333±0.065	4.55±0.89
	IMI	NE	13.3 ±0.7	0.402±0.053	5.32±0.70
MBH	Saline	DA	5.57±0.2	0.77 ±0.06	4.29±0.324
	IMI	DA	6.41±0.2[c]	0.83 ±0.05	5.32±0.321[a]
MBH	Saline	DOPAC	0.51±0.01	–	–
	IMI	DOPAC	0.58±0.02[b]	–	–

We used 7 rats per group for determination of initial concentrations and 21 rats per group for estimation of rate constants and turnover rates.
[a] $0.1 > p < 0.05$; [b] $P < 0.05$; [c] $P < 0.01$.

7 Imipramine Effects on Adrenergic Responsiveness

Male progeny were monitored through 3 months of age for blood pressure. Compared with controls, no effect was observed. Similarly, the chronotropic response of the heart to isoproterenol in vivo was unchanged in drug-treated rats. The responses of aortic rings to a wide dose range of isoproterenol (beta agonist), norepinephrine (alpha agonist), or potassium chloride (a membrane-depolarizing agent) in vitro was not affected by in utero exposure to imipramine. The results indicate that at the dose of IMI used, in utero exposure did not affect blood pressure, cardiac or vascular reactivity in male progeny which survived to adulthood.

8 Conclusions

Our work in animals has demonstrated that a variety of developmental parameters, including reproductive function (estrous cyclicity) and brain neurotransmission (persistent hyperactivity of hypothalamic catecholaminergic neurons), are altered in the adult progeny of imipramine exposed mothers. The effects on reproductive function are particularly significant. It was observed that imipramine enhanced the sensitivity of the brain to the inhibitory feedback effects of estrogens and reduced the sensitivity of the hypothalamus to the stimulatory feedback effects of progesterone on LH release. Thus, the constant estrous state at sexual maturation reflects premature aging of the female reproductive system as a consequence of prenatal IMI exposure. This suggests that a novel teratological consequence of fetal drug exposure is an enhancement of the rate of aging of particular body systems or of the organism itself. Our studies suggest that more caution is warranted in the use of antidepressants during pregnancy than has been previously expressed.

Acknowledgement. The work reported in this paper was supported by NIH grant no. HD 14075.

References

Brodie BB, Costa E, Dlabec A, Neff NH, Smookler HW (1966) Application of steady state kinetics to the stimulation of synthesis rate and turnover time of tissue catecholamines. J Pharmacol Exp Ther 154:493–498

Calabrese JR, Gulledge AD (1985) Psychotropics during pregnancy and lactation: a review. Psychosomatics 26:413–426

Crombie D, Pinsent RJ, Felming D (1972) Imipramine in pregnancy. Br Med J 1:745

Csernansky JG, Hollister LE (1984) Psychotropic medications: the risk of teratogenesis. Hosp Formul Manage 19:718–723

DeVane CL, Simpkins JW (1985) Pharmacokinetics of imipramine and its major metabolites in pregnant rats and their fetuses following a single dose. Drug Metab Dispos 13:438–442

Scanlon FV (1969) Use of antidepressant drugs during the first trimester. Med J Aust 2:1077

Simpkins JW, Geagan GJ (1986) Teratogenic effects of late pregnancy exposure to imipramine in the rat. (submitted for publication)

Simpkins JW, Field FP, Torosian G, Soltis EE (1985) Effects of prenatal exposure to tricyclic antidepressants on adrenergic responses in progeny. Dev Pharmacol Ther 8:17–33

Pharmacological Specificity Is Not the Same as Clinical Selectivity

S. A. Montgomery, D. James, and D. B. Montgomery

1 Introduction

Numerous putative antidepressants are currently being developed on the basis of selective theories of action. Most such theories are derived from experiments in animal pharmacology and extrapolated to the ill human condition. These selective theories continue to be promoted despite the fact that currently available so-called selective antidepressants appear to have comparable levels of efficacy with each other and with the nonselective antidepressants. The long delay between production of compounds and the testing of their clinical efficacy in depressed patients might allow some to think that time-honoured theories could be accepted without proper testing in the clinic.

2 Clinical Efficacy of Selective Reuptake Inhibitors

Few studies have systematically examined the clinical effect of pharmacological specificity under double blind conditions. We tested the theory of a differential effect predicted by the simple amine theory of depression. This theory would predict that a "noradrenaline (NA) deficit depression" should respond selectively to a NA uptake inhibitor and that a "5-hydroxytryptamine (5HT) deficit depression" should respond selectively to a 5HT uptake inhibitor. In our study, maprotiline, a relatively pure NA uptake inhibitor, was compared with zimelidine, which is a relatively pure 5HT uptake inhibitor, as is its metabolite norzimelidine.

Fifty in-patients suffering from moderate to severe primary affective disorder of the depressed type (Feighner et al. 1972) were randomly assigned to treatment with maprotiline 150 mg nocte or zimelidine 200 mg nocte on a double blind basis. Administration of these compounds for a 4-week period was preceded by a 2-week period of placebo treatment, at the end of which CSF was drawn from all patients. The CSF samples were analysed for levels of MHPG and 5HIAA, the principal metabolites of noradrenaline and 5HT, respectively. At the end of the 4 weeks' active treatment, nonresponders were crossed over under double blind conditions to the other treatment for a further 4 weeks.

Patients were rated for the severity of their depression before and after treatment with placebo, and weekly thereafter for 4 weeks during active treatment, us-

St Mary's Hospital, Medical School, London, England.

Clinical Pharmacology in Psychiatry
Editors: Dahl, Gram, Paul, Potter
(Psychopharmacology Series 3)

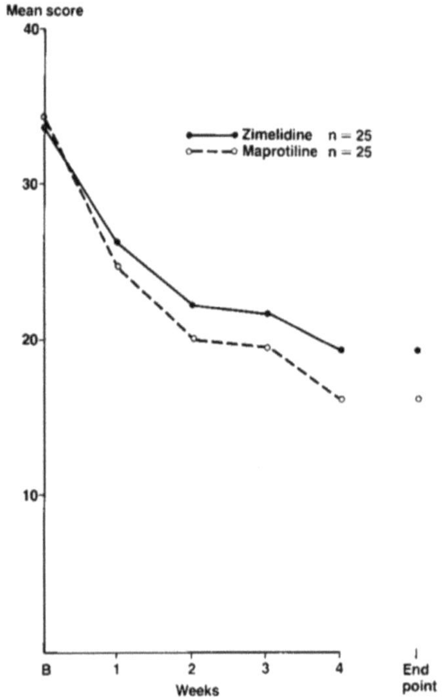

Fig. 1. Mean response (total score on MADRS) to 4 weeks' treatment with zimelidine 200 mg nocte or maprotiline 150 mg nocte

ing the Montgomery and Åsberg Depression Rating Scale (MADRS) (Montgomery and Åsberg 1979) and the Hamilton Rating Scale (HRS) (Hamilton 1967).

There were no significant differences in mean response of the two groups to treatment (Fig. 1) (Montgomery et al. 1984). The overall response rate was not as good as those observed in some other studies, although there was a significant improvement in MADRS and HRS scores compared with baseline. The only significant differences in profile between the two treatment groups appeared early in treatment in two items on the MADRS concerning reduced sleep and reduced appetite; both differences were in favour of maprotiline (Figs. 2 and 3). These differences related directly to the predicted side-effects of the two drugs – a preparation with properties of sedation and appetite stimulation compared with a non-sedative drug that produces feelings of abdominal fullness and nausea. The profile differences were seen only early in treatment and did not persist. Altogether, there was no significant difference between the overall response of the zimelidine-treated group and the maprotiline-treated group at any stage during the study.

Analysis of the metabolite levels showed no relationship between the pretreatment levels of MHPG in the CSF and response to maprotiline. Similarly, there was no significant relationship between the pretreatment levels of 5HIAA in CSF and response to zimelidine (Table 1). Cross-over of nonresponders to the other treatment revealed no subgroup selectively responding to either so-called selective drug.

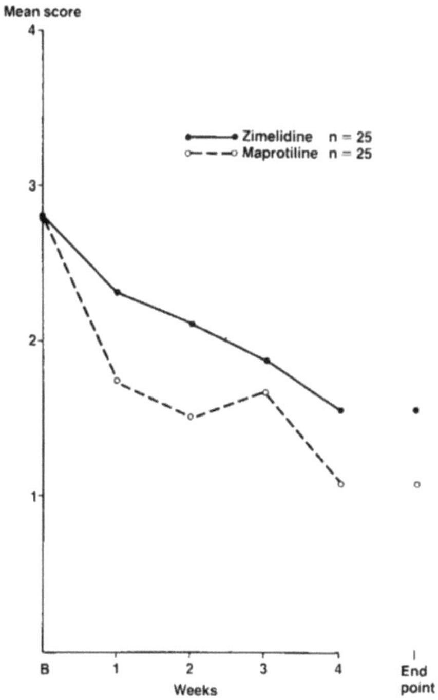

Fig. 2. MADRS reduced sleep item

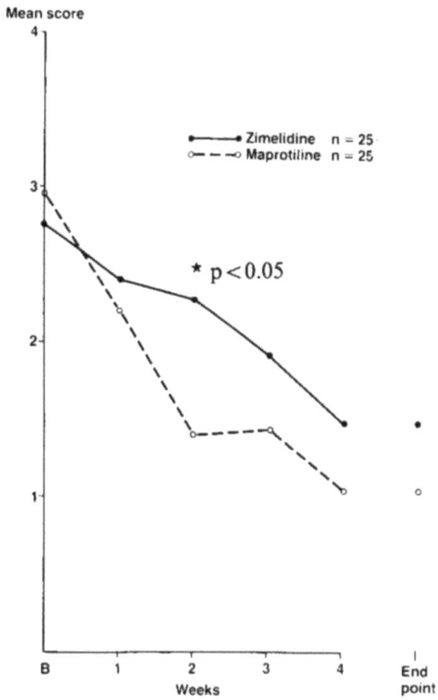

Fig. 3. MADRS reduced appetite item

Table 1. Correlation of pretreatment metabolite levels and response to treatment with zimelidine 200 mg nocte or maprotiline 150 mg nocte

	Pre-treatment CSF metabolite levels (ng/litre)	
	Mean (SD)	Correlation with final HRS score
24 patients treated with zimelidine		
5HIAA	19.4 (15.5)	$r=0.08$, NS
MHPG	10.1 (2.1)	$r=0.34$, NS
24 patients treated with maprotiline		
5HIAA	20.1 (6.7)	$r=0.01$, NS
MHPG	10.2 (2.4)	$r=0.09$, NS

3 Discussion

In this study, three particular aspects of selectivity were investigated.

Firstly, a difference was sought in level of response to an NA uptake inhibitor as opposed to a 5HT uptake inhibitor. No significant difference in overall response was found between the two treatment groups. This result is consistent with other reports (d'Elia et al. 1981; Aberg 1981) and with general clinical experience that effective antidepressants produce rather similar response rates to each other.

The second aspect that we tested was the question of whether pretreatment CSF amine levels predicted response to the relevant selective antidepressant. The low correlation found between 5HIAA levels and response to zimelidine ($r = 0.08$, NS) and the low correlation seen between pretreatment levels of MHPG and response to maprotiline ($r = 0.09$, NS) argue strongly against the existence of subgroups responding to different classes of antidepressants.

The third aspect examined in this study was whether nonresponders to one selective antidepressant would respond to the other treatment. Again there was no evidence in this part of the study for the existence of a selective subgroup.

It is possible that problems of methodology might have contributed to our inability to detect a subgroup responsive selectively to one or other drug. The number of patients in this study was relatively small, and it may be that selective subgroups would emerge in a very much larger study. It is also possible that by chance too few patients admitted to the study happened to be suffering from so-called selective depression. More generally, it may be argued that the levels of monoamine metabolites in CSF are not the best reflectors of subgroups of NA and 5HT depression.

The alternative explanation, which we are inclined to favour, is that the selective theory has little relevance to clinical practice. It may be that any possible selectivity is overwhelmed by general antidepressant response or that the selective subgroups proposed by the simple amine deficit hypothesis do not really exist. More emphasis is now being placed on delayed postsynaptic receptor-mediated events, since it has been observed that chronic treatment with most antidepressants reduces the sensitivity of the NA-sensitive adenylate cyclase system. Current findings suggest that intact serotonergic as well as noradrenergic input is required to bring about this functional change giving rise to a NA-5HT link hypothesis for depression (Sulser et al. 1984). This casts doubt on the possible relevance of selectivity of antidepressants.

The number of double blind studies that have been designed to test selectivity in the clinic is surprisingly small. There is a suggestion in the study of Aberg (1981) that patients with low levels of 5HIAA respond selectively to zimelidine. In our study, we could find no evidence for this at all. The number of studies that have been undertaken in this area overall do not justify the conclusion that the so-called selective antidepressants work selectively in clinical practice. It seems likely that the "simple" amine deficit theory is not as simple as it at first appeared. Claims for selective antidepressants based upon animal studies should be treated with caution until their selectivity has been unequivocally demonstrated in the clinic, and selective theories should not be given greater weight than they deserve.

References

Aberg A (1981) Controlled cross-over study of a 5HT uptake inhibiting and an NA uptake inhibiting antidepressant. Acta Psychiatr Scand [Suppl] 290(63):244–255

D'Elia G, Hallstrom T, Nystrom C, Ottosson JO (1981) Zimelidine vs maprotiline in depressed outpatients. Acta Psychiatr Scand [Suppl] 290(63):225–235

Feighner JP, Robins E, Guze SB, Woodruff RA, Winokur G, Munoz R (1972) Diagnostic criteria for use in psychiatric research. Arch Gen Psychiatry 26:57–63

Hamilton M (1967) Development of a rating scale for primary depressive illness. Br J Soc Clin Psych 6:278–296

Montgomery SA, Åsberg M (1979) A new depression scale designed to be more sensitive to change. Br J Psychiatry 134:382–389

Montgomery SA, Roy DH, Montgomery DB (1984) HVA: a marker for suicidal acts? Prog Neuropsychopharmacol 8:159–166

Sulser F (1984) Antidepressant treatments and regulation of norepinephrine – receptor-coupled adenylate cyclase systems in brain. Front Biochem Pharmacol Res Depression 39:249–261

Pharmacokinetic Considerations Relevant to the Pharmacodynamics of Antidepressants

L. F Gram[1], K. Brøsen[1], P. Christensen[1], and P. Kragh-Sørensen[2]

1 Introduction

In the course of development of new drugs there is a tendency to think and plan, on both conscious and unconscious levels, on the basis of the experience with existing therapeutics. Often, therefore, the development of new antidepressants has been based on knowledge collected with tricyclic antidepressants or MAO inhibitors. The experimental pharmacodynamics of tricyclics in particular has played a dominant role in the development of models for the mode of action of antidepressants and hence in the development of rational drugs with selective effects. On the clinical side our planning is also influenced by earlier experience, when side effects are recorded or when pharmacokinetic studies are designed, for example. Our experience with earlier drugs should be the inspiration and not the limitation of our research on new compounds. What we must do, then, is distil the essence of the earlier experience that can be expected to be relevant for the new drugs.

2 Experimental Pharmacodynamics and Effective Concentrations

Experimental pharmacodynamic results are usually expressed in terms of concentration-effect relationships, but this pharmacokinetic information is normally only used for interdrug comparisons of potency and seldom related to the clinical situation. However, such considerations might be essential when the appropriate dose of a new compound is to be determined.

Tricyclic antidepressants have been shown to possess a number of well-defined pharmacological effects, as listed in Table 1. Newer antidepressants are often characterized by the absence of some or several of these effects. The concentration at which these effects occur varies to some extent between antidepressants, but often occur at the low nanomolar level (Table 2). Usually the concentration measures are calculated from the amount of drug added to the medium, whereas direct concentration measurements often are not reported.

As indicated in Table 1, only a few of the experimental effects have been unequivocally associated with clinical effects (Gram 1983; Hall 1983). These relationships have largely been based on comparisons between the potency of differ-

Departments of [1]Clinical Pharmacology and [2]Psychiatry, Odense University, School of Medicine, J. B. Winsløwsvej 19, DK-5000 Odense, Denkmark.

Clinical Pharmacology in Psychiatry
Editors: Dahl, Gram, Paul, Potter
(Psychopharmacology Series 3)

Table 1. Pharmacodynamics of tricyclic antidepressants

Experimental effects	Related clinical effects
Reuptake inhibition (NA, 5HT)	?
High affinity binding (imip. dmi)	?
Receptor blockade: Muscarine	Dry mouth, blurred vision, etc.
α_1-Adrenoreceptor	Orthostatic hypotension
H_1-Histamine	Sedation
Serotonin	?
Receptor down-regulation	?
?	Antidepressant
?	Antienuretic
?	Analgetic
Membrane effect	Antiarrhythmic

Table 2. Reported effective concentrations (IC_{50}, inhibitor constants, dissociation constants) for the effect of different antidepressants on various receptor systems

Mechanism of action	Relative potency[b]	Effective concentration range (n*M*)	Ref.
Noradrenaline reuptake inhibition	DMI > NT > IP > CI > DX > AT	5–150	Rehavi et al. (1981)
	DMI > NT > IP > DX > AT > CI > MN	1–50	Richelson and Pfenning (1984)
Serotonin reuptake inhibition[a]	CI > IP > AT > NT > DX > DMI	100–3000	Rehavi et al. (1981)
	CI > IP > AT > NT > DX > DMI	5–500	Richelson and Pfenning (1984)
^{3}H-Imipramine high-affinity binding[a]	CI > AT > IP > DMI > NT > DX	15–400	Langer et al. (1980)
	IP > CI > AT > DX > NT > DMI	10–150	Rehavi et al. (1983)
^{3}H-Desipramine high-affinity binding	DMI > NT > IP	10–200	Langer et al. (1981)
	DMI > NT > IP = AT > DX	5–150	Rehavi et al. (1981)
Muscarine receptor blockade	AT > CI > DX > IP > NT > DMI > MN	15–1000	Richelson (1983)
	AT > IP > NT > CI > MN > DMI	50–1000	Hall and Ögren (1981)
H_1-Histamine receptor blockade	AT = MN > IP > NT > CI > DMI	5–500	Hall and Ögren (1981)
	DX > AT > MN > NT = IP > CI > DMI	0.03–250	Richelson (1983)
α_1-Adrenoceptor blockade	DX > AT > MN > CI = NT > IP > DMI	20–500	Tang and Seemann (1980)
	AT > CI > MN > NT > IP > DMI	20–250	Hall and Ögren (1981)
Serotonin receptor blockade	MN > AT > DX > NT > CI > IP > DMI	100–2000	Tang and Seeman (1980)
	MN > NT > AT > CI > DMI > IP	100–1500	Hall and Ögren (1981)

[a] MN only effective at high concentration (> 2000–10000 n*M*).
[b] AT, amitriptyline; CI, clomipramine; DMI, desipramine; DX, doxepine; IP, imipramine; NT, nortriptyline; MN, mianserin.

ent tricyclics in the experimental and the clinical setting. Most clearly a relationship between the muscarinic receptor blocking potency and the tendency to produce anticholinergic side effects such as hyposalivation has been demonstrated (Hall 1983). Sedation is assumed to be related to H_1-histamine receptor blockade, but α_1-adrenoceptor blockade may be a contributing factor (Hall 1983). Orthostatic hypotension may also be related to α_1-adrenoceptor blockade, but interdrug differences between imipramine and nortriptyline do not correspond to differences in potency on this parameter (Nielsen et al. 1983), and reuptake inhibition of noradrenaline (NA) or serotonin may play some role. The analysis of interdrug differences has its limitations. One reason for this is that several tricyclics are partially metabolized into active metabolites with a different effect profile. This is typical of imipramine and its primary metabolite desipramine (see below). Another problem is that the rank order of relative potency is rather similar on several receptor systems (Table 2).

3 Clinical Pharmacokinetics

Pronounced interindividual variability in hepatic clearance is a common characteristic of tricyclic antidepressants and results in a corresponding variability in steady state concentrations when fixed standard doses are used. For imipramine, this variability affects both the parent compound and the main metabolite (desipramine), and also the ratio between the two compounds (Gram et al. 1976, 1977, 1983) (Fig. 1).

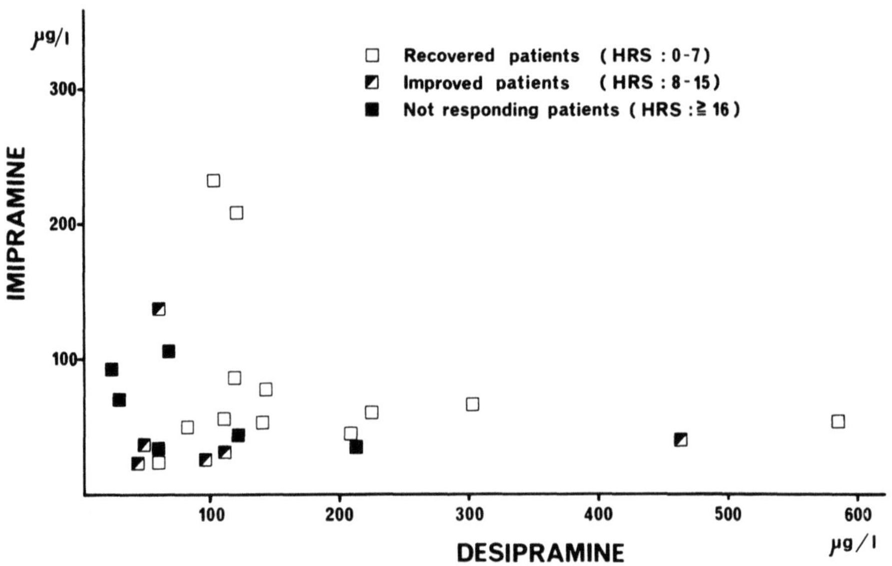

Fig. 1. Corresponding steady state concentrations of imipramine and desipramine in relation to therapeutic outcome in 24 depressed patients treated with imipramine for 4 weeks. (Data from Gram et al. 1976)

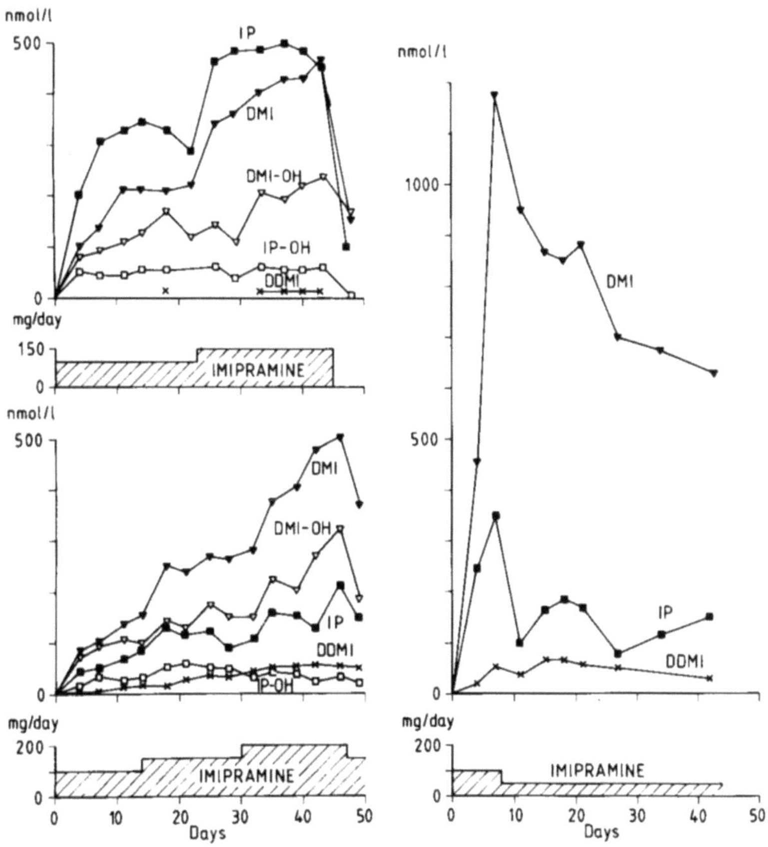

Fig. 2. Concentration of imipramine (*IP*) and its metabolites, desipramine (*DMI*), 2-OH-imipramine (*IP-OH*), 2-OH-desipramine (*DMI-OH*), and didesipramine (*DDMI*) during imipramine treatment in a patient (A7) identified as a poor sparteine metabolizer (*right panel*) and two "normal" patients. (Data from Gram et al. 1983)

There are several sources of this variability in hepatic clearance. The extremes of variability seem to be related to genetic factors. The sparteine/debrisoquine drug oxidation polymorphism thus also relates to the metabolism of antidepressants, including imipramine. Among Caucasians, 7%–9% of the population are poor metabolizers of sparteine/debrisoquine (Brøsen et al. 1985). When poor metabolizers are treated with imipramine they develop extremely high levels of desipramine, in particular, and do not have measurable levels of the 2-OH metabolites (Gram et al. 1983) (Fig. 2). The genetic defect in drug oxidation thus affects the 2-hydroxylation of imipramine and desipramine, but not the demethylation of imipramine.

Family members of the poor metabolizer (69-year-old woman) shown in Fig. 2 have been examined with sparteine tests. As shown in Fig. 3, two of her sons were also identified as poor metabolizers. One of these also suffered from a manic-depressive disorder and had been treated with both neuroleptics and antide-

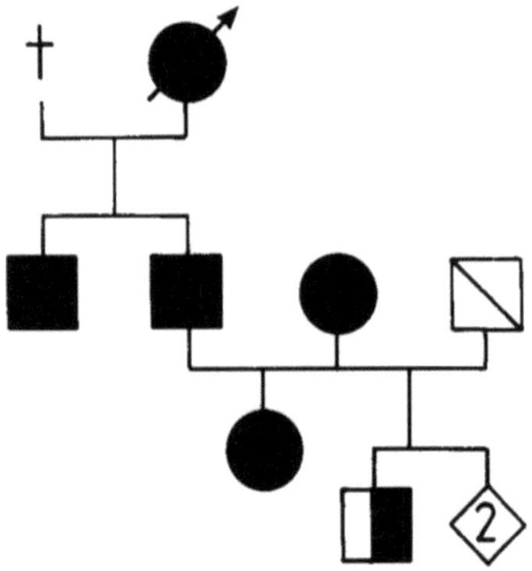

Fig. 3. Sparteine oxidation: pedigree of a 69-year-old woman (patient A7 reported by Gram et al. 1983). Symbols: ●↗, index patient; ●, female poor metabolizer; ■, male poor metabolizer; ◨, male extensive metabolizer (heterozygous); †, decreased; ◇2, two siblings, unknown sex; ⧅, male not sparteine-tested

pressants. With both types of drugs he had experienced considerable anticholinergic and sedative side effects (K. Brøsen, unpublished).

For imipramine, dose-dependent kinetics at therapeutic doses, affecting the 2-hydroxylation also contributes considerably to the interindividual variability (Bjerre et al. 1981; Brøsen et al. 1986). For nortriptyline, linear kinetics at therapeutic doses have been well established (Kragh-Sørensen and Larsen 1980). Other factors contributing to the interindividual variations in steady state levels are plasma protein binding (Kristensen 1983), age (Gram et al. 1977; Abernethy et al. 1985), disease (cardiovascular, hepatic), and drug interactions (neuroleptics) (Gram 1977a). The interaction with neuroleptics is possibly linked to the cytochrome P-450 isoenzyme involved in the sparteine-oxidation polymorphism.

4 Clinical Concentration-Effect Relationships

The relationship between steady state concentrations and antidepressant effect of various tricyclics has been extensively examined in several reviews (Gram 1977b; Gram et al. 1982). In our first report on imipramine we found indications of a separate significance of imipramine and desipramine, in the sense that optimal response appeared to be obtained only when the concentrations of both imipramine and desipramine were above certain levels (45 and 75 µg/liter, respectively). This led us to the tentative hypothesis that "effects on both serotonin and noradrenaline transmitters are needed for the clinical antidepressive effect" (Fig. 2, Gram et al. 1976). Further studies showed that the simple sum of imipramine + desipramine gave about the same level of differentiation between responding and nonresponding patients. The question of a separate significance of the two compounds thus remains unresolved, but future development of selective serotonin or noradrenaline reuptake inhibitors may provide the experimental tool to test this hypothesis.

For imipramine we have also had the oportunity of establishing concentration-effect relationships in two quite different therapeutic situations; nocturnal enuresis and pain in diabetic neuropathy. In both conditions the effective concentrations (imipramine + desipramine > 100 μg/liter) were less than half those optimal for antidepressant effect (> 200–240 μg/liter). This, together with the much faster onset of action, shows that these two conditions are not "depressive equivalents."

Side effects may occur at subtherapeutic levels, e.g., orthostatic hypotension with imipramine (Thayssen et al. 1981) and hyposalivation with nortriptyline (Bertram et al. 1979). The orthostatic hypotensive effect seems to be correlated more closely with the imipramine than with the desipramine concentration (Thayssen et al. 1981). Toxic effects to be avoided by drug level monitoring mainly stem from the CNS and the cardiovascular system. In overdose studies prolongations of the QT_c and QRS intervals are seen at plasma concentrations 2–4 times the therapeutic levels (Pedersen et al. 1982), but some patients may develop partial or complete AV block at lower, even therapeutic, levels (Kragh-Sørensen 1978).

5 Experimental and Clinical Effects and Concentrations

As indicated in Table 1, the relationship between experimental and clinical effects of tricyclic antidepressants are only partly understood. Theoretically some of this confusion might reflect differences in effective concentrations in the experimental and clinical settings. The extrapolation from clinical to experimental concentration (or vice versa) involves a series of problems (Table 3).

Table 3. Confounding factors in extrapolating from clinical to experimental effective concentrations or vice versa

Total plasma concentration	|	Free plasma concentration	|	Receptor concentration	|	Experimetal concentration
	↑ Plasma protein binding		↑ Gradients? Active transport?		↑ Artificial milieu? Binding? Relevant concentration?	
-------- Active metabolites --------						
-------- Multiple receptor systems --------						
-------- Time factor --------						

Table 4. Clinically and experimentally effective concentrations of imipramine and its primary metabolite desipramine

Clinical effect (imipramine + desipramine)	Concentration Free in plasma/IC_{50} (n*M*)	Receptor binding	
		Imipramine	Desipramine
	10	^{3}H-IMIP	^{3}H-DMI
Orthostatic hypotension			
	20		
		H_1-Histamine	
Antienuretic			
Analgetic	50		
	100	α_1-Adreno-	
			^{3}H-IMIP
Antidepressant		Muscarine	
	200		
		^{3}H-DMI	
Negative inotropic			α_1-Adreno-
	500		H_1-Histamine
Conductance disturbances			Muscarine
		Serotonin	
	1000		
		Dopamine	

^{3}H-IMIP, ^{3}H-imipramine high-affinity binding; ^{3}H-DMI, ^{3}H-desipramine high-affinity binding. For references see Table 2.

It seems logical that the free (unbound) drug concentration in plasma most closely approximates the concentration at a certain receptor site in the brain. The clinical concentration measurement to be related to the experimental concentration thus should be corrected to free concentration (imipramine: ~10% of total concentration), and interindividual variations in the free-to-total concentration ratio (usually up to a factor 2; Kristensen 1983) is thus a source of variability.

However, we still do not know whether there are gradients across the blood-brain barrier or whether the concentration measurements reported in experimental studies are relevant to the clinical effect; for example, are IC_{50} or IC_{90} (difference often with a factor of 10, most relevant? The time factor in onset of action, the possible significance of parallel effects on different receptor systems, and the presence of active metabolites with different effect profiles compound the problems. Table 4 gives an example of how one may compare effective concentrations for clinical effects with those producing experimentally demonstrated effects on specific receptors. In general, many of the latter effects have potential clinical relevance. However, the rank order by concentration of the different receptor interactions does not provide a basis for further linking them with clinical effects.

The above considerations, mainly based on the literature on tricyclic antidepressants, are also relevant in the evaluation of the new selective compounds. The introduction of such compounds has opened the way for clinical testing of the relevance for humans of many of the experimentally demonstrated effects of the tricyclics. The use of selective receptor assays may be a different way of addressing the problem by measuring plasma concentrations of antidepressants in relation to a given receptor. We have recently found a significant therapeutic difference between a mixed-action tricyclic, clomipramine, and the selective 5-HT reuptake inhibitor citalopram, the latter being less effective. A common site of action of these two drugs is the serotonin reuptake inhibition, which in turn closely correlates with the high-affinity ^{3}H-imipramine binding (Paul et al. 1981). A receptor assay based on binding to this high-affinity site showed that drug concentrations in the citalopram group were only about one tenth of those in the clomipramine group (Christensen, this volume). However, after correction for differences in protein binding (free fraction: citalopram 20%–30%, clomipramine: 2%–3%) no difference in concentration was found. The difference in therapeutic outcome thus could not be explained in this way, and the results give further support to the assumption that the clinical difference is due to pharmacodynamic differences, e.g., the lack of noradrenaline reuptake-inhibitory properties in the case of citalopram.

References

Abernethy DR, Greenblatt DJ, Shader RI (1985) Imipramine and desipramine disposition in the elderly. J Pharmacol Exp Ther 232:183–188

Bertram U, Kragh-Sørensen P, Rafaelsen OJ, Larsen NE (1979) Saliva secretion following long-term antidepressant treatment with nortriptyline controlled by plasma levels. Scand J Dent Res 87:58–64

Bjerre M, Gram LF, Kragh-Sørensen P, Kristensen CB, Pedersen OL, Møller M, Thayssen P (1981) Dose-dependent kinetics of imipramine in elderly patients. Psychopharmacology (Berlin) 75:354–357

Brøsen K, Otton SV, Gram LF (1985) Sparteine oxidation polymorphism in Denmark. Acta Pharmacol Toxicol 57:357–360

Brøsen K, Gram LF, Klysner R, Bech P (1986) Imipramine and its metabolites during steady-state: significance of dose-dependent kinetics. Eur J Clin Pharmacol 30:43–49

Gram LF (1977a) Factors influencing the metabolism of tricyclic antidepressants. Studies on interactions and first pass elimination. Dan Med Bull 24:81–88

Gram LF (1977b) Plasma level monitoring of tricyclic antidepressants. Clin Pharmacokinet 2:237–251

Gram LF (1983) Antidepressants: receptors, pharmacokinetics and clinical effects. In: Burrows GD, Norman T, Davis B (eds) Antidepressants. Elsevier/North-Holland, Amsterdam, pp 81–96 (Drugs and psychiatry, vol 1)

Gram LF, Reisby N, Ibsen I, Nagy A, Dencker SJ, Bech P, Petersen GO, Christiansen J (1976) Plasma levels and antidepressive effect of imipramine. Clin Pharmacol Ther 19:318–324

Gram LF, Søndergaard I, Christiansen J, Petersen GO, Bech P, Reisby N, Ibsen I, Ortmann J, Nagy A, Dencker SJ, Jacobsen O, Krautwald O (1977) Steady state kinetics of imipramine in patients. Psychopharmacology (Berlin) 54:255–261

Gram LF, Pedersen OL, Kristensen CB, Bjerre M, Kragh-Sørensen P (1982) Drug level monitoring in psychopharmacology: usefulness and clinical problems, with special reference to tricyclic antidepressants. Ther Drug Monit 4:17–25

Gram LF, Bjerre M, Kragh-Sørensen P, Kvinesdal B, Molin J, Pedersen OL, Reisby N (1983) Imipramine metabolites in blood of patients during therapy and after overdose. Clin Pharmacol Ther 33:335–342

Hall H (1983) Relationships between receptor affinities of different antidepressants and their clinical profiles. In: Gram LF, Usdin E, Dahl SG, Kragh-Sørensen P, Sjöqvist F, Morselli PL (eds) Clinical pharmacology in psychiatry, bridging the experimental therapeutic gap. Macmillan, London, pp 251–267

Hall H, Ögren So (1981) Effects of antidepressant drugs on different receptors in the brain. Eur J Pharmacol 70:393–407
Kragh-Sørensen P (1978) Correlation between plasma levels of nortriptyline and clinical effects. Psychopharmacology (Berlin) 2:451–456
Kragh-Sørensen P, Larsen NE (1980) Factors influencing nortriptyline steady-state kinetics: plasma and saliva levels. Clin Pharmacol Ther 28:796–803
Kristensen CB (1983) Serum protein binding of imipramine in healthy subjects. Clin Pharmacol Ther 34:689–694
Langer SZ, Briley MS, Raisman R, Henry JF, Morselli PL (1980) Specific ^{3}H-imipramine binding in human platelets. Naunyn-Schmiedebergs Arch Pharmacol 313:189–194
Langer SZ, Raisman R, Briley M (1981) High-affinity ^{3}H-DMI binding is associated with neuronal noradrenaline uptake in the periphery and the central nervous system. Eur J Pharmacol 72:423–424
Nielsen JR, Johansen T, Arentoft A, Gram LF (1983) Effects of imipramine on the orthostatic changes in blood pressure, heart rate and plasma catecholamines. Clin Exp Pharmacol Physiol 10:497–503
Paul SM, Rehavi M, Rice KC, Ittah Y, Skolnick P (1981) Does high affinity ^{3}H-imipramine binding label serotonin reuptake sites in brain and platelets? Life Sci 28:2753–2760
Pedersen OL, Gram LF, Kristensen CB, Møller M, Thayssen P, Bjerre M, Kragh-Sørensen P, Klitgaard NA, Sindrup E, Hole P, Brinkløv M (1982) Overdosage of antidepressants: clinical and pharmacokinetic aspects. Eur J Clin Pharmacol 23:513–521
Rehavi M, Skolnick P, Hulihan B, Paul SM (1981) High affinity binding of ^{3}H-desipramine to rat cerebral cortex: relationship to tricyclic antidepressant-induced inhibition of norepinephrine uptake. Eur J Pharmacol 70:597–599
Rehavi M, Tracer H, Rice K, Skolnick P, Paul SM (1983) ^{3}H-2-nitroimipramine: a selective "slowly-dissociating" probe of the imipramine binding site ("serotonin transporter") in platelets and brain. Life Sci 32:645–653
Richelson E (1983) Antidepressants: effects on histaminic and muscarinic receptors. In: Gram LF, Usdin E, Dahl SG, Kragh-Sørensen P, Sjöqvist F, Morselli PL (eds) Clinical pharmacology in psychiatry, bridging the experimental therapeutic gap. Macmillan, London, pp 288–300
Richelson E, Pfenning M (1984) Blockade by antidepressants and related compounds of biogenic amine uptake in to rat brain synaptosomes: most antidepressants selectively block norepinephrine uptake. Eur J Pharmacol 104:277–286
Tang SW, Seeman P (1980) Effect of antidepressant drugs on serotonergic and adrenergic receptors. Naunyn-Schmiedebergs Arch Pharmacol 311:255–261
Thayssen P, Bjerre M, Kragh-Sørensen P, Møller M, Pedersen OL, Kristensen CB, Gram LF (1981) Cardiovascular effects of imipramine and nortriptyline in elderly patients. Psychopharmacology (Berlin) 74:360–364

Receptor Assay Based on ^{3}H-Imipramine Binding

P. CHRISTENSEN

1 Introduction

During recent years routine monitoring of plasma levels of cyclic antidepressants has been introduced in many psychiatric institutions, following the demonstration of a relationship between clinical effect and plasma levels of certain antidepressants (Gram 1983; Kragh-Sørensen 1984; Reisby et al. 1979).

Usually the parent compound and the primary desmethyl metabolite have been measured, but this may not be a sufficient measure of the "total" pharmacological activity of the drug. However, since the demonstration of binding sites for cyclic antidepressants on human thrombocytes (Briley et al. 1979; Paul et al. 1980a; Asarch et al. 1980) it has become possible to measure the "total" activity of the antidepressant by using the binding sites in a radiobinding assay (RBA). This measure is considered to represent the effective concentration for reuptake inhibition of serotonin (Briley et al. 1980; Rehavi et al. 1980).

2 Patients and Methods

In total 78 patients joined the study, which was part of a double blind study on the therapeutic effect and side effects of clomipramine 150 mg/day ($n=38$) and citalopram 40 mg/day ($n=40$) (Danish University Antidepressant Group, DUAG 1986). *Inclusion criteria* were a score on the Hamilton rating scale for depression (HDS) of at least 18 after a placebo washout period of 7 days and age between 18 and 65 years. *Exclusion criteria* were duration of the present episode for more than 1 year, schizophrenia, drug or alcohol abuse, dementia, and serious somatic illness. Patients were classified as having endogenous or nonendogenous depression on the basis of their score on the Newcastle scale (N-II) (Gurney et al. 1972). After 5 weeks of active treatment with either clomipramine or citalopram a final HDS rating was carried out.

Blood samples taken after 4 weeks' treatment (steady state) were used for simultaneous measurement of the plasma levels of the parent compound and the desmethyl metabolite quantitative thin-layer chromatography (QTLC) and the total displacing effect on ^{3}H-imipramine-labeled thrombocytes (RBA).

Department of Clinical Pharmacology, and the Danish University Antidepressant Group Odense University, J. B. Winsløwsvej 19, DK-5000 Odense, Denmark.

Clinical Pharmacology in Psychiatry
Editors: Dahl, Gram, Paul, Potter
(Psychopharmacology Series 3)

In ten patients in the clomipramine group and nine patients in the citalopram group, equilibrium dialysis of plasma was carried out to determine the free, non-protein-bound RBA concentration.

3 Results

Initial studies on different antidepressants revealed the IC_{50} values shown in Table 1. Tertiary amines were all potent inhibitors of binding, whereas secondary

Table 1. Inhibition of ^{3}H-imipramine binding to platelet membranes by various antidepressants and their metabolites

Drug	IC_{50} (n*M*) (mean ± SD)
Paroxetin	8 ± 3
Imipramine	14 ± 2
Desmethylclomipramine	17 ± 2
Clomipramine	19 ± 6
Citalopram	25 ± 2
Desmethylcitalopram	25
Nor-femoxitine	25 ± 2
Amitriptyline	27 ± 1
2-Hydroxyimipramine	51 ± 2
Nortriptyline	189 ± 25
Desipramine	203 ± 42
Femoxitine	234 ± 3
2-Hydroxydesipramine	289 ± 32

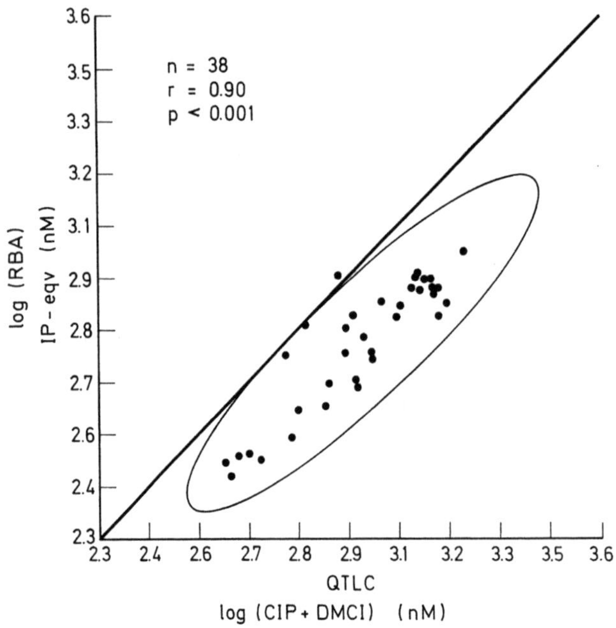

Fig. 1. Plasma levels of clomipramine (*CIP*) + desmethylclomipramine (*DMCI*) (measured by QTLC) in relation to the total displacing effect on ^{3}H-imipramine-labeled thrombocytes (RBA)

amines were less potent. However, both desmethylclomipramine and desmethylcitalopram were quite potent.

When samples from the patients were analyzed, a highly significant correlation was demonstrated between concentrations measured with QTLC (parent compound + desmethyl metabolite) and concentrations measured with RBA (Fig. 1 and 2). As can be seen for both clomipramine and citalopram, the plasma

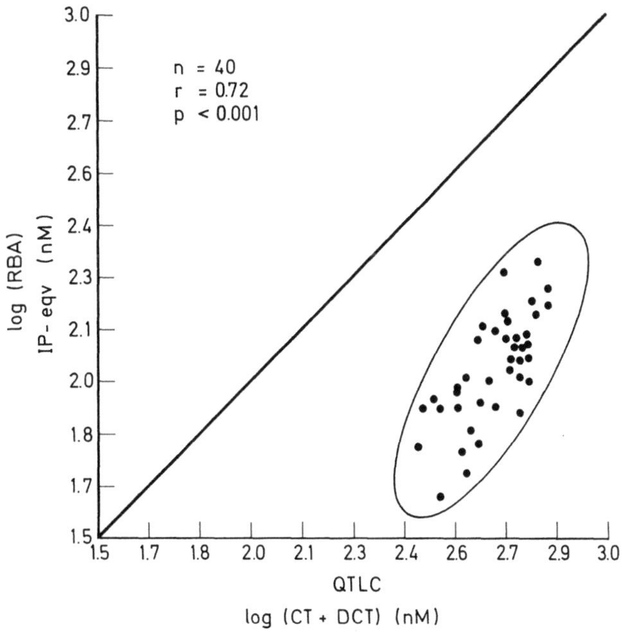

Fig. 2. Plasma levels of citalopram (*CT*) + desmethylcitalopram (*DCT*) (measured by QTLC) in relation to the total displacing effect on ³H-imipramine-labeled thrombocytes (RBA)

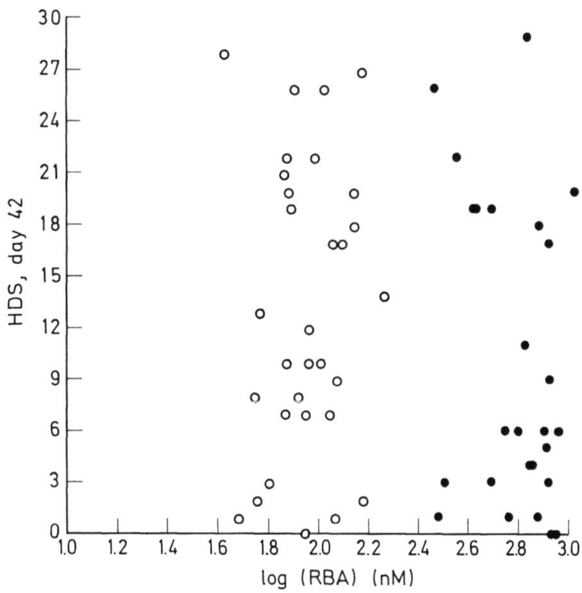

Fig. 3. Plasma levels of clomipramine (●) ($n = 27$) and citalopram (○) ($n = 31$) measured by RBA in relation to therapeutic outcome in patients with endogenous depression

Table 2. Protein binding of antidepressants measured by radiobinding assay

Samples from clomipramine-treated patients	98% ± 1%
Samples from citalopram-treated patients	77% ± 6%
Clomipramine added to plasma	94% ± 3%
Desmethylclomipramine added to plasma	99% ± 1%
Citalopram added to plasma	55% ± 13%
Desmethylcitalopram added to plasma	32% ± 2%

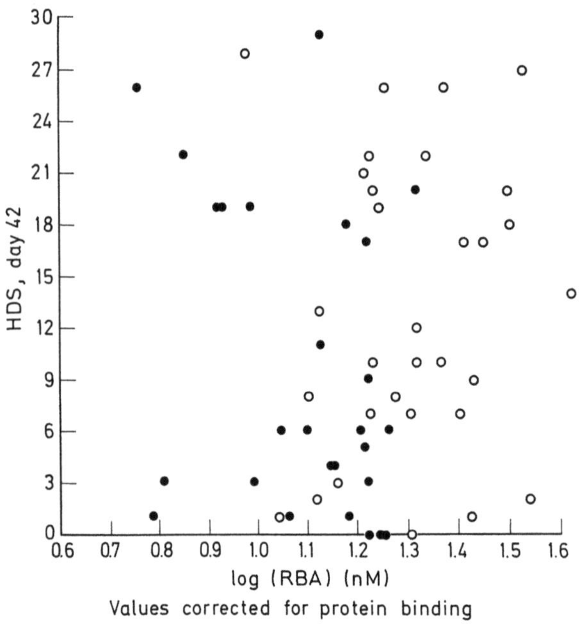

Fig. 4. Plasma levels of clomipramine (●) ($n=27$) and citalopram (o) ($n=31$) (values corrected for protein binding) in relation to therapeutic outcome in patients with endogenous depression

levels measured by RBA were lower than the corresponding QTLC levels, and this was most pronounced for citalopram. Plasma levels of the clomipramine patients were higher compared to the citalopram patients (Fig. 3), but when results were corrected for protein binding (Table 2) the highest free fraction was found for the citalopram group (Fig. 4). When plasma levels were related to the therapeutic effect in the patients with endogenous depression a rather poor correlation was found for both groups of patients (Fig. 3 and 4). This was also found with QTLC, although there were some suggestions that patients with total levels of clomipramine + desmethylclomipramine above 750 nmol/liter responded somewhat better than those patients with lower levels.

4 Discussion

When applied for the determination of clomipramine and citalopram, which are tertiary amines, the RBA yields results comparable to those obtained with QTLC. The RBA method is rapid, sensitive, and inexpensive. The latter method does not measure parent compound and metabolite separately, and for the two drugs examined the desmethyl metabolite was about equally active according to ^{3}H-imipramine binding. Desmethylclomipramine also has an effect on noradrenaline reuptake, which might be quantitated by use of the high-affinity binding sites for ^{3}H-desipramine (Paul et al. 1980 b).

The protein binding levels determined for citalopram were in the same range as found earlier (Fredricson Overø 1982). However, both the parent compound and all metabolites were measured. Experiments with only one active compound yielded slightly lower levels (Table 2). The method may, however, be of value for determination of the protein binding of antidepressants with a high protein binding, such as clomipramine and desmethylclomipramine (Bertilsson et al. 1979).

In the patients with endogenous depression a poor relationship between therapeutic effect and plasma levels measured by RBA was demonstrated. One possible reason for this is that the serotonin system is not the only essential one in the treatment of depression. It has been shown that "pure" serotonin reuptake inhibitors, such as citalopram, in fact also have effects on the noradrenergic system (Gjerris 1984), but these effects are not seen until after several weeks of treatment. In the study on clomipramine and citalopram (DUAG 1986) it was shown that the antidepressant action of citalopram was slower than that of clomipramine, which is also a noradrenaline reuptake inhibitor.

References

Asarch KB, Shih JC, Kulscar A (1980) Decreased ^{3}H-imipramine binding in depressed males and females. Commun Psychopharmacol 4:425–432

Bertilsson L, Braithwaite R, Tybring G, Garle M, Borgå O (1979) Techniques for plasma protein binding of desmethylchlorimipramine. Clin Pharmacol Ther 26:265–271

Briley MS, Raisman R, Langer SZ (1979) Human platelets possess high-affinity binding sites for ^{3}H-imipramine. Eur J Pharmacol 58:347–348

Briley MA, Raisman R, Sechter D, Zarifian E, Langer SZ (1980) (^{3}H)-imipramine binding in human platelets: a new biochemical parameter in depression. Neuropharmacology 19:1209–1210

Danish University Antidepressant Group (DUAG) (1986): Citalopram: Clinical effect profile in comparison with clomipramine. A controlled multicenter study. Psychopharmacology (Berlin) 90:131–138

Fredricson Overø K (1982) Kinetics of citalopram in man; plasma levels in patients. Progr Neuropsychopharmacol Biol Psychiatry 6:311–318

Gjerris A, Rafaelsen OJ, Christensen NJ (1984) Antidepressivas indvirkning på centralt adrenalin og noradrenalin. (Effects of antidepressants on central adrenaline and noradrenaline.) Paper Presented at the Annual Meeting of the Scandinavian Society for Biological Psychiatry, Skokloster 24–26 May, 1984

Gram LF (1983) Antidepressants: receptors, pharmacokinetics and clinical effects. In: Burrows GD, Norman TR, Davis B (eds) Antidepressants. Elsevier/North-Holland, Amsterdam, pp 81–96 (Drugs in psychiatry, vol 1)

Gurney C, Roth M, Garside RF, Kerr TA, Schapira K (1972) Studies in the classification of affective disorders. The relationship between anxiety states and depressive illnesses. J Psychiatr Res 121:162–166
Kragh-Sørensen P (1984) Monitoring plasma concentration of nortriptyline. Methodological, pharmacokinetic and clinical aspects. Dan Med Bull 32:29–53
Paul SM, Rehavi M, Skolnick P, Goodwin FK (1980a) Demonstration of specific high affinity binding sites for (^{3}H)-imipramine on human platelets. Life Sci 26:953–959
Paul SM, Rehavi M, Hulihan B, Skolnick P, Goodwin FK (1980b) A rapid and sensitive radio receptor assay for tertiary amine tricyclic antidepressants. Commun Psychopharmacol 4:487–494
Rehavi M, Paul SM, Skolnick P, Goodwin FK (1980) Demonstration of specific high affinity binding sites for (^{3}H)-imipramine in human brain. Life Sci 26:2273–2279
Reisby N, Gram LF, Bech P, Sihm F, Krautwald O, Elley J, Ortmann J, Christiansen J (1979) Climipramine: plasma levels and clinical effects. Commun Psychopharmacol 3:341–351

Neuroleptics

Pharmacological Validation of the Two-Dopamine-Receptor Hypothesis

M. E. GOLDMAN[1] and J. W. KEBABIAN[2]

1 Introduction

Stimulation of dopamine receptors by dopamine receptor agonists has proven effective in the treatment of Parkinson's disease, hyperprolactinemia, amenorrhea/galactorrhea, acromegaly, pituitary adenomas, shock, and hypertension (Calne and Larsen 1983). Conversely, blockade of dopamine receptors by dopamine receptor antagonists is effective in the treatment of psychoses, Huntington's chorea, emesis, and hiccough. The major drawback in the use of these agents is that most dopaminergic agonists or antagonists nonspecifically stimulate or block, respectively, dopamine receptors and, as a result, cause many unwanted side effects. For example, dopamine receptor agonists may cause nausea, emesis, or elevated growth hormone levels. Dopamine receptor antagonists frequently cause hyperprolactinemia and dystonic reactions, such as extrapyramidal symptoms, akathisia and tardive dyskinesia. By designing pharmacological agents that selectively stimulate or inhibit specific dopamine receptors, it should be possible to induce maximum therapeutic benefit with minimum side effects. One approach to the attainment of this goal relies on categorizing dopamine receptors into different groups and then developing selective pharmacological agents which act specifically on the subpopulation of therapeutically relevant receptors.

Dopamine receptors have been categorized on the basis of many criteria, including pharmacological, biochemical, and electrophysiological differences following receptor stimulation or inhibition and anatomical location (presynaptic vs postsynaptic) and receptor binding affinities. This article reviews the biochemical and pharmacological evidence for the existence of two categories of dopamine receptors as proposed by Kebabian and Calne (1979). The pharmacological properties of the first generation of selective agents that occupy each category of receptor are also examined.

2 The Two-Dopamine-Receptor Hypothesis

The two-dopamine-receptor hypothesis was proposed to account for (a) the distinct biochemical consequences of dopamine receptor stimulation in various tis-

[1] Section on Molecular Pharmacology, Clinical Neuroscience Branch, National Institute of Menthal Health, Bethesda, MD 20892, USA. (Present address: Merck Sharp and Dohme Research Laboratories, West Point, PA 19486, USA.)
[2] Biochemical Neuropharmacology Section, Experimental Therapeutics Branch, National Institute of Neurological and Communicative Disorders and Stroke, Bethesda, MD 20892, USA.

Clinical Pharmacology in Psychiatry
Editors: Dahl, Gram, Paul, Potter
(Psychopharmacology Series 3)

sues and (b) the divergent pharmacological responses that certain drugs produce in these tissues. In particular, lergotrile, which had been demonstrated to mimic the ability of dopamine to inhibit prolactin secretion from the anterior pituitary gland both in vivo and in vitro (an effect not related to dopamine-stimulated cAMP synthesis), was found to block the dopamine-stimulated formation of cAMP in striatal homogenates (Kebabian et al. 1977). These findings led Kebabian and Calne (1979) to propose that two categories of dopamine receptors exist, which, when stimulated, either increase cAMP synthesis or do not increase cAMP synthesis and that certain drugs can discriminate between these receptors.

Stimulation of the D-1 dopamine receptor results in an enhancement of adenylate cyclase activity and subsequently an enhanced formation of cAMP. Tests performed with parenchymal cells of the bovine parathyroid gland have yielded a strong body of evidence demonstrating that enhanced formation of cAMP is causally related to enhanced release of parathyroid hormone (for a review, see Brown and Dawson-Hughes 1983). Horizontal cells of the carp retina also possess D-1 dopamine receptors. Recent evidence suggests that enhanced cAMP synthesis in this tissue reduces electrical coupling and responsiveness of these cells (Teranishi et al. 1983; Mangel and Dowling 1985). R(−)Apomorphine was a partial agonist upon this D-1 receptor, whereas R(−)*N*-*n*-propylnorapomorphine was a full agonist with a similar potency to dopamine (Goldman and Kebabian 1984). Fluphenazine, *cis*-flupenthixol, (+)butaclamol, chlorpromazine, S(+)apomorphine and dopaminergic ergots (lisuride, lergotrile and β-ergocriptine) were antagonists upon this receptor (Watling and Dowling 1981; Goldman and Kebabian 1984).

The mammotroph of the anterior pituitary gland was considered in 1979 to be the prototypical location of the D-2 dopamine receptor. Stimulation of this receptor by full D-2 agonists such as apomorphine or dopaminergic ergots resulted in a potent dose-dependent diminution of prolactin release (Caron et al. 1978). Conversely, antagonists of the dopamine receptor blocked the agonist-induced inhibition of prolactin secretion.

The role of the D-2 receptor in the modulation of adenylate cyclase activity was not clear in 1979. The anterior lobe of the pituitary gland contains many cell types, and therefore, studies attempting to correlate changes in dopamine-modulated adenylate cyclase activity and prolactin release directly could not readily be carried out. Since cholera toxin, a specific activator of adenylate cyclase, did not decrease prolactin release, and since dopamine inhibited adenylate cyclase activity from prolactin-secreting human pituitary adenoma cells, it was concluded that stimulation of the D-2 dopamine receptor was not linked to enhanced adenylate cyclase activity.

The intermediate lobe (IL) of the rat pituitary gland is an ideal tissue for investigation of the pharmacology of D-2 dopamine receptors. This tissue is composed of a single cell type, the melanotroph. The cell membranes of most (or all) melanotrophs possess D-2 dopamine receptors (Lightman et al. 1982). The melanotroph synthesizes and stores the melanotropic peptides desacetyl αMSH (melanocyte-stimulating hormone), αMSH, and *N,O*-diacetyl αMSH (Goldman et al. 1983). The calcium-dependent release of these peptides can be measured in vitro by radioimmunoassay as total immunoreactive αMSH (IR-αMSH) in the incubation medium (Munemura et al. 1980a; Tsuruta et al. 1982).

In addition to possessing D-2 dopamine receptors, the melanotroph also contains β-adrenoceptors, which may be exploited methodologically in studies of the D-2 dopamine receptor. This site may be labeled directly with $[^{125}I]$hydroxybenzylpindolol (HYP) (Cote et al. 1980). The order of potency of a series of β-adrenergic agonists for competition with this ligand was *l*-isoprotenenol > *l*-epinephrine > *l*-norepinephrine > *d*-isoproterenol, which demonstrated that $[^{125}I]$HYP labeled a β_2-adrenoceptor.

Stimulation of the IL β_2-adrenoceptor by β_2-adrenergic agonists resulted in enhanced activity of adenylate cyclase (Munemura et al. 1980b). The rank order of potency for stimulation of IL adenylate cyclase activity was the same as for inhibition of specific binding of $[^{125}I]$HYP to homogenates of IL tissue (Cote et al. 1980). The guanine nucleotide GTP was obligatory for maximal enhancement of adenylate cyclase activity (Cote et al. 1982a). β_2-Adrenergic agonists also enhanced the synthesis of cAMP and the release of IR-αMSH from dispersed IL cells in vitro (Munemura et al. 1980a).

Several lines of evidence suggest that there is a causal relationship between enhanced cAMP formation and IR-αMSH release. First, agents (other than β-adrenergic agonists) that enhanced cAMp formation also stimulated IR-αMSH release. For example, corticotropin-releasing factor stimulated the formation of cAMP and IR-αMSH release by binding to a membrane receptor distinct from the β-adrenoceptor (Meunier and Labrie 1983). In addition, cholera toxin enhanced cAMP formation and IR-αMSH release by inhibiting GTPase activity associated with the hypothetical stimulatory guanine nucleotide regulatory protein (N_s) (Cote et al. 1982a; Rodbell 1980). Forskolin is thought to stimulate the catalytic component of adenylate cyclase directly, with resultant enhanced formation of cAMP and enhanced release of IR-αMSH (Miyazaki et al. 1984). Second, inhibitors of cAMP metabolism enhanced the release of IR-αMSH (Munemura et al. 1980a). Third, analogues of cAMP that cross the cell membrane enhanced IR-αMSH release (Tsuruta et al. 1982).

Stimulation of the IL D-2 dopamine receptor attenuated both basal adenylate cyclase activity and adenylate cyclase activity stimulated by agents such as isoproterenol, corticotropin-releasing factor, cholera toxin, or forskolin (Munemura et al. 1980b; Cote et al. 1981; Miyazaki et al. 1984; Meunier and Labrie 1983). GTP was obligatory for the inhibition of adenylate cyclase activity (Cote et al. 1982a). The hypothesis has been proposed that GTP binds to the inhibitory guanine nucleotide regulatory protein (N_i) (Rodbell 1980). The N_i also recognized GppNHp, a nonhydrolyzable analogue of GTP (Cote et al. 1982b). Unlike GTP, in the absence of a dopamine agonist GppNHp can interact with N_i to inhibit adenylate cyclase activity. In the presence of dopamine agonists, however, GTP cannot reverse the GppNHp-induced inhibition of adenylate cyclase activity (Cote et al. 1982b). The GppNHp-induced inhibition of adenylate cyclase activity was not reversed by dopamine receptor antagonists, suggesting that GppNHp acted at a site distinct from the dopamine receptor.

The dopamine receptor in the IL can be labeled with the antagonist $[^3H]$spiroperidol or the agonist $[^3H]$*N*-*n*-propyl norapomorphine (Frey et al. 1982; Sibley and Creese 1980). Since significant differences were found between the number of binding sites with each ligand, it was proposed that the D-2 dopamine receptor can exist in two interconvertible states differing in affinity towards agonists and antagonists (Sibley and Creese 1980). When the same incubation medium was used for the [^{3}H]spiroperidol binding assay and the adenylate cyclase assay, it was possible to compare the effects of a series of dopamine agonists and antagonists directly on both parameters. The results demonstrated that there was a close correlation between the potency of dopaminergic drugs displacing [^{3}H]spiroperidol and the potency of drugs altering adenylate cyclase activity (Frei et al. 1982).

Dopamine agonists inhibited the accumulation of cAMP within dispersed IL cells and the release of cAMP and IR-αMSH from dispersed IL cells. The rank order of potency of the drugs to inhibit basal IR-αMSH was lisuride > bromocriptine(CB-154) > lergotrile > apomorphine = dopamine (Munemura et al. 1980b). The effect of dopamine agonists on the inhibition of adenylate cyclase-mediated events can be reversed competitively by dopamine receptor antagonists, including substituted benzamides, butyrophenones, and many nonselective antagonists such as chlorpromazine, fluphenazine, S(+)apomorphine and *cis*-flupenthixol (Munemura et al. 1980b; Beaulieu et al. 1984; Goldman and Kebabian 1984).

3 Selective Pharmacology of the Two Dopamine Receptors

Since the two-dopamine-receptor hypothesis was proposed in 1979, a series of selective agonists and antagonists for each receptor have been synthesized and evaluated (for related reviews, see Stoof and Kebabian 1984; Kaiser and Jain 1985). These agents are summarized in Table 1. In the sections that follow the pharmacology of these agents will be discussed with particular attention to the concepts of potency, relative selectivity for each dopamine receptor, structure-activity relationships, and stereoisomerism.

Table 1. Selective ligands of each dopamine receptor

	D-1	D-2
Agonists	SKF-38393 (S)-3′,4′-Dihydroxy-nomifensine	Quinpirole LY-149632 RU-24926 RU-24123 RU-28251
Antagonists	SCH-23390 SKF-83509	YM-09151-2 (-) Sulpiride Metoclopramide Spiroperidol Haloperidol Domperidone Piquindone

3.1 D-1 Dopamine Receptor Agonists

3.1.1 SKF-38393

Rigidification of the ethylamine moiety of dopamine is a common method of studying stereochemical orientations of this side chain (Kaiser and Jain 1985). The tetrahydro-3-benzazepines are cyclic dopamine analogues containing an ethylene bridge between the 6-position of the catechol ring and the primary amine. Tetrahydro-3-benzazepine, the parent molecule, was a weak partial dopamine agonist in biochemical and behavioral tests (Kaiser and Jain 1985). Incorporation of a phenyl group into the 1-position of this molecule (SKF-38393; Fig. 1) resulted in a significant enhancement of dopaminergic agonist activity (Setler et al. 1978). SKF-38393 stimulated parathyroid hormone secretion from dispersed parathyroid cells to almost the same extent as dopamine (Brown et al. 1980). SKF-38393 mimicked the ability of dopamine to increase cAMP accumulation in these cells, although the maximal stimulation was only 80% that of dopamine. In the carp retinal dopamine-stimulated adenylate cyclase assay, SKF-38393 was not a full agonist (Watling and Dowling 1981). Similarly, in the rat striatal adenylate cyclase assay SKF-38393 was a partial agonist, causing a maximum stimulation of 68% relative to dopamine (Kaiser et al. 1982). The pharmacological activity of this agent resides almost exclusively in the R-enantioner (Kaiser et al. 1982).

The effects of SKF-38393 on the D-2 dopamine receptor vary with different assay systems. In vivo, this agent did not alter serum prolactin levels (Selter et al. 1978). Similarly, in dispersed IL cells SKF-38393 did not inhibit IR-αMSH release at concentrations up to 10 μM (Goldman and Kebabian, unpublished observations). This agent did, however, weakly inhibit *l*-isoproterenol-stimulated IL cAMP accumulation (Munemura et al. 1980b). Also, SKF-38393 inhibited [^{3}H]spiroperidol binding to rat striatal membranes (although it was over 100-fold more potent at displacing [^{3}H]flupenthixol, a D-1 ligand) (Sibley et al. 1982).

3.1.2 3′,4′-Dihydroxynomifensine

3′,4′-Dihydroxynomifensine (Fig. 2) bears several similarities to SKF-38393. First, both agents are selective D-1 receptor agonists. Second, unlike most other dopamine agonists, the asymmetric center of each molecule is located on the *β* carbon of the dopamine skeleton. The enantiomers of 3′,4′-dihydroxynomifensine have been resolved and characterized pharmacologically (Danridge et al. 1984). The S-enantiomer was 45-fold more potent in the stimulation of striatal adenylate cyclase activity than in the inhibition of striatal [^{3}H]spiroperidol binding ($EC_{50} = 1.9$ μM for cyclase; $IC_{50} = 85$ μM for binding). In the carp retinal ad-

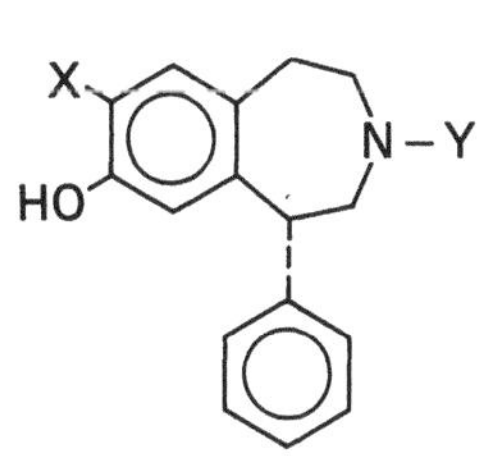

X	Y	
OH	H	SKF 38393
OH	CH_3	SKF 75670
Cl	H	SKF 83509
Cl	CH_3	SCH 23390

Fig. 1. Chemical structures of selected tetrahydro-3-benzazepines

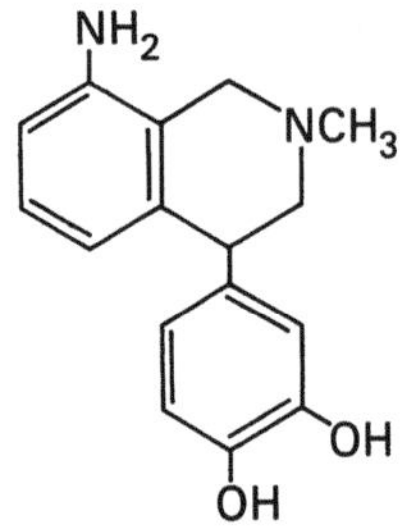

Fig. 2. Chemical structure of 3′,4′-dihydroxynomifensine

enylate cyclase assay this agent was a partial dopamine agonist, causing approximately 50% stimulation relative to dopamine (Watling and Dowling 1981). The R-enantiomer was devoid of activity upon the D-1 receptor at concentrations up to 100 μ*M*.

3.2 D-1 Dopamine Receptor Antagonists

3.2.1 SCH-23390 and Analogues

The tetrahydro-3-benzazepine analogue, SCH-23390 (Fig. 1) was the first selective D-1 dopamine receptor antagonist. SCH-23390 was over 2000-fold more potent in the inhibition of striatal dopamine-stimulated adenylate cyclase activity than in the displacement of [^{3}H]spiroperidol from striatal homogenates (IC_{50} = 10 n*M* and 24 μ*M*, respectively) (Iorio et al. 1983). In the carp retinal adenylate cyclase assay, SCH-23390 blocked the stimulatory effects of dopamine (K_i = 4.1 n*M*) (Itoh et al. 1984). The *N*-desmethyl analogue (SKF-83509; Fig. 1) was significantly less potent in the carp assay (K_i = 70 n*M*) but remained a full antagonist upon the D-1 receptor. The 7-hydroxy analogue of SCH-23390 (SKF-75670; Fig. 1) was a weak partial agonist upon the D-1 receptor. SCH-23390 and SKF-75670 were weak partial D-2 agonists in the IL adenylate cyclase assay. SKF-83509 was devoid of activity in this biochemical model of the D-2 receptor. These data verify that SCH-23390 is a potent and selective D-1 receptor antagonist. Since the 7-hydroxy analogue (SKF-75670) was a partial agonist upon this receptor, it may be concluded that the 7-chloro substituent contributed to the D-1 antagonist activity. Because the *N*-desmethyl analogue of SCH-23390 (SKF-83509) was still a selective D-1 antagonist, although less potent than SCH-23390, it may be concluded that the *N*-methyl substituent was not essential for D-1 antagonist activity but did play a role in increasing the affinity of the ligand for the receptor.

3.3 D-2 Dopamine Receptor Agonists

3.3.1 LY-141865 and Related Compounds

LY-141865 contains the BCD ring (Fig. 3) of the azaergoline nucleus (Bach et al. 1980). This compound mimicked the ability of dopamine to inhibit IR-αMSH release from the IL. The EC_{50} for this response was approximately 30 n*M* (Tsuruta et al. 1981). The half-maximum inhibition of IL adenylate cyclase activity by LY-

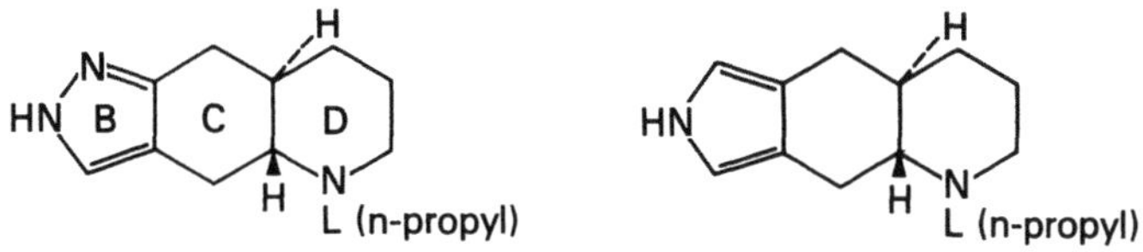

Quinpirole LY-149632

Fig. 3. Chemical structures of quinpirole and LY-149632

141865 was approximately 30 μ*M*. The effects of LY-141865 were reversed by fluphenazine or (−)sulpiride. In carp retinal homogenates, LY-141865 at concentrations up to 100 μ*M* did not stimulate adenylate cyclase activity or inhibit the ability of dopamine (10 μ*M*) to stimulate adenylate cyclase activity. These results demonstrate that LY-141865 is a potent and selective D-2 dopamine receptor agonist.

The dopaminergic activity of LY-141865 resides in the (−)stereoisomer (Quinpirole, LY-171555) whose absolute configuration is known (Fig. 3) (Titus et al. 1983). Quinpirole was an agonist upon the D-2 receptor in the rat IL (Itoh et al. 1985). This compound inhibited the release of IR-αMSH from dispersed IL cells with an EC_{50} of 30 n*M*. This inhibitory effect was abolished by the selective D-2 antagonist, YM-09151-2. Quinpirole was devoid of activity (either as an agonist or antagonist) upon the D-1 receptor in the carp retina. Both nitrogens in the pyrazole ring were not necessary for D-2 agonist activity since LY-149632 (compound 25, R = pro in Bach et al. 1980) was also a selective D-2 agonist (Itoh et al. 1985).

The *n*-propyl group on the quinoline nitrogen of quinpirole or LY-149632 resulted in greater dopaminergic agonist activity than equivalent hydroxyl or methyl substitution (Bach et al. 1980). Similarly, *n*-propyl substitution of a series of octahydrobenzoquinolines yielded greater dopaminergic agonist activity than corresponding molecules with hydrogen or ethyl substitutions (Cannon et al. 1980). This effect of the *n*-propyl group has been dubbed the "*n*-propyl phenomenon" by Nichols (1983).

3.3.2 RU-24926 and RU-24213

The *N*-diphenethylamine derivatives RU-24926 and RU-24213 (Fig. 4) are specific D-2 dopamine receptor agonists (Euvrard et al. 1980). These compounds dis-

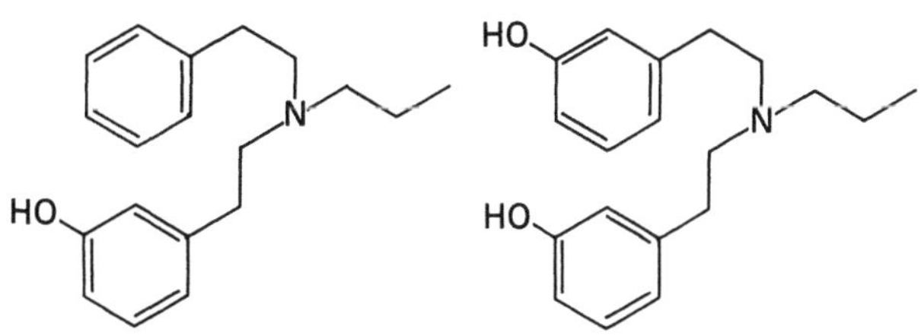

RU-24213 RU-24926

Fig. 4. Chemical structures of RU-24213 and RU-24926

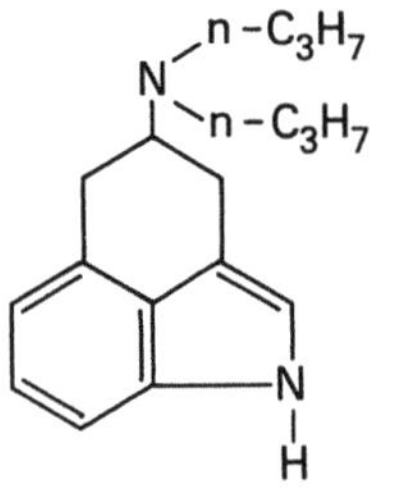

Fig. 5. Chemical structure of RU-28251

placed [^{3}H]dihydroergocriptine from bovine anterior lobe membranes in a dose-dependent manner with K_d values of 100 n*M* and 150 n*M*, respectively. These compounds also inhibited prolactin secretion from anterior lobe cells in vitro, with EC_{50} values of 3 and 5 n*M*, respectively. At concentrations up to 10 μ*M*, however, these drugs did not stimulate the D-1 receptor in the striatum.

RU-24926 and RU-24213 bear several structural similarities to the previously-mentioned D-2 dopamine receptor agonists. These compounds possess hydrated di-secoquinoline skeletons, which are related to the hydrated quinoline structures of quinpirole and LY-149632. In addition, the nitrogen residue of the RU compounds possess *n*-propyl groups as do quinpirole and LY-149632.

3.3.3 RU-28251

RU-28251, a partial ergoline containing a tricyclic ergoline ring (Fig. 5), was both a potent inhibitor of [^{3}H]spiroperidol binding and an inhibitor of prolactin secretion (Bach et al. 1980; Euvrard et al. 1981). In addition, this agent caused contralateral rotation in lesioned rats (Bach et al. 1980). RU-28251, however, did not alter striatal adenylate cyclase activity (Euvrard et al. 1981). As with the other D-2 agonists, replacement of the *n*-propyl with a methyl or hydrogen resulted in decreased agonist activity.

3.4 D-2 Dopamine Receptor Antagonists

3.4.1 Substituted Benzamides

The dopamine receptor blocking properties of substituted benzamides were discovered during structure-activity relationship studies of procainamide derivatives (for a review, see Angrist 1982). In 1957, it was noted that orthochloroprocainamide had an antiemetic action without causing significant autonomic or sedative effects such as are seen following the administration of chlorpromazine or haloperidol. Another substituted benzamide, metoclopramide, was found to be 35 times more potent than chlorpromazine at antagonizing apomorphine-induced emesis. The benzamide sulpiride was subsequently shown to be 150 times more potent than chlorpromazine as an antiemetic. Further evidence for the dopamine receptor as the site of action of the substituted benzamides came from studies on the abilities of these drugs to mimic the effects of chlorpromazine and haloperidol on DOPAC and HVA levels. Metoclopramide and sulpiride were

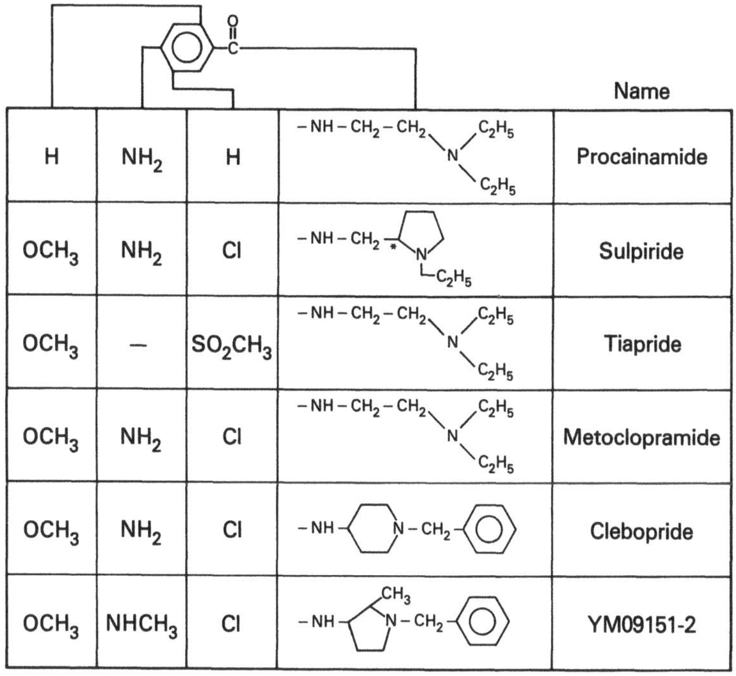

Fig. 6. Chemical structures of selected substituted benzamides

then shown to be clinically effective antipsychotics. It had been demonstrated as early as 1976 that these agents did not block dopamine-sensitive adenylate cyclase activity.

The substituted benzamides listed in Fig. 6 are potent D-2 dopamine receptor antagonists (Grewe et al. 1982). These agents reversed dopamine-induced inhibition of cholera toxin-stimulated adenylate cyclase activity. YM-09151-2 was the most potent benzamide tested and was equipotent with fluphenazine. The other benzamides were less potent than YM-09151-2. The (−)isomer of sulpiride was 18 times more potent than the (+)isomer of sulpiride.

YM-09151-2 did not possess significant activity upon the D-1 dopamine receptor. At concentrations up to 30 μ*M*, this agent did not inhibit dopamine-stimulated adenylate cyclase activity. YM-09151-2 was 100-fold less potent than fluphenazine in the inhibition of the dopamine-stimulated formation of cAMP in dispersed carp retinal cells.

3.4.2 Spiroperidol and Haloperidol

Spiroperidol and haloperidol are members of the butyrophenone class of dopamine receptor antagonists (Fig. 7). These agents were potent inhibitors of dopamine-induced inhibition of isoproterenol- or cholera toxin-stimulated adenylate cyclase activity and cAMP accumulation (Munemura et al. 1980b; Frey et al. 1982; Meunier and Labrie 1983). These agents were also potent inhibitors of [^{3}H]spiroperidol binding to striatal and anterior pituitary membranes and potent

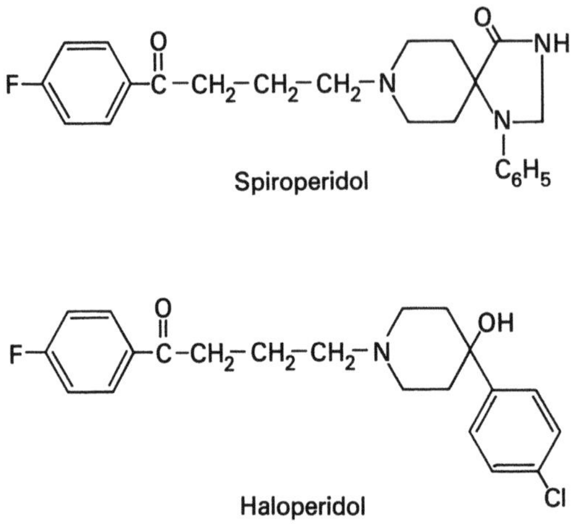

Fig. 7. Chemical structures of spiroperidol and haloperidol

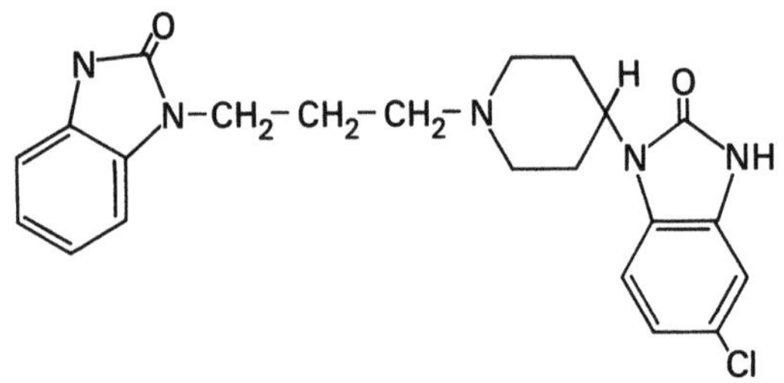

Fig. 8. Chemical structure of domperidone

enhancers of serum prolactin levels (Meltzer et al. 1983; Iorio et al. 1983). Conversely, these butyrophenones were much weaker inhibitors of striatal and retinal dopamine-stimulated adenylate cyclase activities (Kebabian et al. 1972; Watling and Dowling 1981; Iorio et al. 1983). These results, therefore, demonstrate that spiroperidol and haloperidol are selective D-2 antagonists.

3.4.3 Domperidone

The benzimidazolone derivative domperidone (Fig. 8) possessed activities very similar to the butyrophenones. Domperidone reversed the dopamine-induced inhibition of cAMP accumulation in dispersed IL cells with a K_d of 0.01 nM (Meunier and Labrie 1983). The K_d for inhibition of carp retinal dopamine-stimulated adenylate cyclase activity was greater than 1 μM (Watling and Dowling 1981). Like spiroperidol and haloperidol, therefore, domperidone is a selective D-2 antagonist. Unlike spiroperidol and haloperidol, however, domperidone does not cross the blood-brain barrier.

3.4.4 Piquindone

Piquindone (Fig. 9) is a pyrroloisoquinoline derivative of molindone (Olson et al. 1981). Piquindone was a potent inhibitor of avoidance and escape behaviors and [^{3}H]spiroperidol binding (Olson et al. 1981; Davidson et al. 1983; Nakajima and

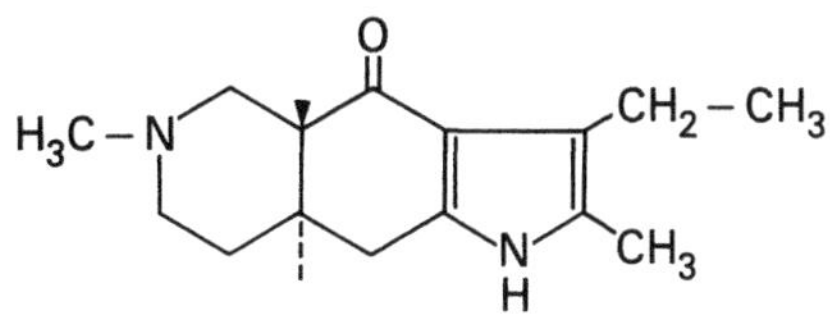

Fig. 9. Chemical structure of piquindone

Iwata 1984). This agent did not inhibit dopamine-sensitive adenylate cyclase activity and is therefore a selective D-2 receptor antagonist. Only the (−)enantiomer was pharmacologically active (Nakajima and Iwata 1984).

4 Conclusions

The two-dopamine-receptor hypothesis was proposed in 1979 to account for the contrasting effects of certain drugs upon dopamine receptors. When the hypothesis was proposed, few drugs were available that selectively stimulated or inhibited these receptors. Since that time, the "first generation" of selective agonists and antagonists acting upon each receptor has been discovered, thus validating the hypothesis. The next goal is to use the two-dopamine-receptor hypothesis as the basis to develop drugs with actions upon specific subpopulations of therapeutically relevant receptors.

References

Angrist BM (1982) The neurobiologically active benzamides and related compounds: some historical aspects. In: Rotrosen J, Stanley M (eds) The Benzamides: pharmacology, neurobiology and clinical aspects. Raven, New York, pp 1–6

Bach NJ, Kornfeld EC, Jones ND, Chaney MO, Dorman DE, Paschal JW, Clemens JA, Smalstig EB (1980) Bicyclic and tricyclic ergoline partial structures. Rigid 3-(2-aminoethyl) pyrroles and 3- and 4-(2-aminoethyl) pyrazoles as dopamine agonists. J Med Chem 23:481–491

Beaulieu M, Goldman ME, Miyazaki K, Frey EA, Eskay RL, Kebabian JW, Cote TE (1984) Bromocriptine-induced changes in the biochemistry, physiology and histology of the intermediate lobe of the rat pituitary gland. Endocrinology 114:1871–1884

Brown EM, Dawson-Hughes B (1983) D-1 dopamine receptor-mediated activation of adenylate cyclase, cAMP accumulation and PTH release in dispersed parathyroid cells. Am Chem Soc Symp Ser 224:1–21

Brown EM, Attie MF, Gardner DG, Kebabian J, Aurbach GD (1980) Characterization of dopaminergic receptors in dispersed bovine parathyroid cells. Mol Pharmacol 18:335–340

Calne DB, Larsen TA (1983) Potential therapeutic uses of dopamine receptor agonists and antagonists. Am Chem Soc Symp Ser 224:147–153

Cannon JG, Lee T, Hsu FL, Long JP, Flynn JR (1980) Congeners of the α-conformer of dopamine derived from octahydrobenz[h]isoquinoline. J Med Chem 23:502–505

Caron MG, Beaulieu M, Raymond V, Gagne B, Dorwin J, Lefkowitz RJ, Labrie F (1978) Dopaminergic receptors in the anterior pituitary gland. J Biol Chem 253:2244–2253

Cote TE, Munemura M, Eskay RL, Kebabian JW (1980) Biochemical identification of the β-adrenoceptor and evidence for the involvement of an adenosine 3′,5′-monophosphate system in the β-adrenergically induced release of α-melanocyte-stimulating hormone in the intermediate lobe of the rat pituitary gland. Endocrinology 107:108–116

Cote TE, Grewe CW, Kebabian JW (1981) Stimulation of a D-2 dopamine receptor in the intermediate lobe of the rat pituitary gland decreases the responsiveness of the β-adrenoceptor: biochemical mechanism. Endocrinology 108:420–426
Cote TE, Grewe CW, Kebabian JW (1982a) Guanyl nucleotides participate in the β-adrenergic stimulation of adenylate cyclase activity in the intermediate lobe of the rat pituitary gland. Endocrinology 110:805–811
Cote TE, Grewe CW, Tsuruta K, Stoof JC, Eskay RL, Kebabian JW (1982b) D-2 dopamine receptor-mediated inhibition of adenylate cyclase activity in the intermediate lobe of the rat pituitary gland requires guanosine 5′-triphosphate. Endocrinology 110:812–819
Dandridge PA, Kaiser C, Brenner M, Gaitanopoulos D, Davis LD, Webb RL, Foley JJ, Sarau HM (1984) Synthesis resolution, absolute stereochemistry and enantioselectivity of 3′,4′-dihydroxynomifensine. J Med Chem 27:28–35
Davidson AB, Boff E, MacNeil A, Wenger J, Cook L (1983) Pharmacological effects of Ro 22-1319: a new antipsychotic agent. Psychopharmacology (Berlin) 79:32–39
Euvrard C, Ferland L, DiPaolo T, Beaulieu M, Labrie F, Oberlander C, Raynaud JP, Boissier JR (1980) Activity of two new potent dopaminergic agonists at the striatal and anterior pituitary levels. Neuropharmacology 19:379–386
Euvrard C, Ferland L, Fortin M, Oberlander C, Labrie F, Boissier JR (1981) Dopaminergic activity of some simplified ergoline derivatives. Drug Dev Res 1:151–161
Frey EA, Cote TE, Grewe CW, Kebabian JW (1982) [^{3}H]Spiroperidol identifies a D-2 dopamine receptor inhibiting adenylate cyclase activity in the intermediate lobe of the rat pituitary gland. Endocrinology 110:1897–1904
Goldman ME, Kebabian JW (1984) Aporphine enantiomers: interactions with D-1 and D-2 dopamine receptors. Mol Pharmacol 25:18–23
Goldman ME, Beaulieu M, Kebabian JW, Eskay RL (1983) α-Melanocyte-stimulating hormone-like peptides in the intermediate lobe of the rat pituitary gland: characterization of content and release in vitro. Endocrinology 112:435–441
Grewe CW, Frey EA, Cote TE, Kebabian JW (1982) YM-09151-2: a potent antagonist for a peripheral D_2-dopamine receptor. Eur J Pharmacol 81:149–152
Iorio LC, Barnett A, Leitz FH, Houser VP, Korduba CA (1983) SCH 23390, a potential benzazepine antipsychotic with unique interactions on dopaminergic systems. J Pharmacol Exp Ther 226:462–468
Itoh Y, Beaulieu M, Kebabian JW (1984) The chemical basis for the blockade of the D-1 dopamine receptor by SCH 23390. Eur J Pharmacol 100:119–122
Itoh Y, Goldman ME, Kebabian JW (1985) TL333, a benzhydro[g]guinoline, stimulates both D-1 and D-2 dopamine receptors: implications for the selectivity of LY 141865 towards the D-2 receptor. Eur J Pharmacol 108:99–101
Kaiser C, Jain T (1985) Dopamine receptors: functions, subtypes and emerging concepts. Med Res Rev 5:145–229
Kaiser C, Dandrige PA, Garvey E, Hahn RA, Sarau HM, Setler PE, Bass LS, Clardy J (1982) Absolute stereochemistry and dopaminergic activity of enantiomers of 2,3,4,5-tetrahydro-7,8-dihydroxy-1-phenyl-1H-3-benzazepine. J Med Chem 25:697–703
Kebabian JW, Calne DB (1979) Multiple receptors for dopamine. Nature 277:93–96
Kebabian JW, Petzold GL, Greengard P (1972) Dopamine-sensitive adenylate cyclase in caudate nucleus of rat brain and its similarity to the "dopamine receptor." Proc Natl Acad Sci USA 69:2145–2149
Kebabian JW, Calne DC, Kebabian PR (1977) Lergotride mesylate: an in vivo dopamine agonist which blocks dopamine receptors in vitro. Commun Psychopharmacol 1:311–318
Lightman SL, Ninkovic M, Hunt SP (1982) Localization of [^{3}H]spiperone binding sites in the intermediate lobe of the rat pituitary gland. Neurosci Lett 32:99–102
Mangel SC, Dowling JE (1985) Responsiveness and receptive field size of carp horizontal cells are reduced by prolonged darkness and dopamine. Science 229:1107–1109
Meltzer HY, Simonovic M, So R (1983) Effects of a series of substituted benzamides on rat prolactin secretion and ^{3}H-spiperone binding to bovine anterior pituitary membranes. Life Sci 32:2877–2886
Meunier H, Labrie F (1983) Multiple hormonal control of pars intermedia cell activity. Can J Biochem Cell Biol 61:516–531

Miyazaki K, Goldman ME, Kebabian JW (1984) Forskolin stimulated adenylate cyclase activity, adenosine 3′,5′-monophosphate production and peptide release from the intermediate lobe of the rat pituitary gland. Endocrinology 114:761–766
Munemura M, Eskay RL, Kebabian JW (1980a) Release of α-melanocyte-stimulating hormone from dispersed cells of the intermediate lobe of the rat pituitary gland: involvement of catecholamines and adenosine 3′,5′-monophosphate. Endocrinology 106:1795–1803
Munemura M, Cote TE, Tsuruta K, Eskay RL, Kebabian JW (1980b) The dopamine receptor in the intermediate lobe of the rat pituitary gland: pharmacological characterization. Endocrinology 107:1676–1683
Nakajima T, Iwata K (1984) [^{3}H] Ro-22-1319 (Piquindone) binds to the D_2 dopaminergic receptor subtype in a sodium-dependent manner. Mol Pharmacol 26:430–438
Nichols DE (1983) The development of novel dopamine agonists. In Dopamine Receptors. Am Chem Soc Symp Ser 224:201–218
Olson GL, Cheung HC, Morgan CD, Blount JF, Tadaro L, Berger L, Davidson AB, Boff D (1981) Dopamine receptor model and its application in the design of a new class of rigid pyrrolo[2,3-g]isoquinoline antipsychotics. J Med Chem 24:1026–1034
Rodbell M (1980) The role of hormone receptors and GTP-regulatory proteins in membrane transduction. Nature 284:17–22
Setler PE, Sarau HM, Zirkle CL, Saunders HL (1978) The central effects of a novel dopamine agonist. Eur J Pharmacol 50:419–430
Sibley DR, Creese I (1980) Dopamine receptor binding in bovine intermediate pituitary membranes. Endocrinology 107:1405–1409
Sibley DR, Leff SE, Creese I (1982) Interactions of novel dopaminergic ligands with D-1 and D-2 dopamine receptors. Life Sci 637–645
Stoof JC, Kebabian JW (1984) Two dopamine receptors: biochemistry, physiology and pharmacology. Life Sci 35:2281–2296
Teranishi T, Negishi K, Kato S (1983) Dopamine modulates S-potential amplitude and dye coupling between external horizontal cells in carp retina. Nature 301:243–246
Titus RD, Kornfeld EC, Jones ND, Clemens JA, Smalstig EB, Fuller RW, Hahn RA, Hynes MD, Mason NR, Wong DT, Foreman MM (1983) The resolution and absolute configuration of an ergoline-related dopamine agonist, *trans* 4,4a,5,6,7,8,8a,9-octahydro-5-propyl-1H (or 2H)-pyrazolo[3,4]quinoline. J Med Chem 26:1112–1116
Tsuruta K, Frey EA, Grewe CW, Cote TE, Eskay RL, Kebabian JW (1981) Evidence that LY-141865 specifically stimulates the D-2 dopamine receptor. Nature 292:463–465
Tsuruta K, Grewe CW, Cote TE, Eskay RL, Kebabian JW (1982) Coordinated action of calcium and adenosine 3′,5′-monophosphate upon the release of α-melanocyte stimulating hormone from the intermediate lobe of the rat pituitary gland. Endocrinology 110:1133–1140
Watling KJ, Dowling JE (1981) Dopaminergic mechanisms in the teleost retina. J Neurochem 36:559–568

Differential Regulation of Dopamine-D_2 and Serotonin-S_2 Receptors by Chronic Treatment with the Serotonin-S_2 Antagonists, Ritanserin, and Setoperone

J. E. LEYSEN, P. VAN GOMPEL, W. GOMMEREN, and P. M. LADURON

1 Introduction

Serotonin-S_2 receptor sites were first described in studies in which ^{3}H-spiperone was used in frontal cortical membrane preparations (Leysen et al. 1978; Peroutka and Snyder 1979). The receptor binding sites were further characterized and could be better distinguished by using the more selective serotonin antagonist ^{3}H-ketanserin (Leysen et al. 1982). Serotonin-S_2 receptors were shown to have a role in serotonin agonist-induced behavioral excitation and discriminative stimulus effects in rodents, and also to mediate serotonin-induced vasoconstriction and platelet function. Recently it has been shown that inositol phospholipid turnover forms part of the signal transducing system coupled to serotonin-S_2 receptor sites (for review see Leysen et al. 1984).

The observation that chronic treatment of rats with the antidepressant amitriptyline caused down-regulation of the frontal cortical serotonin-S_2 receptor sites led to the hypothesis that the receptors may be involved in the pathology of depressive illness (Peroutka and Snyder 1980; Snyder and Peroutka 1982). According to the then current theory that receptor down-regulation occurs following persistent receptor stimulation, the observation was interpreted as being a consequence of the inhibition by amitriptyline of serotonin uptake. However, the theory has been challenged by a number of recent findings. Chronic treatment of rats with serotonin antagonists such as mianserin, cyproheptadine, and ketanserin was reported to cause apparently a serotonin-S_2 down-regulation (Blackshear et al. 1983; Blackshear and Sanders-Bush 1982; Gandolfi et al. 1984, 1985). In contrast, serotonin-S_2 receptor numbers were not decreased following chronic treatment with selective serotonin uptake inhibitors such as citalopram, zimelidine, and alaproclate (Hall et al. 1984; Hyttel et al. 1984).

In this study, we investigated serotonin-S_2 receptor alteration following treatment of rats with the new serotonin-antagonists ritanserin and setoperone. In-vivo, ritanserin is a particularly selective and long-acting serotonin-S_2 antagonist (Leysen et al. 1985a; Niemegeers et al. 1984; Colpaert et al. 1985). Clinical studies have revealed therapeutic activity of ritanserin in dysthymic disorders (Reyntjens et al. 1984). Setoperone is primarily a serotonin-S_2 antagonist, but has dopamine-antagonistic properties in addition (Niemegeers et al. 1984). Accordingly, neuro-

Department of Biochemical Pharmacology, Janssen Pharmaceutica Research Laboratories, B-2340 Beerse, Belgium.

Clinical Pharmacology in Psychiatry
Editors: Dahl, Gram, Paul, Potter
(Psychopharmacology Series 3)

leptic-like activity has been observed (Ceulemans et al. 1985). Because of the dual action of setoperone, chronic treatment with this drug allowed the investigation of both serotonin-S_2 and dopamine-D_2 receptor alterations.

2 Materials and Methods

2.1 Drug Treatment

Male Wistar rats with body weight 150 g at the beginning of drug treatment were used. For acute treatment an oral bolus dose (1 ml per 100 g body weight) of ritanserin (suspended in 20% polypropylene glycol) or setoperone (dissolved in lightly acidified water) was given. For chronic treatment drugs were mixed with powdered food (10 or 100 mg drug/kg food for treatment with 1 mg kg^{-1} day^{-1} or 10 mg kg^{-1} day^{-1}, respectively). Body weight and food consumption were measured weekly. Chronic drug treatment (25 or 28 days) was followed by a drug-free period of 1–18 day's duration, after which animals were sacrificed. Control rats were given solvent or powdered food without drug and were kept under exactly the same conditions as the drug-treated animals.

2.2 Receptor Binding and Neurotransmitter Uptake Assays

Following the treatment period, rats were killed by decapitation, brains were immediately removed from the skull, and various brain areas were dissected. Tissues were either processed immediately or frozen in liquid nitrogen and kept in a biofreezer at -80 °C until assayed. Small brain areas (frontal cortex for serotonin-S_2 receptor binding, striatum for dopamine-D_2 receptor binding) were pooled (3 rats) to provide sufficient tissue for assaying saturation binding curves.

Tissue homogenization, membrane fraction preparation, assay conditions for receptor binding and neurotransmitter uptake in in vitro and ex vivo binding experiments were as described by Leysen et al. (1986). Drug receptor dissociation was measured as described by Leysen et al. (1986).

In vivo receptor binding was performed with ^3H-spiperone and the prevention of labeling technique described by Laduron et al. (1982) was used.

3 Results

The in vitro receptor binding and neurotransmitter uptake inhibition properties of ritanserin and setoperone are presented in Table 1. Both drugs show as their most prominent activity high affinity binding to serotonin-S_2 receptor sites. In vitro, they bind weakly to moderately to histamine-H_1, dopamine-D_2, and adrenergic-α_1, and adrenergic-α_2 receptor sites and show only very weak interactions with serotonin-S_1 binding sites and effects on noradrenaline and serotonin uptake. The drugs differ markedly in their in vitro dissociation rate from serotonin-S_2 receptors; this is extremely slow for ritanserin and rapid for setoperone. Accordingly, ritanserin exerted a mixed, partially noncompetitive inhibition of ^3H-

Table 1. In vitro profile of ritanserin and setoperone for binding to receptor sites and for inhibition of neurotransmitter uptake in brain tissue preparations

Receptor	^{3}H-Ligand	Conc.	Ritanserin		Setoperone	
			IC_{50} n*M*	Dissociation $t_{1/2}$ (min)	IC_{50} n*M*	Dissociation $t_{1/2}$ (min)
Serotonin-S_2	Ketanserin	1 n*M*	1.0 ± 0.5 (5)	160 ± 20 (10)	1.3 ± 0.3 (3)	6.8 ± 0.7 (6)
Histamine-H_1	Pyrilamine	1 n*M*	35 ± 10 (4)	77 ± 4 (7)	100 ± 40 (5)	5.1 ± 0.3 (5)
Dopamine-D_2	Haloperidol	2 n*M*	70 ± 60 (4)	11 ± 1 (3)	70 ± 30 (3)	4.8 ± 0.4 (6)
Adrenergic-α_1	WB-4101	0.5 n*M*	100 ± 25 (4)	18 ± 1 (10)	38 ± 17 (4)	4.3 ± 0.6 (3)
Adrenergic-α_2	Clonidine	3 n*M*	150 ± 40 (3)	26 ± 3 (7)	60 ± 40 (5)	–
Serotonin-S_1	Serotonin	3 n*M*	6500 ± 2000 (2)	–	2600 ± 800 (2)	–
Uptake						
Noradrenaline	Noradrenaline	3 n*M*	500 ± 300 (2)		5100 ± 1600 (2)	
Serotonin	Serotonin	3 n*M*	650 ± 200 (2)		2400 ± 200 (2)	

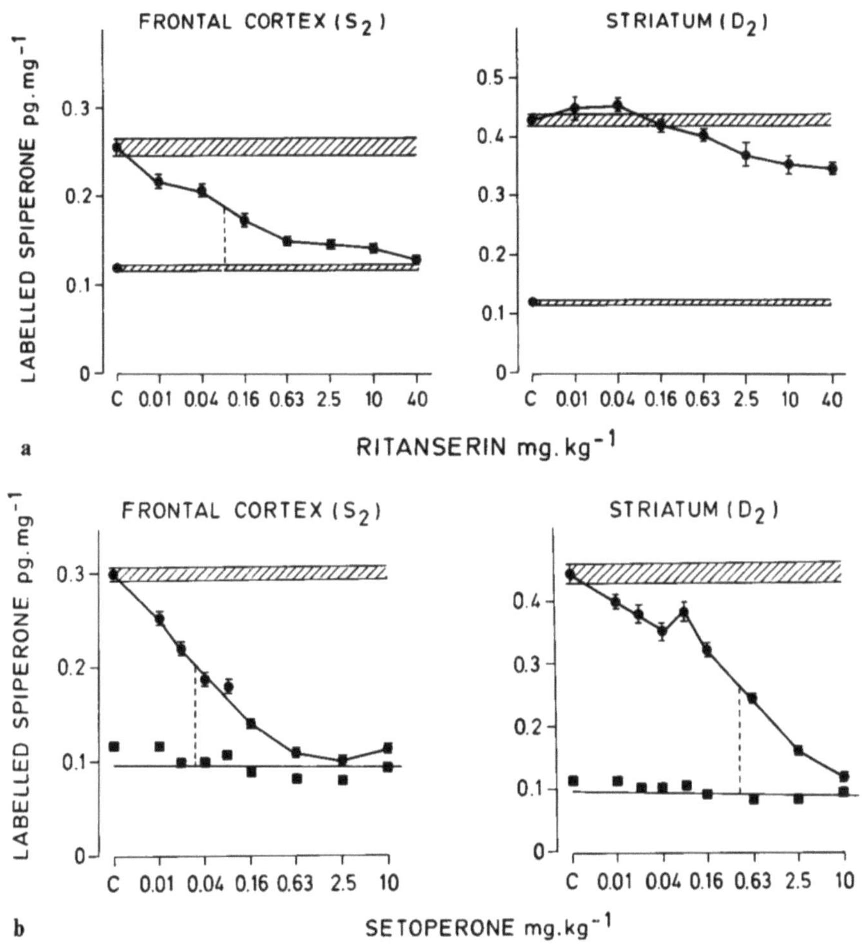

Fig. 1 a, b. In vivo inhibition by ritanserin (**a**) and setoperone (**b**) of labeling of serotonin-S_2 receptors in the frontal cortex and dopamine-D_2 receptors in the striatum of rats. Rat brain receptors were labeled in vivo with ^{3}H-spiperone (0.5 µg/kg i.v.) administered 60 min after a dose of ritanserin or setoperone; the radioactivity in the dissected brain regions was measured 60 min after ^{3}H-spiperone injection ($n=6$, mean values ± SEM)

ketanserin binding to serotonin-S_2 sites in vitro, whereas the inhibition by setoperone was fully competitive (Leysen et al. 1985, 1986).

In spite of the similarities in the in vitro receptor binding profiles of ritanserin and setoperone, the drugs behaved differently on in vivo binding. At low doses (ED_{50} 0.08 mg/kg s.c.) ritanserin prevented the in vivo labeling by ^{3}H-spiperone of frontal cortical serotonin-S_2 receptors, but up to 40 mg/kg the drug did not inhibit dopamine-D_2 receptor labeling in the striatum (Fig. 1 a). Setoperone also potently inhibited in vivo serotonin-S_2 receptor labeling (ED_{50} 0.03 mg/kg), but at a 10 times higher dose it inhibited the labeling of striatal dopamine-D_2 receptors (Fig. 1 b).

Table 2. Effect of treatment of rats with ritanserin, single dose of 5 mg/kg p.o. or 10 mg p.o. daily for 25 days on serotonin-S_2 receptor sites labeled with ^{3}H-ketanserin in the frontal cortex and dopamine-D_2 receptor sites labeled with ^{3}H-spiperone in the striatum

	Acute treatment		Mean values ± SD (*n*)	Chronic treatment		%
	K_D n*M*	B_{max} fmol/mg tissue		K_D n*M*	B_{max} fmol/mg tissue	
^{3}*H-Ketanserin binding*[a]						
Control	0.36 ± 0.08	22.7 ± 2.6 (19)	Control	0.37 ± 0.04	19.7 ± 1.9 (3)	100
Time after drug administration			Drug-free period			
2 h	Complete inhibition		1 day	0.51 ± 0.07[b]	9.8 ± 0.6[d] (3)	50
4 h	1.0 ± 0.3[d]	6.6 ± 1.5[d] (4)	3 days	0.43 ± 0.05	13.0 ± 0.7[d] (3)	66
6 h	0.76 ± 0.18[d]	8.1 ± 1.3[d] (4)	6 days	0.37 ± 0.01	16.1 ± 0.4[d] (3)	82
8 h	0.52 ± 0.11[b]	7.6 ± 1.3[d] (3)	12 days	0.44 ± 0.07	17.8 ± 1.3 (3)	91
12 h	0.30 ± 0.06	15.1 ± 1.3[c] (4)	18 days	0.42 ± 0.04	18.7 ± 0.9 (3)	95
18 h	0.37 ± 0.03	18.4 ± 2.0 (3)				
24 h	0.43 ± 0.18	21.2 ± 3.1 (8)				
48 h	0.41 ± 0.05	24.2 ± 2.4 (4)				
^{3}*H-Spiperone binding*[a]						
Control	0.046 ± 0.010	28.2 ± 3.1 (33)	Control	0.046 ± 0.010	28.2 ± 3.1 (33)	100
Time after drug administration			Drug-free period			
2 h	0.053 ± 0.006	27.6 ± 1.3 (4)	3 days	0.045 ± 0.009	29.4 ± 3.4 (7)	100

[a] ^{3}H-Ketanserin binding to serotonin-S_2 sites in washed frontal cortical membranes and ^{3}H-spiperone binding to dopamine-D_2 sites in washed striatal membranes and analysis of the binding in Scatchard plots was as described in Leysen et al. (1985b).
Significance of difference from controls according to Student's *t*-test: [b] $P<0.05$; [c] $P<0.01$; [d] $P<0.001$.

Table 3. Effect of setoperone treatment of rats with single dose of 5 mg/kg p. o. or 1 mg/kg and 10 mg/kg daily p. o. for 28 days on serotonin-S_2 receptor sites labeled with ^{3}H-ketanserin in the frontal cortex and dopamine-D_2 receptor sites labeled with ^{3}H-spiperone in the striatum

	Acute treatment		Mean values ± SD (*n*)	Chronic treatment		%
	K_D n*M*	B_{max} fmol/mg tissue		K_D n*M*	B_{max} fmol/mg tissue	
^{3}*H-Ketanserin binding*[a]						
Control	0.60 ± 0.06	24.6 ± 2.2 (4)	Control	0.5 ± 0.2	20.5 ± 1.9 (7)	100
Setoperone 5 mg/kg			*Setoperone 1 mg/kg*			
Time after drug administration			Drug-free period			
2 h	0.82 ± 0.03[d]	18.0 ± 0.7[c] (4)	5 days	0.4 ± 0.1	18.5 ± 1.6 (4)	90
			Setoperone 10 mg/kg			
			Drug-free period			
			5 days	0.6 ± 0.1	16.1 ± 3.0[b] (7)	78
^{3}*H-Spiperone binding*[a]						
Control	0.046 ± 0.010	28.2 ± 3.1 (33)	Control	0.043 ± 0.009	24.2 ± 2.6 (24)	100
Setoperone 5 mg/kg			*Setoperone 10 mg/kg*			
Time after drug administration			Drug-free period			
2 h	0.050 ± 0.007	28.5 ± 0.9 (4)	1 day	0.047 ± 0.004	37.3 ± 2.5[d] (4)	154
			3 days	0.040 ± 0.003	36.9 ± 1.4[d] (4)	153
			5 days	0.046 ± 0.007	34.3 ± 3.0[d] (4)	142
			7 days	0.041 ± 0.004	37.9 ± 2.7[d] (4)	157
			9 days	0.042 ± 0.007	37.2 ± 1.3[d] (4)	154
			12 days	0.035 ± 0.006	30.4 ± 2.8[c] (4)	126

[a] See legend to Table 2.
Significance of difference from controls according to Student's *t*-test: [b]$P < 0.05$; [c]$P < 0.01$; [d]$P < 0.001$.

Serotonin-S_2 and dopamine-D_2 receptor inhibition were investigated in washed frontal cortex and striatal membranes, respectively, following acute oral administration of ritanserin and setoperone at doses of 5 mg/kg. Results are shown in Tables 2 and 3. In rats treated with ritanserin, ^{3}H-ketanserin binding to serotonin-S_2 receptors was inhibited in a mixed noncompetitive fashion, i.e., the K_D value was increased and the B_{max} value was markedly reduced. Receptors remained significantly inhibited for 12 h; ^{3}H-ketanserin binding was normalized 24 h after ritanserin administration (Table 2). Ex vivo ^{3}H-spiperone binding to striatal dopamine-D_2 receptor sites was not affected by ritanserin treatment. Two hours after acute setoperone administration ^{3}H-ketanserin binding in washed frontal cortical membranes was also partially noncompetitively inhibited, but the inhibition was less marked and reversible to a greater extent than following ritanserin treatment. Under these conditions no inhibition of ^{3}H-spiperone binding to dopamine-D_2 sites in washed striatal membranes was observed (Table 3).

Chronic treatment of rats with ritanserin (10 mg kg^{-1} day^{-1} mixed with food) for 25 days produced a marked reduction in the number of serotonin-S_2 receptor sites labelled with ^{3}H-ketanserin in washed frontal cortical membranes (see Table 2). After a 1-day drug-free period the K_D-value of ^{3}H-ketanserin was slightly increased and the B_{max} was reduced by 50%. After drug-free periods of 3 and 6 days a significant reduction in B_{max} was found, but no change in K_D. After 12- and 18-day drug-free periods ^{3}H-ketanserin binding had returned to control values. Chronic ritanserin treatment did not affect ^{3}H-spiperone binding to striatal dopamine-D_2 receptors (Table 2), nor did it affect α_1-, α_2- and β-adrenergic receptors, benzodiazepine receptors, or substance-P receptors measured in brain tissue. Chronic treatment with setoperone 1 mg kg^{-1} day^{-1} for 28 days did not markedly affect ^{3}H-ketanserin binding to serotonin-S_2 receptor sites, but the numbers of striatal dopamine-D_2 receptor sites labeled with ^{3}H-spiperone were significantly increased to 115% of controls. Chronic treatment with setoperone 10 mg kg^{-1} day^{-1} for 28 days produced a significant reduction in the number of frontal cortical serotonin-S_2 receptor sites and a marked increase in striatal dopamine-D_2 receptor sites (Table 3). ^{3}H-Ligand K_D-values were unchanged. The increase up to about 150% in the number of striatal dopamine-D_2 receptor sites was maintained between 1 day and 9 days after the discontinuation of drug treatment, while after a 12-day drug-free interval the increase in B_{max} was diminished.

Drug levels in whole brain extracts were measured by HPLC (Leysen et al. 1985b). Following oral treatment with 5 mg/kg 2 h prior to sacrifice ritanserin levels were 3.4–26.2 ng/g and setoperone levels 114–316 ng/g (lowest and highest value from determinations in 9 animals). Following chronic drug tratment and a drug-free period of 1 day, whole brain levels of both drugs were below detection level, i.e., <1 ng/g.

4 Discussion

Ritanserin and setoperone both bind with high affinity to frontal cortical serotonin-S_2 receptors under in vitro and in vivo conditions. Although both drugs show moderate in vitro binding to dopamine-D_2 receptors, these receptors are not occupied by ritanserin in vivo even after prolonged administration of a high dose of the drug. In vivo, setoperone occupies both serotonin-S_2 and dopamine-D_2 receptors in relation to the in vitro binding affinities of the drug. Since after acute administration of a high dose ritanserin levels were about 20 times lower than setoperone levels, it is assumed that the free ritanserin concentration in the vicinity of striatal dopamine-D_2 receptors is never sufficiently high to yield receptor occupation.

Chronic treatment studies with ritanserin were of interest because of its pronounced in vivo selectivity for serotonin-S_2 receptors and its long-acting receptor occupation. Chronic treatment with setoperone allowed investigation of differential alterations of serotonin-S_2 and dopamine-D_2 receptors with the same drug, and since the drug dissociates rapidly from the receptors as shown in vitro, it avoided misinterpretation of data resulting from persistent binding of the drug to the receptors.

Acute drug treatment followed by receptor binding assays in washed membrane preparations yielded unexpected findings regarding drug interactions with the serotonin-S_2 receptors, which were different from those recorded with dopamine-D_2 receptors. Not surprisingly, following acute oral treatment with ritanserin, ^{3}H-ketanserin binding to serotonin-S_2 receptors was very markedly inhibited in a partially noncompetitive way (K_D increased, B_{max} decreased) for several hours.

Hence, in accordance with the slow dissociation of ritanserin, the drug seemed not to be washed away from the membranes during the tissue preparation. Dissociation in vivo, however, was complete within 24 h. Surprisingly, a partially noncompetitive inhibition of ^{3}H-ketanserin binding was also observed following acute setoperone administration. This could not have been predicted from the in vitro serotonin-S_2 receptor binding studies of setoperone, which showed rapid dissociation and fully competitive inhibition (Leysen et al. 1985 b). In contrast to the apparent persistence of setoperone on serotonin-S_2 receptors following acute drug administration, the drug was found to be completely removed from the striatal dopamine-D_2 receptors by tissue washing.

It seems that when drugs hit serotonin-S_2 receptors under in vivo conditions they are "captured" by the receptors in such a way that they become difficult to wash out, a phenomenon which is not observed for the dopamine-D_2 receptor.

Following chronic administration of a high dose of ritanserin and setoperone (10 mg kg^{-1} day^{1-}) serotonin-S_2 receptors became apparently down-regulated. ^{3}H-Ketanserin binding in washed frontal cortical membranes was fully noncompetitively inhibited, i.e., the B_{max} value was reduced and the K_D value was unchanged. Following chronic treatment with ritanserin, the reduction in B_{max} value was observed for several days after stopping the drug, control values not being reached again for a further 12–18 days. This is in contrast to the observation, following acute treatment with ritanserin, that ^{3}H-ketanserin binding was normalized 24 h after drug administration. The fully noncompetitive type of inhibition, the similar observations with ritanserin and setoperone, the slow reappearance of receptor numbers, and the fact that 1 day after stopping drug treatment drug levels in the brain were too low for detection (<1 ng/g) suggest that the observed reduction in B_{max} really represents a receptor down-regulation and is probably not due to persistence of the drug at the receptor site.

A different pattern of regulation of dopamine-D_2 receptors was clearly apparent in the setoperone-treated animals. Dopamine-D_2 receptors became up-regulated in proportion to the dose and dopamine-D_2 receptor binding affinity of the drug. The up-regulation was already fully apparent 1 day after discontinuation of the drug (no persistence of drug in striatal tissue) and was maintained at the same level for at least 9 days; the up-regulation did not start to diminish until after 12 days. This is in contrast to the down-regulation of serotonin-S_2 receptors for which high drug dosages were required and which was gradually reversed over a period of between 1 and 12 days after discontinuation of the drug.

The dopamine-D_2 receptor regulation is in agreement with current theories that persistent receptor blockade results in an increase in receptor numbers probably because of inhibition of receptor internalization when occupied by an antagonist. Serotonin-S_2 receptor regulation does not obey this rule, and the mechanisms involved seem to be quite complex. The serotonin-S_2 receptor down-regulation appears to be a specific effect of serotonin antagonists; drugs which have been reported to be effective all bind with moderate to high affinity to serotonin-S_2 receptors. This is illustrated in Fig. 2, where reported serotonin-S_2 receptor down-regulation of drugs (effective, +; ineffective, −: conflicting reports, ±) is related to serotonin-S_2 receptor binding affinity and inhibition of serotonin up-

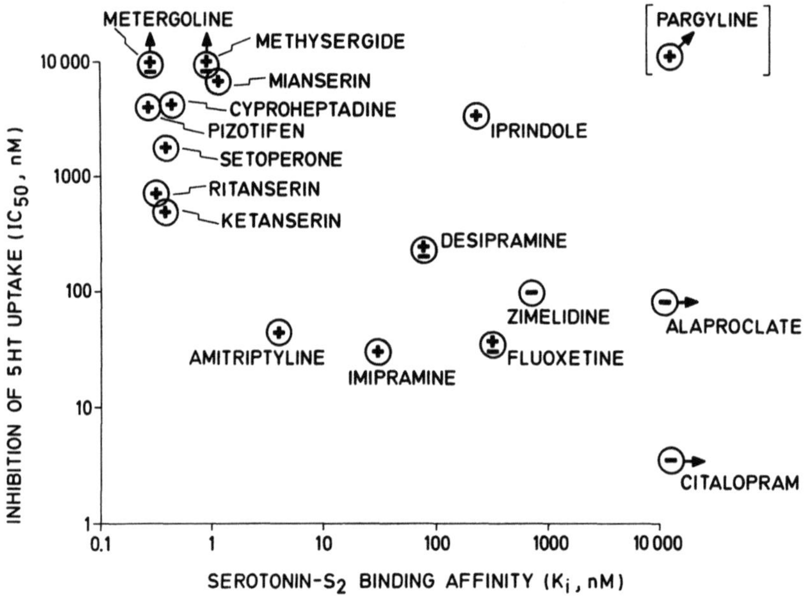

Fig. 2. Plot of drugs reported to be effective ⊕ or ineffective ⊖ (conflicting reports ±) in down-regulating serotonin-S_2 receptor sites following chronic treatment. The positions of the *points* shows the in vitro drug-binding affinity for serotonin-S_2 receptor sites on the *abscissa* and the potency of the drugs to inhibit serotonin uptake on the *ordinate*. (Data on drug receptor down-regulation are from Blackshear et al. [1983], Gandolfi et al. [1984, 1985], Hall et al. [1984], Hyttel et al. [1984], Snyder and Peroutka [1982], Crews et al. [1983], Stolz et al. [1983], and this study)

take. Selective serotonin uptake inhibitors are ineffective. The only exception to an association with affinity for serotonin-S_2 receptors is the monoamine oxidase inhibitor pargyline, which reportedly causes serotonin-S_2 receptor down-regulation and does not bind to serotonin-S_2 receptors or inhibit serotonin uptake.

Since many of the effective drugs have histamine-antagonistic properties, we performed preliminary studies with a potent and selective centrally active histamine antagonist (levocabastine) and found no serotonin-S_2 down-regulation following chronic treatment with a dose of 10 mg kg^{-1} day^{-1}. Although detailed studies have not yet been performed, the dosage required for serotonin-S_2 receptor down-regulation seemed to be high and therefore not in direct proportion to the serotonin-S_2 receptor binding affinity of the drugs. Nevertheless, the effect is specifically restricted to serotonin-S_2 receptors, since in this study other receptors such as α_1-, α_2-, and β-adrenergic, dopamine-D_2, benzodiazepine and substance-P receptors were not affected by ritanserin treatment. Gandolfi et al. (1985) who observed serotonin-S_2 receptor down regulation with ketanserin and mianserin, hypothesized that the drugs mimic an unknown, probably peptidergic endogenous agonist acting on the serotonin-S_2 receptors, and that after all down-regulation would be a consequence of agonistic action. Since there is no evidence for the existence of such an endogenous substance, we favor another hypothesis. In view of both the acute and the chronic drug effects, it seems that serotonin antagonists affect membranous processes in an uncommon way. They may not prevent, and may probably even promote, receptor internalization and consequently enhance receptor degradation. Such a mechanism would agree with the observed slow time-course of receptor reappearance. Other explanations would be that the serotonin antagonists cause alterations in the conformation, aggregation or chemical (e.g., phosphorylation) state of the receptor in such a way that the receptor loses its drug-binding properties. Such mechanisms would, however, be expected to be more readily reversible.

Regardless of the mechanism, the question remains as to the significance of receptor regulation for long-term drug treatment. The dopamine-D_2 receptor up-regulation has tentatively been related to phenomena of receptor supersensitivity and side effects such as tardive dyskinesia. Down-regulation of serotonin-S_2 receptors was originally proposed to be involved in the therapeutic effect of antidepressants (Snyder and Peroutka 1982). A role of serotonin-S_2 receptors in mood disorders seems to be supported by the present studies, since the selective serotonin-S_2 antagonist ritanserin is reported to be effective in the treatment of dysthymic disorders (Reyntjens et al. 1984). The acute and chronic effects of the serotonin antagonist would be complementary, and the drug may treat pathology caused by receptor supersensitivity.

References

Blackshear MA, Sanders-Bush E (1982) Serotonin receptor sensitivity after acute and chronic treatment with mianserin. J Pharmacol Exp Ther 221:303–308

Blackshear MA, Friedman RL, Sanders-Bush E (1983) Acute and chronic effects of serotonin (5-HT) antagonists on serotonin binding sites. Naunyn-Schmiedebergs Arch Pharmacol 324:125–129

Ceulemans DLS, Gelders YG, Hoppenbrouwers MLJA, Reyntjens ASM, Janssen PAJ (1985) Effect of serotonin antagonism in schizophrenia: a pilot study with setoperone. Psychopharmacology (Berlin) 85:329–339
Colpaert FC, Meert TF, Niemegeers CJE, Janssen PAJ (1985) Behavioral and 5-HT antagonist effects of ritanserin: a pure and selective antagonist of LSD discrimination in rat. Psychopharmacology (Berlin) 86:45–54
Crews FT, Scott JA, Shorstein NH (1983) Rapid down-regulation of serotonin-S_2 receptor binding during combined administration of tricyclic antidepressant drugs and α_2 antagonists. Neuropharmacology 22:1203–1209
Gandolfi O, Barbaccia ML, Costa E (1984) Comparison of iprindole, imipramine and mianserin action on brain serotonergic and beta adrenergic receptors. J Pharmacol Exp Ther 229:782–876
Gandolfi O, Barbaccia ML, Costa E (1985) Different effects of serotonin antagonists on ^{3}H-mianserin and ^{3}H-ketanserin recognition sites. Life Sci 36:713–721
Hall H, Ross SB, Sällemark M (1984) Effect of destruction of central noradrenergic and serotonergic nerve terminals by systemic neurotoxins on the long-term effects of antidepressants on β-adrenoceptors and 5-HT_2 binding sites in the rat cerebral cortex. J Neural Transm 59:9–23
Hyttel J, Fredericson Overø K, Arnt J (1984) Biochemical effects and drug levels in rats after long-term treatment with the specific 5-HT-uptake inhibitor, citalopram. Psychopharmacology (Berlin) 83:20–27
Laduron PM, Janssen PFM, Leysen JE (1982) In vivo binding of [^{3}H]ketanserin on serotonin-S_2 receptors in rat brain. Eur J Pharmacol 81:43–48
Leysen JE, Niemegeers CJE, Tollenaere JP, Laduron PM (1978) Serotonergic component of neuroleptic receptors. Nature 272:168–171
Leysen JE, Niemegeers CJE, Van Nueten JM, Laduron PM (1982) [^{3}H]Ketanserin (R 41 468), a selective ^{3}H-ligand for serotonin$_2$ receptor binding sites. Mol Pharmacol 21:301–314
Leysen JE, de Chaffoy de Courcelles D, De Clerck F, Niemegeers CJE, Van Nueten JM (1984) Serotonin-S_2 receptor binding sites and functional correlates. Neuropharmacology 23:1493–1501
Leysen JE, Gommeren W, Van Gompel P, Wynants J, Jansen PFM, Laduron PM (1985 a) Receptor-binding properties in vitro and in vivo of ritanserin. A very potent and long-acting serotonin-S_2 antagonist. Mol Pharmacol 27:600–611
Leysen JE, Van Gompel P, Gommeren W, Woestenborghs R, Janssen PAJ (1986) Down regulation of serotonin-S_2 receptor sites in rat brain by chronic treatment with the serotonin-S_2 antagonists: ritanserin and setoperone. Psychopharmacology (Berlin) 88:434–444
Niemegeers CJE, Leysen JE, Laduron PM, Janssen PAJ (1984) Differential pharmacological and biochemical profiles of serotonin-S_2 antagonists. Collegium Internationale Neuro-Psychopharmacologicum, 14th Congress, 16–19 June, Firenze, pp 889 (Abstracts)
Peroutka SJ, Snyder SH (1979) Multiple serotonin receptors differential binding of [^{3}H] 5-hydroxytryptamine, [^{3}H] lysergic acid diethylamide, and [^{3}H] spiroperidol. Mol Pharmacol 16:687–699
Peroutka SJ, Snyder SH (1980) Regulation of serotonin$_2$ (5-HT_2) receptors labeled with [^{3}H] spiroperidol by chronic treatment with the antidepressant amitriptyline. J Pharmacol Exp Ther 215:582–587
Reyntjens A, Waelkens J, Gelders Y, Ceulemans D, Janssen PAJ (1984) A novel approach for psychosomatic normalization: a placebo-controlled pilot trial of R 55667, a potent indolamine antagonist. Collegium Internationale Neuro-Psychopharmacologicum, 14th Congress, 16–19 June, Firenze, pp 566 (Abstracts)
Snyder SH, Peroutka SJ (1982) A possible role of serotonin receptors in antidepressant drug action. Pharmacopsychiatry 15:131–134
Stolz JF, Marsden CA, Middlemiss DN (1983) Effect of chronic antidepressant treatment and subsequent withdrawal on [^{3}H]5-hydroxytryptamine and [^{3}H]spiperone binding in rat frontal cortex and serotonin receptor-mediated behaviour. Psychopharmacology (Berlin) 80:150–155

Chronic Neuroleptic Effects on Dopamine Neuron Activity: A Model for Predicting Therapeutic Efficacy and Side Effects?

A. S. Freeman and B. S. Bunney

1 Introduction

The treatment for most psychotic patients was largely ineffectual and care primarily custodial until the discovery of the antipsychotic properties of chlorpromazine in 1953. Ten years later Carlsson and Lindqvist (1963) discovered that antipsychotic drugs (neuroleptics) exert a specific action on central catecholamine systems, and hypothesized that they produced their effects by blocking catecholamine receptors in catecholamine-innervated sites. They further posited that the receptor blockade resulted in an increase in catecholamine neuronal activity which was mediated through long-loop feedback pathways from forebrain regions innervated by catecholamine neurons (Carlsson and Lindqvist 1963). This concept was a major impetus behind the last two decades of research on the mode of action of neuroleptics. During this time the dopamine (DA) system has been the primary focus of attention and DA receptor blockers have continued to be the treatment of choice for the major symptoms of psychosis (Klein et al. 1980).

Since the pioneering work of Carlsson and Lindqvist (1963) the research effort to determine the mechanism of action of antipsychotic drugs has focused mainly on DA system of the *midbrain*. Anatomical studies provided researchers with detailed maps of the location of brain monoamine cell bodies and projection sites (Dahlström and Fuxe 1964; Ungerstedt 1971). The cell bodies of DA neurons were shown to be concentrated in the zona compacta of the substantia nigra (A9 of Dahlström and Fuxe) and in the adjacent ventral tegmental area (A10) of the midbrain. Electrophysiological recordings from putative DA cells in these areas were first obtained in 1973 with the use of single unit recording techniques in rats (Bunney et al. 1973). The tentative identification of these cells as DA was based on several indirect findings. Direct proof of their DA identity was later provided by in vivo intracellular recording and the subsequent visualization of the heightened histofluorescence resulting from injection of L-dopa (precursor of DA), tetrahydrobiopterin (cofactor for tyrosine hydroxylase), or colchicine (blocks axoplasmic transport of DA and synthesizing enzymes) into the cells recorded (Grace and Bunney 1980, 1983; Chiodo et al. 1984). These directly identified DA cells were found to have electrophysiological characteristics identical to those attributed to DA cells identified by indirect methods. In recent years the technique of single unit recording in freely moving animals has been applied to

Departments of Psychiatry and Pharmacology, Yale University School of Medicine, New Haven, CT 06510-8066, USA.

Clinical Pharmacology in Psychiatry
Editors: Dahl, Gram, Paul, Potter
(Psychopharmacology Series 3)

the study of DA neurons. The extracellularly recorded firing properties of presumed A9 and A10 DA neurons in freely moving rats have been found to be indistinguishable from those of identified DA cells (Meltzer and Bunney 1981; Miller et al. 1983; Freeman and Bunney 1985; Freeman et al. 1985). With the electrophysiological identification of these neurons it was possible to begin studying the effects of DA agonists and antagonists on their activity.

2 Acute Administration

Directly and indirectly acting DA agonists have been found to decrease the activity of A9 and A10 DA cells. For example, depression of unit firing results from the systemic administration of *d*-amphetamine, apomorphine, and a variety of other drugs with DA-agonist properties (for reviews see Bunney 1979; Wang et al. 1984). Numerous electrophysiological studies have demonstrated that neuroleptics increase the activity of A9 and A10 DA neurons when acutely administered to anesthetized or paralyzed rats (Bunney et al. 1973; for reviews see Bunney 1979; Chiodo and Bunney 1984). Similar findings have been obtained in freely moving rats (Freeman et al. 1985). Although these drugs are able to block DA autoreceptors, it appears that their rate-increasing effects on A9 DA neurons are primarily related to the blockade of postsynaptic DA receptors and subsequent feedback activation as originally proposed by Carlsson in 1963 (see Bunney 1979; Kondo and Iwatsubo 1980; Chiodo and Bunney 1984).

These studies also noted that all neuroleptics tested were able to block or reverse the reduction in DA neuronal activity produced by DA agonists in both A9 and A10 areas. Only the weakly antipsychotic phenothiazine analog mepazine was able to discriminate between these two regions. That is, mepazine reversed the d-amphetamine-induced inhibition of A9 but *not* A10 DA neuronal firing (Bunney and Aghajanian 1975 a). The ability to reverse DA agonist-induced depression of DA cell firing appeared to be specific to antipsychotic drugs, since the phenothiazine promethazine (which lacks antipsychotic efficacy and does not produce neurological side effects) did not affect the firing of these neurons.

By the late 1970s it had been demonstrated that neuroleptics which were associated with a high incidence of extrapyramidal side effects (e.g., haloperidol and perphenazine) readily reversed agonist-induced suppression of A9 and A10 cell activity to above baseline levels, while the antipsychotic compounds associated with a low incidence of extrapyramidal side effects (e.g., clozapine and thioridazine) returned A9 cell activity only to predrug baseline (see Bunney 1979; Chiodo and Bunney 1984). Thus, this pattern of response of A9 and A10 DA neurons to acute neuroleptic administration appeared to provide a predictive model for screening antipsychotic drugs. Unfortunately, "false-positives" were soon discovered. For example, the γ-aminobutyric acid (GABA) receptor antagonist picrotoxin (Bunney and Aghajanian 1976), the GABA facilitator diazepam (Bunney and Aghajanian 1975 b) and α-adrenergic drugs (Bunney and DeReimer 1982), none of which has antipsychotic activity, also reversed DA agonist-induced decreases in DA neuronal activity. Therefore, even though these electrophysiological studies confirmed the earlier hypothesis based on biochemical data that acute DA antagonists increase DA cell activity, they were unable to establish a reliable model that would differentiate between clinical efficacy and neurological side effect potential.

3 Chronic Administration

The therapeutic action and many of the neurological side effects of antipsychotic drugs usually take days or even weeks to develop (Klein and Davis 1969; Crane 1973; Beckman et al. 1979). This delayed onset of clinical responses has spurred research into the effects of repeated drug treatment on central neurons. Biochemical studies carried out in several laboratories have revealed marked differences between the effects of acute and chronic neuroleptic treatment on DA turnover. For example, with repeated treatment tolerance develops in several DA-innervated areas to the increase in DA turnover associated with the acute administration of antipsychotic drugs (for reviews see Roth 1983; Bannon et al. 1986).

Several studies have investigated the effects of repeated neuroleptic treatment on the *electrophysiology* of midbrain DA cells. In one study rats were treated with two subcutaneous (s.c.) injections of the depot neuroleptic fluphenazine decanoate (Nowycky and Roth 1977). One day after the second injection A9 DA neuronal firing rates were no different from controls, suggesting that the acute increase in activity induced by this drug disappears during chronic exposure. In another study A9 DA autoreceptor sensitivity was increased when assessed 7 days after cessation of repeated haloperidol (21 days, i.p.) treatment (Gallager et al. 1978). The co-administration of lithium with haloperidol prevented the development of supersensitivity (Gallager et al. 1978).

We now know that all A9 and A10 DA neurons are not homogeneous with respect to their projection sites (for a review see Björklund and Lindvall 1985) or their biochemical and electrophysiological characteristics (Chiodo et al. 1984). Since current electrophysiological techniques do not allow us to record from the same neuron continuously during the entire period of chronic drug administration, it was necessary to devise alternative methods with which to assess the effects of repeated neuroleptic administration on the firing properties of DA cells. A technique was developed by which an index of the activity of populations of DA cells could be determined. The technique involves counting the number of DA cells encountered per electrode track while repeatedly lowering the electrode (in a predetermined fashion) through a stereotaxically defined block of the rat midbrain known to contain DA neurons (Bunney and Grace 1978). Careful employment of the cells/track technique allows one to make quantitative measures of the response of a given population of DA neurons to both acute and chronic drug treatment.

This population sampling technique has been applied in several studies of neuroleptics. The first of these studies sampled the A9 area of animals either one hour after a single s.c. injection of haloperidol (0.5 mg/kg) or on day 22 of repeated treatment (Bunney and Grace 1978). Relative to controls, the acute treatment resulted in a significantly higher number of spontaneously active DA neurons in A9. These results suggested that there was a population of DA cells that was inactive ("silent") under control conditions but which was activated by acute haloperidol administration. This interpretation was supported by the finding that direct iontophoretic application of an excitatory amino acid, glutamate, activated silent DA cells which could subsequently be activated by i.v. haloperidol. The fact that these inactive DA cells could be induced to fire by local application of glutamate suggested that they were in a hyperpolarized state. In contrast to the results obtained from acutely treated animals, chronic haloperidol treatment resulted in significantly fewer cells/track (90% reduction) than in saline-treated controls. Moreover, the DA neurons which were not firing in the chronically treated animals appeared to be inactive due to excessive *depolarization* (i.e., depolarization block). Thus, the silent DA neurons in chronically treated animals could not be made to fire by the iontophoretic application of glutamate, but would begin to fire after the local application of the inhibitory substance GABA (Fig. 1) (Bunney and Grace 1978; Chiodo and Bunney 1983). In vivo intracellular recordings have confirmed that chronic administration of antipsychotic drugs results in a reduction (10–15 mV) in the resting membrane potential of DA cells (Grace and Bunney 1986). In addition, in vivo voltammetric techniques have recently provided evidence that nerve terminal DA release is greatly reduced in animals receiving chronic haloperidol treatment (Bunney et al. 1985).

Using a similar population sampling design, White and Wang (1983a) later confirmed that chronic s.c. haloperidol treatment results in a reduction in A9 DA cell incidence as a result of apparent depolarization inactivation. In addition,

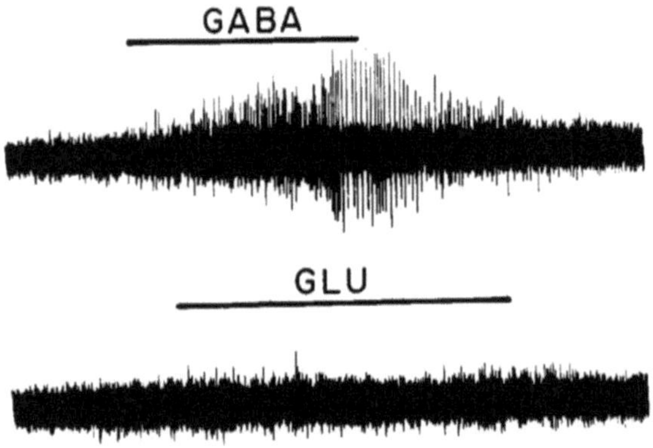

Fig. 1. Oscillograph tracings showing typical responses of a "silent" A10 DA neuron to glutamic acid (GLU) and γ-aminobutyric acid (GABA) in an animal chronically treated with chlorpromazine. *Top:* This cell was activated by the microiontophoretic application of GABA (3 nA). After a short delay GABA caused spikes to appear out of the background noise. Continued application resulted in a decrease in activity (action potential amplitude increased and duration decreased). When the GABA was turned off the firing rate increased markedly (amplitude decreased and duration markedly increased) and the spikes disappeared back into the noise. (The changes in spike duration are not visible owing to the paper speed.) These changes in action potential amplitude and duration are identical to those observed in untreated animals when the spontaneous activity of a DA cell increases or decreases. The *lower trace* shows that the excitatory amino acid GLU (ejected at 12 nA 1 min after the GABA ejection shown in the *upper trace*) was unable to activate the silent DA neuron. *Horizontal bars* represent onset and duration of the microiontophoretic drug application. Calibration equals 400 μV and 2 s. (From Chiodo and Bunney 1983, with permission)

Table 1. Changes in the number of spontaneously active midbrain DA neurons following acute and chronic drug treatment

Drug	A9		A10	
	Acute	Chronic	Acute	Chronic
Haloperidol[a–f]	↑	↓	↑	↓
Chlorpromazine[a, b]	↑	↓	↑	↓
l-Sulpiride[a]	↑	↓	↑	↓
d-Sulpiride[a]	o	o	o	o
dl-Sulpiride[b, *]	o	o	↑	↓
Clozapine[a, c]	↑	↑	↑	↓
Clozapine[b]	o	o	↑	↓
Thioridazine[b]	o	o	↑	↓
Mesoridazine[c]	↑	↑	↑	↓
Molindone[b]	o	o	↑	↓
Promethazine[a]	o	o	o	o
Metoclopramide[b]	↑	↓	o	o
Desmethylimipramine[a]	o	↑	o	↑
Trihexyphenidyl[c]	o	o	o	o
Prazosin[c]	↑	o	o	o
Idazoxan[c]	↑	o	o	o
Proglumide[f]	o	↑	o	↑
Haloperidol + Trihexyphenidyl[c]	↑	↑	↑	↓
Prazosin[c]	↑	↑	↑	↓
Idazoxan[c]	↑	↓	↑	↓
Acute proglumide[f]		↑		↑
Acute muscimol[f]		↑		↑
Acute naloxone[f]		↓		↓

↑ = increase; ↓ = decrease; o = no change.
[a] Chiodo and Bunney (1983). [b] White and Wang (1983a). [c] Chiodo and Bunney (1985b). [d] Bunney and Grace (1978). [e] White and Wang (1983b). [f] Chiodo and Bunney (1985a).
* Racemic mixture assumed, since specific isomer not designated.

these investigators reported a reduced number of DA cells/track in A10. The decline in A10 DA cell incidence (70% reduction at 1 week) occurred earlier and to a greater extent than that which occurred in A9 (40% reduction at 3 weeks).

Chronic studies have now been extended to include an investigation of the effects of repeated *oral* neuroleptic administration on the activity of both A9 and A10 DA neurons (Chiodo and Bunney 1982, 1983, 1985a, b). In these studies animals were studied either 1 h after a single gavage or on day 21 or after 7 months of continuous administration via the drinking water. To date all neuroleptics studied which are associated with a moderate to high incidence of extrapyramidal side effects (e.g., haloperidol, chlorpromazine, *l*-sulpiride) acutely increase the number of cells/track, but induce a state of depolarization inactivation (a decreased number of active DA neurons) in both A9 and A10 when given chronically. In contrast, those antipsychotic drugs associated with a low incidence of extrapyramidal side effects (e.g., the atypical neuroleptics clozapine and mesoridazine) acutely increase the cells/track in both areas and inactivate A10, but *not* A9, DA neurons when given chronically (Table 1). Similar results have been reported by White and Wang (1983b), who chronically treated rats s.c. with a variety of neuroleptics. Thus, all neuroleptics produced a reduction in the number of cells/track in A10 upon repeated administration; haloperidol and chlorpromazine also decreased A9 DA cell incidence. In addition, two more atypical neuroleptics, thioridazine and molindone, were found to selectively inactivate A10 DA cells with chronic treatment. However, in contrast to the results obtained by Chiodo and Bunney (1983), neither acute nor chronic treatment with sulpiride produced any change in the A9 cells/track ratio (White and Wang 1983b). The reason for this discrepancy between the two studies is not readily apparent but may be due to differences in the regions of A9 sampled, the doses employed and the use of racemic sulpiride in the latter study instead of the active isomer. The induction of depolarization inactivation appears to be a property specific to neuroleptics, since a non-neuroleptic phenothiazine (promethazine), the inactive isomer of sulpiride (*d*-sulpiride), an antidepressant (desmethylimipramine) and α-noradrenergic receptor blockers (prazosin and idazoxan) did not inactivate A9 or A10 DA neurons when chronically administered (Chiodo and Bunney 1982–1984; White and Wang 1983b).

4 A Model System?

Combined, the above studies suggest that by examining the population response of both A9 and A10 DA neurons to chronic treatment it may be possible to predict whether or not a new compound will exert an antipsychotic action (because of the correlation between A10 DA cell inactivation and clinical efficacy) or induce extrapyramidal side effects (because of the correlation between inactivation of A9 DA cells and induction of neurological side effects) or produce both effects. The inability of the atypical antipsychotic drugs to inactivate A9 DA neurons provides hope that new drugs or drug combinations can be developed which lack the neurological side effects which plague the patient receiving typical neuroleptics. However, for rational development of such new drugs, we need to understand the mechanisms responsible for making the atypical antipsychotic drugs different from classical neuroleptics. Several suggestions have been offered as to why clozapine lacks the ability to induce extrapyramidal side effects. These include a central anticholinergic action (Snyder et al. 1974; Miller and Hiley 1974; Andén and Stock 1973; Marco et al. 1976; Pelham and Munsat 1979; Racagni et al. 1980); α-noradrenergic blocking action (Bartholini et al. 1972; Burki et al. 1974; McMillen and Shore 1978; Souto et al. 1979); and a differential DA receptor blocking action in limbic versus striatal areas (Bunney and Aghajanian 1978; Kohler et al. 1981).

The first two possibilities have been tested with the use of the DA cell sampling procedure. Repeated co-administration of the anticholinergic drug trihexyphenidyl or the α_1-noradrenergic receptor antagonist prazosin with haloperidol (via the drinking water) resulted in changes in A9 and A10 DA cell activity similar to those produced by clozapine alone (Chiodo and Bunney 1984; Chiodo and Bunney 1985b). Thus, chronic treatment with haloperidol and trihexyphenidyl or prazosin inactivated only A10 DA neurons (Table 1). However, the mechanisms responsible for this induction of depolarization inactivation may be very complex, as recent evidence suggests other endogenous neurotransmitter or neuromodulator systems may be involved in its development and/or maintenance. For example, the acute administration of either the GABA agonist muscimol or the cholecystokinin antagonist proglumide reversed the haloperidol-induced depolarization inactivation of A9 and A10 DA cells (Table 1) (Chiodo and Bunney 1985a).

In both the A9 and A10 regions the presence of long-loop feedback pathways are necessary for the induction of depolarization inactivation by chronic neuroleptics. Thus, kainic acid lesions of the striatum and globus pallidus (which eliminate the striato-nigral and pallido-nigral feedback pathways) prior to chronic haloperidol treatment result in no change in the number of A9 DA cells/track encountered when compared to controls (Bunney and Grace 1978). Similarly, ibotenic acid lesions of the nucleus accumbens prevents, to a large degree, the decline in A10 DA cell incidence (White and Wang 1983a). However, there may be a difference between the two areas in the importance of such feedback regulation in the maintenance of depolarization block once it has been induced (Chiodo and Bunney 1983, 1984). That is, hemitransection of the forebrain (which destroys all long-loop feedback pathways from anterior structures) on day 21 of neuroleptic treatment abolishes the inactivation of A9, but not A10, DA neurons.

Not all DA neurons respond in the same manner when an animal is repeatedly treated with even a typical antipsychotic drug. Thus, though most midbrain DA neurons enter a state of depolarization inactivation during repeated treatment with neuroleptics, a small number of cells are found to remain active. The majority of these DA cells have been identified as mesocortical cells which project to the prefrontal or cingulate cortices (Chiodo and Bunney 1983). This finding is consistent with biochemical studies which show that tolerance to the effects of DA antagonists does not develop in the prefrontal cortex (for review see Bannon et al. 1985). However, the relationship of this finding to the therapeutic effects of neuroleptics remains obscure at this time.

5 Clinical Speculations

It may be clinically significant that the time-dependent changes in DA neuron functioning during repeated neuroleptic administration occurs with a time course similar to that associated with the emergence of some of the therapeutic and neurological side-effects of these drugs. Antipsychotic drugs are competitive postsynaptic DA receptor blockers. With acute neuroleptic administration the increased activity of DA systems – increased number of active cells and increased firing rate – combined with the demonstrated ability of these drugs to block autoreceptors would lead to a significant increase in DA release. [This hypothesized increase in DA release has recently been demonstrated in vivo with the use of push-pull, dialysis and voltametric techniques (Nieoullon et al. 1977; Schenk and Bunney 1983; Imperato and DiChiara 1985; Blaha and Lane 1984).] Thus, a greater amount of DA would be available to compete with neuroleptic molecules for postsynaptic DA receptors. Under these circumstances receptor blockade may not be very effective. If this is the case, it might explain why immediate clinical effects of these drugs are not seen. However, with repeated treatment the large decrease in the number of spontaneously active DA cells due to depolarization inactivation likely leads to a decrease in depolarization-dependent DA release from nerve terminals (as recently demonstrated with the use of in vivo voltammetry; Schenk and Bunney 1983). Thus, as depolarization inactivation develops, the number of DA molecules available to compete with the antipsychotic drug would decrease. At the same time, repeated treatment should cause the number of antipsychotic drug molecules to increase. These time-dependent events should lead to increasingly effective blockade of postsynaptic DA receptors and, as a result, the emergence of clinical improvement and/or neurological side effects. The finding that antipsychotic drugs apparently devoid of neurological side effects (e.g., clozapine) fail to inactivate A9 DA cells but, like all antipsychotic drugs, inactivate A10 DA cells would support this hypothesis.

6 Conclusions

Recent advances in the application of electrophysiological techniques have begun to contribute to our understanding of the mechanism of action of antipsychotic drugs. The combination of anatomical, biochemical, behavioral, and electrophysiological techniques has enabled us to begin formulating hypotheses which are testable. For example, if neuroleptic-induced depolarization block of A9 DA cells can be selectively prevented or reversed pharmacologically, such new drugs might provide new treatments for the neurological side effects of antipsychotic agents and make clinical testing of the mechanisms for side effect induction hypothesized above possible. Furthermore, the fact that all antipsychotic drugs tested to date inactivate most A10 DA neurons when given repeatedly, while only those neuroleptics associated with a high to moderate incidence of neurological side effects inactivate A9 DA cells, suggests that determining the ability of new putative neuroleptics to produce DA neuron inactivation in these two regions may predict therapeutic efficacy and severity of neurological side effects.

Acknowledgments. We thank S. Mulready for manuscript preparation and C.-L. Pun for technical assistance. The work reported in this paper was supported by National Institutes of Health grants MH-08987 (ASF), MH-25642 (BSB), MH-28849 (BSB), the Robert Alwin Hay Fund for Schizophrenia Research, and the State of Connecticut.

References

Andén NE, Stock G (1973) Effects of clozapine on the turnover of dopamine in the corpus striatum and in the limbic system. J Pharm Pharmacol 25:346–348

Bannon MJ, Reinhard JF Jr, Bunney EB, Roth RH (1982) Unique response to antipsychotic drugs is due to the absence of terminal autoreceptors in mesocortical dopamine neurons. Nature 296:444–446

Bannon MJ, Freeman AS, Chiodo LA, Bunney BS, Roth RH (1986) The electrophysiological and biochemical pharmacology of the mesolimbic and mesocortical dopamine neurons. In: Iversen LL, Iversen SD, Snyder SH (eds) Handbook of psychopharmacology, vol 19. Plenum, New York (in press)

Bartholini G, Haefely W, Jalfre M, Keller HH, Pletscher A (1972) Effects of clozapine on central catecholaminergic neurone systems. Br J Pharmacol 46:736

Beckman B, Hippius H, Ruther E (1979) Treatment of schizophrenia. Prog Neuropsychopharmacol Biol Psychiatry 3:47–52

Björklund A, Lindvall O (1985) Dopamine-containing systems in the CNS. In: Björklund A, Hökfelt T (eds) Handbook of chemical neuronanatomy, vol 2, part 1. Elsevier, Amsterdam, pp 55–122

Blaha CD, Lane RF (1984) Direct in vivo electrochemical monitoring of dopamine release in response to neuroleptic drug. Eur J Pharmacol 98:113–117

Bunney BS (1979) The electrophysiological pharmacology of midbrain dopaminergic systems. In: Horn AS, Korf J, Westerink BHC (eds) The neurobiology of dopamine. Academic, New York, pp 417–452

Bunney BS, Aghajanian GK (1975a) Antipsychotic drugs and central dopaminergic neurons: a model for predicting therapeutic efficacy and incidence of extrapyramidal side effects. In: Sudilovsky A, Gershon S, Beer B (eds) Predictability in psychopharmacology: preclinical and clinical correlations. Raven, New York, pp 225–245

Bunney BS, Aghajanian GK (1975b) The effect of antipsychotic drugs on the firing of dopaminergic neurons: a reappraisal. In: Sedvall G (ed) Antipsychotic drugs, pharmacodynamics and pharmacokinetics. Pergamon, New York, pp 305–318

Bunney BS, Aghajanian GK (1976) Dopaminergic influence in the basal ganglia: evidence for striatonigral feedback regulation. In: Yahr MD (ed) The basal ganglia. Raven, New York, pp 249–267

Bunney BS, Aghajanian GK (1978) Mesolimbic and mesocortical dopaminergic systems: physiology and pharmacology. In: Lipton MA, DiMascio A, Killam KF (eds) Psychopharmacology: a generation of progress. Raven, New York, pp 159–169

Bunney BS, DeRiemer S (1982) Effects of clonidine on dopaminergic neuron activity in the substantia nigra: possible indirect mediation by noradrenergic regulation of the serotonergic raphe system. In: Friedhoff AJ, Chase TN (eds) Gilles de la Tourette Syndrome. Raven, New York, pp 99–104

Bunney BS, Grace AA (1978) Acute and chronic haloperidol treatment: comparison of effects on nigral dopaminergic cell activity. Life Sci 23:1715–1728

Bunney BS, Walters JR, Roth RH, Aghajanian GK (1973) Dopaminergic neurons: effect of antipsychotic drugs and amphetamine on single cell activity. J Pharmacol Exp Ther 185:560–571

Bunney BS, Chiodo LA, Grace AA, Schenk JO (1985) In vivo effects of acute and chronic antipsychotic drug administration on midbrain dopaminergic neuron activity. In: Seiden LS, Balster RL (eds) Behavioral pharmacology: the current status. Liss, New York, pp 205–220

Burki HR, Ruch W, Asper H, Baggiolini M, Stille G (1974) Effect of single and repeated administration of clozapine on the metabolism of dopamine and noradrenaline in the brain of the rat. Eur J Pharmacol 27:180–190

Carlsson A, Lindqvist M (1963) Effects of chlorpromazine and haloperidol on formation of 3-methoxytyramine and normetanephrine in mouse brain. Acta Pharmacol Toxicol 20:140–144

Chiodo LA, Bunney BS (1982) Effects of chronic neuroleptic treatments on nigral dopamine cell activity. Soc Neurosci 8:482 (Abstract)

Chiodo LA, Bunney BS (1983) Typical and atypical neuroleptics: differential effects of chronic administration on the activity of A9 and A10 midbrain dopaminergic neurons. J Neurosci 3:1607–1619

Chiodo LA, Bunney BS (1984) Effects of dopamine antagonists on midbrain dopamine cell activity. In: Usdin E, Carlsson A, Dahlström A, Engel J (eds) Catecholamines. Pergamon, Elmsford, pp 369–391

Chiodo LA, Bunney BS (1985) Possible mechanisms by which repeated clozapine administration differentially affects the activity of two subpopulations of midbrain dopamine neurons. J Neurosci 5:2539–2544

Chiodo LA, Bunney BS (1986) Pharmacological alterations of chronic neuroleptic-induced depolarization of midbrain dopamine-containing neurons. J Neurosci (in press)

Ciodo LA, Bannon MJ, Grace AA, Roth RH, Bunney BS (1984) Evidence for the absence of impulse-regulating somatodendritic and synthesis-modulating nerve terminal autoreceptors on subpopulations of mesocortical dopamine neurons. Neuroscience 12:1–16
Crane GE (1973) Persistent dyskinesia. Br J Psychiatry 122:395–405
Dahlström A, Fuxe K (1964) Evidence for the existence of monoamine-containing neurons in the central nervous system: I. Demonstration of monoamines in the cell bodies of brain stem neurons. Acta Physiol Scand [Suppl]62(232):1–55
Freeman AS, Bunney BS (1985) Characterization of putative dopaminergic neuronal firing in the ventral tegmental area (A10) of unrestrained rats. Soc Neurosci 11:1074 (Abstract)
Freeman AS, Meltzer LT, Bunney BS (1985) Firing properties of substantia nigra dopaminergic neurons in freely moving rats. Life Sci 36:1983–1994
Gallager DW, Pert A, Bunney WE Jr (1978) Haloperidol-induced presynaptic dopamine supersensitivity is blocked by chronic lithium. Nature 273:309–312
Grace AA, Bunney BS (1980) Nigral dopamine neurons: intracellular recording and identification with L-DOPA injection and histofluorescence. Science 210:654–656
Grace AA, Bunney BS (1983) Intracellular and extracellular electrophysiology of nigral dopaminergic neurons: I. Identification and characterization. Neuroscience 10:301–315
Grace AA, Bunney BS (1986) Induction of depolarization block in midbrain dopamine neurons by repeated administration of haloperidol-analysis using in vivo intracellular recording. J Pharm Exp Ther 238:1092–1100
Imperato A, DiChiara G (1985) Dopamine release and metabolism in awake rats after systemic neuroleptics as studied by trans-striatal dialysis. J Neurosci 5:297–306
Klein DE, Davis JM (1969) Diagnosis and drug treatment of psychiatric disorders. Williams and Wilkins, Baltimore
Kohler C, Haglund L, Ogren O, Angeby T (1981) Regional blockade by neuroleptic drugs of in vivo ^{3}H-spiperone binding in the rat brain. Relation to blockade of apomorphine induced hyperactivity and stereotypies. J Neural Transm 52:163–173
Klein DF, Gittelman R, Quitkin F, Rifkin A (1980) Diagnosis and drug treatment of psychiatric disorders: adults and children, 2nd edn. Williams and Wilkins, Baltimore
Kondo Y, Iwatsubo K (1980) Diminished responses of nigral dopaminergic neurons to haloperidol and morphine following lesions of the striatum. Brain Res 181:237–240
Marco E, Mao CC, Cheney DL, Revuelta A, Costa E (1976) The effects of antipsychotics on the turnover rate of GABA and acetylcholine in rat brain nuclei. Nature 264:363–365
McMillen BA, Shore PA (1978) Comparative effects of clozapine and alpha adrenoceptor blocking drugs on regional noradrenaline metabolism in rat brain. Eur J Pharmacol 52:225–230
Meltzer LT, Bunney BS (1981) Nigral dopaminergic neurons: single unit activity in the awake, unrestrained rat. Soc Neurosci 113:341 (Abstract)
Miller JD, Farber J, Gotz P, Roffwarg H, German DC (1983) Activity of mesencephalic dopamine and non-dopamine neurons across stages of sleep and waking in the rat. Brain Res 273:133–141
Miller RJ, Hiley CR (1974) Anti-muscarinic properties of neuroleptics and drug induced parkinsonism. Nature 248:596–597
Nieoullon A, Cheramy A, Glowinski J (1977) An adaptation of the push-pull cannula method to study the in vivo release of ^{3}H-dopamine synthesized from ^{3}H-tyrosine in the cat caudate nucleus: effect of various physical and pharmacological treatments. J Neurochem 28:819–828
Nowycky MC, Roth RH (1977) Presynaptic dopamine receptors: development of supersensitivity following treatment with fluphenazine decanoate. Naunyn-Schmiedebergs Arch Pharmacol 300:247–254
Pelham RW, Munsat TL (1979) Identification of direct competition for, and direct influences on, striatal muscarinic cholinergic receptors: in vivo (^{3}H)-quinuclidinyl benzilate binding in rats. Brain Res 171:473–480
Racagni G, Bruno F, Bugatti A, Parenti M, Apud JA, Santini V, Carenzi A, Groppetti A, Catabeni F (1980) Behavioral and biochemical correlates after haloperidol and clozapine long-term treatment. Adv Biochem Psychopharmacol 24:45–51
Roth RH (1983) Neuroleptics: functional neurochemistry. In: Coyle JT, Enna SJ (eds) Neuroleptics: neurochemical, behavioral and clinical perspectives. Raven, New York, pp 119–156

Schenk JO, Bunney BS (1983) The effect of repeated haloperidol treatment on K^+ stimulated "release" in the rat striatum measured by in vivo electrochemistry. Soc Neurosci 9:1006 (Abstract)
Snyder SH, Bannerjee SP, Yamamura HI, Greenberg D (1974) Drugs, neurotransmitters and schizophrenia. Science 184:1243–1253
Souto M, Monti JM, Alter H (1979) Effects of clozapine on the activity of central dopaminergic and noradrenergic neurons. Pharmacol Biochem Behav 10:5–9
Ungerstedt U (1971) Stereotaxic mapping of the monoamine pathways in the rat brain. Acta Physiol Scand [Suppl]367:1–48
Wang RY, White FJ, Voigt MM (1984) Effects of dopamine agonists on midbrain dopamine cell activity. In: Usdin E, Carlsson A, Dahlström A, Engel J (eds) Catecholamines. Pergamon, Elmsford, pp 359–367
White FJ, Wang RY (1983 a) Comparison of the effects of chronic haloperidol treatment on A9 and A10 dopamine neurons in the rat. Life Sci 32:983–993
White FJ, Wang RY (1983 b) Differential effects of classical and atypical antipsychotic drugs on A9 and A10 dopamine neurons. Science 221:1054–1057

Effect of Selective D_1 and D_2 Dopamine Receptor Antagonists and Agonists in Cebus Monkeys: Implications for Acute and Tardive Dyskinesias

A Preliminary Report

J. Gerlach, K. Kistrup, and S. Korsgaard

1 Introduction

The discovery of two distinct, but closely related dopamine (DA) receptors [D_1 and D_2 (Kebabian and Calne 1979)] has opened new possibilities for research in the pathophysiology of extrapyramidal syndromes (EPS), including tardive dyskinesia, and may lead to new treatments not only of EPS, but also of psychotic disorders. From a clinical point of view, the primary task is to identify the behavioral consequences of stimulation and inhibition of the D_1 and D_2 DA receptors.

In untreated rodents D_1 and D_2 DA antagonists produce almost the same behavioral effects, including catalepsy and stereotypy antagonism (Christensen et al. 1985). However, the antistereotypy effect of D_2 antagonists can be attenutated by concomitant administration of anticholinergics, while the antistereotypy effect of D_1 antagonists, both the selective D_1 antagonist SCH 23.390 and the mixed D_1/D_2 antagonists such as flupenthixol, has been found to remain unchanged following a supplementary anticholinergic treatment (Christensen et al. 1985; Hyttel et al. 1985). In rats pretreated with reserpine or 6-OH DA, other signs of a differentiation between D_1 and D_2 effects have been found (Arnt 1985; Arnt and Hyttel 1985; Breese and Mueller 1985; Molloy and Waddington 1985). The question is whether such distinct D_1/D_2 effects, including the different response to anticholinergics, can be found in higher species.

An especially interesting aspect of the D_1/D_2 receptor discovery is the characterization of complex interactions between the two receptor functions. Thus, a few studies in rodents suggest that D_1 agonists and D_2 antagonists interact in a synergistic way, while D_1 agonists and D_2 agonists may antagonize each other (Stoof and Kebabian 1981; Rosengarten et al. 1983; Saller and Salama 1985). Although these findings have been challenged by other observations (Arnt 1985), they suggest that perhaps selective D_1 and D_2 drugs may be used to modify the classic D_2 receptor blocking treatment of psychotic patients, to potentiate the antipsychotic effect and prevent or treat the EPS.

Unfortunately, clinical research in this area is hampered by the lack of clinically available selective D_1 DA drugs. Therefore, as an alternative approach to exploring the problems we have used Cebus monkeys which have been treated with haloperidol for 4 years and are primed to develop acute and tardive EPS

Sct. Hans Mental Hospital, Dept. 2, Roskilde, Denmark.

Clinical Pharmacology in Psychiatry
Editors: Dahl, Gram, Paul, Potter
(Psychopharmacology Series 3)

similar to the corresponding syndromes in humans. This paper is a preliminary report on the effect of D_1 and D_2 DA antagonists and agonists, given alone and in combination to four of these Cebus monkeys.

2 Methods

2.1 Subjects

Four male *Cebus apella* monkeys 8–10 years old and weighing 3.4–3.8 kg were used. For the preceding 4 years the monkeys had received a daily oral dose of haloperidol. The initial dose for all monkeys was 0.10 mg/kg. Due to an increasing vulnerability to dystonic reactions, the dose was individually decreased to 0.0125–0.10 mg/kg (mean 0.0575 mg/kg).

After withdrawal of this 4-year treatment, one monkey developed a typical tardive dyskinesia syndrome consisting of tongue protrusions and slight mouth openings. As in humans the syndrome was markedly aggravated (faster movements and bigger amplitudes) whenever the monkey was activated or stressed.

2.2 Drugs

The drugs were freshly prepared in sterile water just prior to s.c. administration. Drugs were SCH 23.390 (D_1 antagonist) (Schering, Bloomfield NJ, USA), raclopride (D_2 antagonist) (Astra, Södertälje, Sweden), SKF 38.393 (D_1 agonist) (Smith, Kline and French, Philadelphia PA, USA), LY 171.555 (D_2 agonist) (Lilly, USA), biperiden (anticholinergic drug) (Knoll, Ludwigshafen, FRG), and apomorphine. The drugs were given at 3- to 4-day intervals.

The study started 3 weeks after withdrawal of the long-term haloperidol treatment. To test the possible changes in haloperidol-induced DA supersensitivity that might have occurred during the study, apomorphine (0.25 mg/kg) was given before, in the middle, and at the end. No significant changes could be detected.

The different drugs were given alone and in combination. In the combined test, SKF 38.393 and LY 171.555 (the drugs with the most prolonged action) were given 45 min before the DA antagonists.

2.3 Evaluation

The effect was evaluated by a rater blind to the drugs given. A specially designed rating scale was used. This scale measures two types of behavior, (a) dystonia and (b) hyperactive behavior, including stereotyped repetitive movements of head, neck, limbs, and trunk and oral hyperkinesia (for details, see Korsgaard et al. 1985). The behavior was rated every 10 min during the first 90 min (135 min in the case of 2 injections), and thereafter at 30-min intervals up to 6 h after drug injection.

Owing to the preliminary nature of this report and the small number of animals included until now, no statistical analysis has been performed. All values are given as mean values.

3 Results

3.1 Effect of SCH 23.390 (D_1 Antagonist) and Raclopride (D_2 Antagonist)

SCH 23.390 (0.025–0.05 mg/kg) and raclopride (0.025–0.05 mg/kg) induced an indistinguishable dystonic syndrome including opening of the mouth, torticollis of head and neck, torsion and flexion of the limbs, and twisting of the trunk. This syndrome was similar to the dystonia induced by other neuroleptics, such as haloperidol.

In three of the four monkeys, dyskinetic repeated mouth opening and tongue protrusion were seen. Especially when the dystonic features diminished, the oral movements became relaxed and similar to tardive dyskinesia. The animals made chewing and licking movements, partly on the cage. This oral hyperkinesia syndrome disappeared soon after the dystonia.

The time-course and the intensity of the dystonia induced by 0.05 and 0.025 mg/kg are shown for both SCH 23.390 and raclopride in Fig. 1. The SCH response was over within 1 h, while the raclopride response lasted approximately 1 h.

3.2 Effect of LY 171.555 (D_2 Agonist) and Biperiden (an Anticholinergic) in Dystonia Induced by SCH 23.390 and Raclopride

As seen in Fig. 2, LY 171.555 (0.1–0.25 mg/kg) markedly reduced or abolished the dystonia induced by the two DA antagonists. The antagonistic effect of LY 171.555 was the same in the SCH 23.390-induced dystonia as in raclopride-induced dystonia. The only difference that could be detected was a pronounced sedation seen during the combined treatment with LY 171.555 and SCH 23.390. This was not seen during LY 171.555-raclopride treatment.

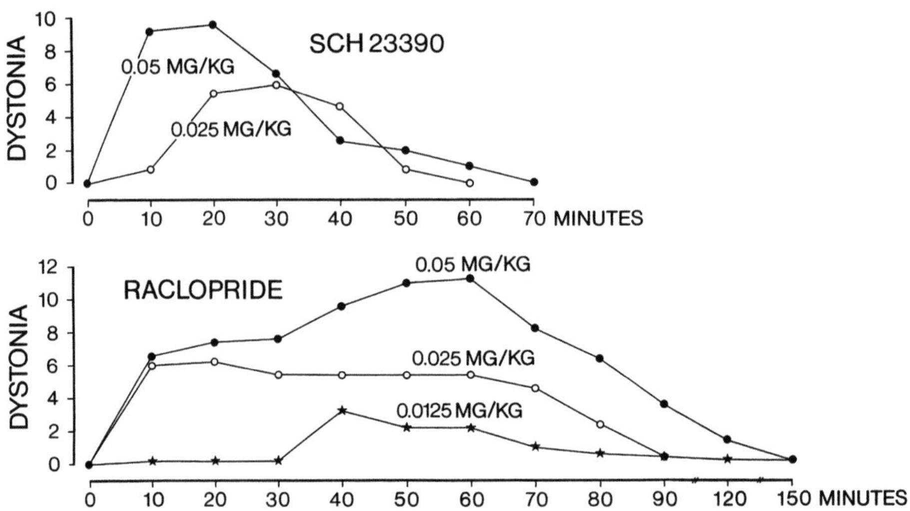

Fig. 1. Dystonia induced by SCH 23.390 and raclopride injected subcutaneously. The values are means from four Cebus monkeys. For rating scale, see Korsgaard et al. (1985)

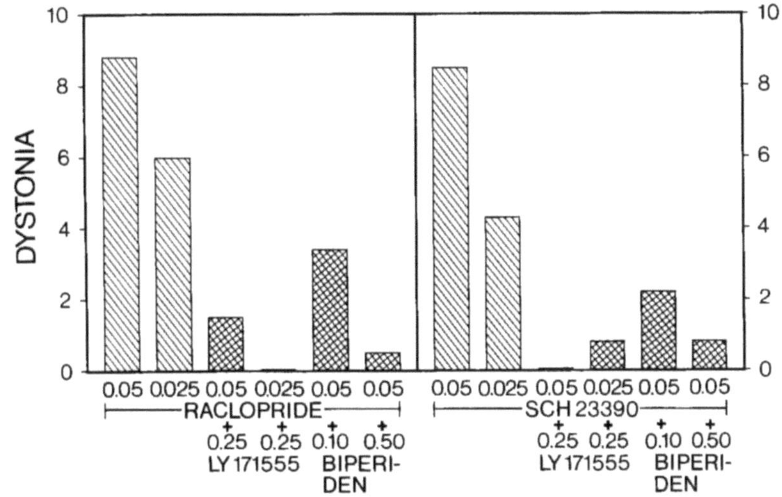

Fig. 2. Effect of Ly 171.555 (D_1 agonist) and biperiden (anticholinergic drug) in dystonia induced by raclopride (D_2 antagonist) and SCH 23.390 (D_1 antagonist) in four Cebus monkeys. Raclopride values are means of 6 scores from 10–60 min after s.c. raclopride injection, while the SCH 23.390 values are means of three scores from 10–30 min after injection. LY 171.555 and biperiden were given s.c. 30 min before the DA antagonists. *Figures* under the *columns* give doses in milligrams per kilogram of body weight

Also, biperiden induced marked reduction/abolishment of dystonia induced by both DA antagonists, and no difference was found between the effect in SCH 23.390-induced dystonia and the effect in raclopride-induced dystonia. No sedation was seen. Otherwise the effect of biperiden was similar to the effect of LY 171.555 (Fig. 2).

3.3 Effect of SKF 38.393 (D_1 Agonist) in Dystonia Induced by SCH 23.390 and Raclopride

SKF 38.393 (5 and 10 mg/kg) given alone had no effect on extrapyramidal motor parameters. SKF 38.393 (10 mg/kg) inhibited the dystonia induced by SCH 23.390 0.05 mg/kg and 0.025 mg/kg. The score was reduced from 8.3 to 6.3, and from 4.3 to 1.1, respectively.

On the other hand, SKF 38.393 increased the dystonia induced by relatively small doses of raclopride. The mean dystonia score increased from 1.5 (raclopride 0.0125 mg/kg) to 3.5 (SKF 38.393 10 mg/kg + raclopride 0.0125 mg/kg).

3.4 Effect of LY 171.555 and SKF 38.393 Alone and in Combination

As seen in Fig. 3, LY 171.555 induced a marked stereotyped behavior characterized by repetitive movements of head, legs, and body. Oral hyperkinesia was not induced and it was not changed in the monkey with oral tardive dyskinesia. The monkeys were aroused and reactive to what was going on outside the cage. As

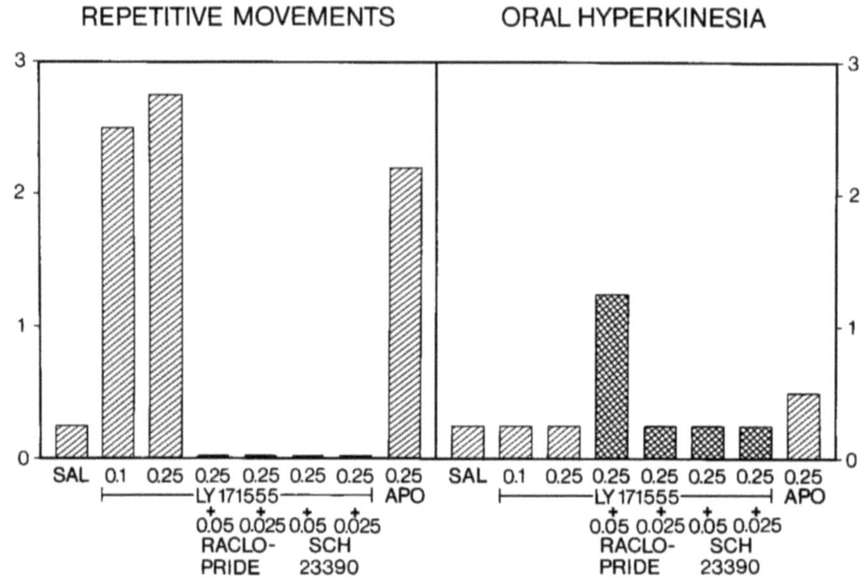

Fig. 3. Repetitive movements and oral hyperkinesia (tardive dyskinesia) induced by LY 171.555 and counteracted by raclopride and SCH 23.390. The effect of apomorphine is included for comparison. The columns represent means of three scores 40–60 min after s.c. LY injections, 20–30 min after injection of SCH and raclopride. *Figures* under the *columns* give doses in milligrams per kilogram of body weight. SAL, saline

seen from Fig. 3, the 2-DA antagonists completely abolished the repetitive movements.

SKF 38.393 (10 mg/kg) induced slight oral hyperkinetic movements in two monkeys and aggravated the syndrome in the monkey with preexisting tardive dyskinesia, but did not induce repetitive movements. On the contrary, SKF 38.393 (10 mg/kg) antagonized the repetitive movements induced by LY 171.555 (0.05 mg/kg) from 2–0.3 (mean scores). At the same time yawning was seen in the monkey with preexisting oral tardive dyskinesia.

Apomorphine induced repetitive movements corresponding to the effect of LY 171.555, but at the same time apomorphine slightly aggravated the tardive dyskinesia-like hyperkinesias (Fig. 3).

4 Discussion

This study indicates that dystonia induced by the D_1 DA antagonist SCH 23.390 in Cebus monkeys is identical to dystonia induced by D_2 DA antagonists. This is in agreement with the observations in rodents (see *Introduction*). Furthermore, the study indicates that LY 171.555 and biperiden have the same antagonistic effect in the D_1 dystonia as in the D_2 dystonia. These observations suggest that, with respect to EPS-inducing capacity, the D_1 antagonists do not possess clinical advantages over traditional D_2 antagonist neuroleptics.

The observation of a similar effect of D_1 and D_2 antagonists and the complete antagonistic effect of a D_2 agonist against both the D_1 and D_2-mediated dystonia indicates that the D_1 and D_2 receptors are closely related and interacting (see also Meller et al. 1985; Molloy and Waddington 1985). The exact nature of this interaction is not clarified, but on the basis on new data from a radiation inactivation study at this laboratory, it has been proposed that some DA D_1 receptors are associated with D_2 receptors as two separate molecules coupled to a common third unit (Gredal and Nielsen 1987).

The sedation observed during treatment with a D_2 agonist plus a D_1 antagonist (in contrast to the effect of a D_2 agonist plus a D_2 antagonist) corresponds to results obtained with apomorphine and SCH 23.390 in rats (Gessa et al. 1985). This sedative effect may be caused by SCH 23.390, but it is more likely to be an effect of LY 171.555 on certain D_2 receptors which are not included in the above-mentioned D_1/D_2 receptor complex and therefore are not influenced by the D_1 receptor blocker. As suggested by Gessa et al. (1985), this subpopulation of D_2 receptors may be the DA autoreceptors which have been attributed to the sedation induced by small doses of DA agonists. Perhaps D_1 antagonists could be clinically useful in this context as blockers of certain unwanted effects of D_2 agonists (hyperactivity and stereotypies) allowing disclosure of potential therapeutic effects such as sedation induced by D_2 agonists.

SKF 38.393 was an interesting drug in this study, although some of the effects were less pronounced than the effects of the other drugs. SKF 38.393 slightly decreased reactivity, counteracted hyperactivity and stereotypies induced by LY 171.555, and aggravated dystonia elicited by raclopride. These observations suggest that agonists may have therapeutic properties, perhaps including antipsychotic effects. The oral hyperkinesias developed during SKF 38.393 treatment have to be evaluated more closely.

The DA antagonists induced dystonia and tardive dyskinesia-like hyperkinetic movements. The hyperkinetic movements were particularly obvious when the dystonic features were diminishing. Although the DA antagonist-induced oral hyperkinesia had a different appearance than the tardive dyskinesia in the untreated animal, it included the same movement qualities and appeared to develop in continuation of the preexisting tardive dyskinesia. D_2 DA agonist treatment did not significantly influence the tardive dyskinesia level. These observations suggest that tardive dyskinesia, or at least a form of tardive dyskinesia, is more related to an antidopaminergic treatment (or maybe stimulation of D_1 receptors) than to D_2 receptor supersensitivity and cholinergic hypofunction which may contribute to the syndrome only by decreasing parkinsonism (for further discussion, see Gerlach 1985).

5 Clinical Implications

The observations reported here may have the following clinical implications: (a) Given alone, D_1 antagonists do not appear to have any clinical advantages over the traditional D_2 DA-blocking antipsychotic drugs, but it may be that D_1 antagonists can be used for neutralizing the stimulating activities of D_2 agonists to disclose a sedating effect of these drugs (mediated by a subgroup of D_2 receptors). (b) The antidyskinetic effect of selective D_2 agonists is equal to the effect of traditional anticholinergic drugs, and perhaps selective D_2 agonists could be used to antagonize some extrapyramidal side effects (e.g., akathisia) of neuroleptic drugs. (c) D_1 agonists may potentiate the effects of traditional D_2 blocking neuroleptics and counteract some effects of D_2 agonists. D_1 agonists should, therefore, be tested for antipsychotic effects. (d) Tardive dyskinesia appears to be more related to the blockade of DA receptors (and maybe stimulation of D_1 receptors) than to a stimulation of D_2 receptors.

References

Arnt J (1985) Behavioural stimulation is induced by separate dopamine D-1 and D-2 receptor sites in reserpine-pretreated but not in normal rats. Eur J Pharmacol 113:79–88

Arnt J, Hyttel J (1985) Differential involvement of dopamine D-1 and D-2 receptors in the circling behaviour induced by apomorphine, SK and F 38.393, pergolide and LY 171.555 in 6-hydroxydopamine-lesioned rats. Psychopharmacology (Berlin) 85:346–352

Breese GR, Mueller RA (1985) SCH 23.390 antagonism of a D-2 dopamine agonist depends upon catecholaminergic neurons. Eur J Pharmacol 113:109–114

Christensen AV, Arnt J, Svendsen O (1985) Pharmacological differentiation of dopamine D-1 and D-2 antagonists after single and repeated administration. In: Casey DE, Chase TN, Christensen AV, Gerlach J (eds) Dyskinesia, research and treatment. Psychopharmacology (New York) [Suppl]2:182–190

Gerlach J (1985) Pathophysiological mechanisms underlying tardive dyskinesia. In: Casey DE, Chase TN, Christensen AV, Gerlach J (eds) Dyskinesia, research and treatment. Psychopharmacology (New York) [Suppl]2:98–103

Gessa GL, Porceddu ML, Collu M, Mereu G, Serra M, Ongini E, Biggio G (1985) Sedation and sleep induced by high doses of apomorphine after blockade of D_1 receptors by SCH 23.390. Eur J Pharmacol 109:269–274.

Gredal O, Nielsen M (1987) Binding of ^{3}H-SKF 38.393 to dopamine D-1 receptors in rat striatum in vitro; estimation of receptor molecular size by radiation inactivation. J Neurochem (in press)

Hyttel J, Larsen J-J, Christensen AV, Arnt J (1985) Receptor-binding profiles of neuroleptics. In: Casey DE, Chase TN, Christensen AV, Gerlach J (eds) Dyskinesia, research and treatment. Psychopharmacology (New York) [Suppl]2:9–18

Kebabian JW, Calne DB (1979) Multiple receptors for dopamine. Nature 277:93–96

Korsgaard S, Gerlach J, Christensson E (1985) Behavioral aspects of serotonin-dopamine interaction in the monkey. Eur J Pharmacol 118:245–252

Meller E, Kuga S, Friedhoff AJ, Goldstein M (1985) Selective D_2 dopamine receptor agonists prevent catalepsy induced by SCH 23.390, a selective D_1 antagonist. Life Sci 36:1857–1864

Molloy AG, Waddington JL (1985) Sniffing, rearing and locomotor responses to the D-1 dopamine agonist R-SK&F 38.393 and to apomorphine: differential interactions with the selective D-1 and D-2 antagonists SCH 23.390, and metoclopramide. Eur J Pharmacol 108:305–308

Rosengarten H, Schweitzer JW, Friedhoff AJ (1983) Induction of oral dyskinesias in naive rats by D_1 stimulation. Life Sci 33:2479–2482

Saller CF, Salama AI (1985) Dopamine receptor subtypes: in vivo biochemical evidence for functional interaction. Eur J Pharmacol 109:297–300

Stoof JC, Kebabian JW (1981) Opposing roles for D-1 and D-2 dopamine receptors in efflux of cyclic AMP from rat neostriatum. Nature 294:366–368

Neuroleptic-Induced Parkinsonism Increases with Repeated Treatment in Monkeys

D. E. CASEY

1 Introduction

Neuroleptic-induced extrapyramidal symptoms (dystonia, parkinsonism, and akathisia) are frequent side effect problems in managing acute psychosis. The prevalence of these neurological syndromes varies widely from 2.2%–95% (Sovner and DiMascio 1978). This broad range is undoubtedly influenced by multiple variables, including patient characteristics (age, sex, previous extrapyramidal symptoms), drug parameters (dose, milligram-potency), and temporal aspects (early, intermediate, late) (Keepers et al. 1983; Casey and Keepers 1985; Keepers and Casey 1985). For example, low-milligram high-potency neuroleptics produce more extrapyramidal symptoms than high-milligram low-potency drugs. Drug dosage is also a factor which correlates positively with symptom prevalence and severity. However, even when these factors are kept constant, some patients may develop symptoms while others do not. These differences are currently attributed to variations in individual vulnerability.

The natural history of neuroleptic-induced parkinsonism is a gradual onset in the first few weeks of treatment, with increasing symptoms in the next 2–6 weeks, followed by slow resolution in many patients over the next few months (Ayd 1961; Sovner and DiMascio 1978). However, this tolerance to drug-induced parkinsonism occurs along a continuum; some patients have symptoms fully resolved, and others require extended antiparkinson drug therapy to control these side effects. Current knowledge about the course of this syndrome within a single treatment period has been derived by extrapolating data from several different reports. Because of the clinical exigencies of alleviating side effects, no studies have evaluted neuroleptic-induced parkinsonism in patients whose symptoms were left untreated.

Similarly, very litte is known about the natural history of drug-induced parkinsonism over the long-term course of repeated neuroleptic therapy which has been interrupted by periods of drug discontinuation. Though this is a very common treatment pattern when managing chronic psychosis, the response to drug-induced side effects has not been carefully charted. The absence of data is understandable when one is faced with the realities of conducting such research in the clinical setting. Seldom are the same patients seen, and treated by the same investigators on successive episodes of acute psychosis using the same drug and dosage schedule, and the effects monitored with the same assessment techniques.

VA Medical Center, Portland, OR; Oregon Health Sciences University, Portland, OR, and Oregon Regional Primate Research Center, Portland, OR 97261, USA.

Clinical Pharmacology in Psychiatry
Editors: Dahl, Gram, Paul, Potter
(Psychopharmacology Series 3)

Since virtually no clinical data exist to elucidate whether extrapyramidal symptoms change over many years of treatment, this problem was studied in Cebus monkeys receiving fixed doses of a single neuroleptic over long-term interrupted treatment.

2 Materials and Methods

2.1 Subjects

Eleven male *Cebus albifrons* monkeys 15–18 years old, were tested.

2.2 Drugs

Oral haloperidol 0.25 mg/kg in 30 ml apple juice was given each morning 7 days a week for 2 months. This was followed by 2 months (1 month during and 1 month after oral haloperidol) of periodic dopamine agonist challenges (apomorphine, D-amphetamine, bromocriptine, pergolide) and then 1 month of no drug treatment. Prior to the oral haloperidol, i.m. haloperidol challenges were also tested. This cycle was repeated five times.

2.3 Rating

Parkinsonism was scored twice weekly (3- and 4-day intervals) 24 h after the last oral haloperidol dose. Separate items of tremor, rigidity, and bradykinesia were scored. The rating scale was 0 = normal; 1 = occasionally present; 2 = regularly present; and 3 = continually present.

2.4 Statistics

Group mean scores across the full 2-month period of oral haloperidol were statistically analyzed with the Wilcoxon paired test.

3 Results

The temporal sequence of symptom changes was similar in all treatment cycles. In the first 2 weeks of oral haloperidol, typical bradykinesia, rigidity (a stiff uncurled tail), and occasional parkinsonian tremor developed. Symptoms peaked during the 2nd to 4th week of treatment, and then partially or fully resolved.

With each subsequent cycle, the mean group score significantly increased ($P < 0.01$) from 2.2 ± 0.4 (standard error of the mean, SEM) up to 4.7 ± 0.5. Across the treatment cycles there was an increasingly rapid onset of symptoms with higher peak scores and less symptom resolution. This increase was due to both an increase in the number of animals affected (3/11 = 27% during the first cycle to 8/11 = 73% during the fifth cycle) and an increase in the severity of symptoms in the affected animals.

4 Discussion

The neuroleptic-induced parkinsonian syndrome in non-human primates replicates the patient, drug, and temporal aspects of the clinical syndrome. Some individuals develop symptoms while others do not. Haloperidol, a low-milligram high-potency neuroleptic, reliably produces the classical symptoms of tremor, rigidity, and bradykinesia at clinically relevant doses and prevalence rates. The time course is also similar, with initial onset in the 2nd week of treatment, increasing symptoms in the first few months, and gradual partial or full resolution of symptoms.

This study delineates in monkeys the time course of parkinsonian symptoms within a treatment cycle which has only been approximated in patients. The dynamically changing course of symptoms in monkeys is particularly relevant in the phase where tolerance to drug-induced parkinsonism develops. This parallels the widely held but seldom studied belief that tolerance to extrapyramidal syndromes also occurs in the clinical setting and may correlate with the observation that antiparkinson agents can eventually be discontinued in some patients who required them earlier to control drug-induced side effects (DiMascio and Demirgian 1970; Klett and Caffey 1972; Casey et al. 1981). However, the decreasing tolerance to neuroleptic-induced parkinsonism over repeated treatment cycles in monkeys may also support the observation that some patients continue to require maintenance antiparkinson drugs for neurological side effects (Rifkin et al. 1975; Casey et al. 1981).

The increasing sensitivity to parkinsonism with repeated neuroleptic treatment was both clinically and statistically significant. This phenomenon has only rarely been assessed in the clinic. One study testing two different dosing schedules of a neuroleptic in the same patients also reported that during the second treatment period increased extrapyramidal symptoms were more difficult to manage, even though this treatment phase used the lower neuroleptic dose (Simpson and Laska 1968). Inability to study the natural history of symptoms in patients is legitimately limited by the need to manage treatment-emergent neurological syndromes. A relevant study would require that the same investigators assess the same patients with the same procedures at the initial and repeated episodes of acute psychoses which are managed with the same drug and dosage schedule. Furthermore, a prohibition against antiparkinson drugs, either prophylactically or when symptoms develop, is highly unlikely and clinically unreasonable. However, this phenomenon could be studied in treatment settings with stable patient populations receiving interrupted neuroleptic therapy. Other intervening variables, such as other drug types and dosage, could be used consistently or statistically controlled for across treatment periods.

It is also possible that the additional drug exposure these monkeys received (periodic dopamine agonist challenges) produced the increased sensitivity to parkinsonism. This is doubtful, though, because other studies with only parenteral or oral administration of haloperidol or other pharmacological classes of neuroleptics (chlorpromazine, fluphenazine) have shown similar increasing sensitivity to acute dystonia (Paulson 1973; Gunne and Barany 1976; Weiss et al. 1977; Casey et al. 1980; Neale et al. 1982; Kovacic and Domino 1984; Porsolt 1984).

In these studies increased symptom severity correlated positively with longer periods of drug exposure. Therefore, this related neuroleptic-induced extrapyramidal syndrome of parkinsonism is also most probably due primarily to increasing periods of drug exposure.

If this clinical syndrome of increasing sensitization to neurological side effects does occur in the clinic it must be more carefully studied. Monitoring of such parameters, as is in progress in this prospective study, will provide answers to the current question of whether vulnerability to drug-induced parkinsonism and other extrapyramidal syndromes is a predictor of the eventual development of tardive dyskinesia. The results of these investigations indicate that prior neuroleptic treatment influences the response to subsequent treatment, and that these findings need to be incorporated in our explanations of the long-term effects of neuroleptics in patients.

5 Conclusions

The natural course of neuroleptic-induced parkinsonism is poorly understood, in part because antiparkinson medications are initiated when symptoms develop. Furthermore, virtually no clinical data are available to elucidate whether the parkinsonian syndrome changes over many years of treatment in patients starting and stopping neuroleptic drugs.

The results reported here suggest that prior neuroleptic treatment strongly influences the expression of drug-induced parkinsonism in subsequent treatment, and has implications for considering interrupted versus continuous neuroleptic therapy.

Acknowledgments. This research was supported in part by funds from the Veterans Administration, National Institute of Mental Health Grant MH36657, and Core Grant RR-00163 at the Oregon Regional Primate Research Center. Haloperidol was supplied by McNeil Laboratories. Marian Karr prepared the typescript.

References

Ayd FJ (1961) A survey of drug-induced extrapyramidal reactions. JAMA 75:1054–1060

Casey DE, Gerlach J, Christensson E (1980) Dopamine, acetylcholine, and GABA effects in acute dystonia in primates. Psychopharmacology (Berlin) 70:83–87

Casey DE, Clappison VJ, Keepers GA (1981) Anticholinergics in acute extrapyramidal symptoms. (Abstract) Proc American Psychiatric Association 22D:50

DiMascio A, Demirgian E (1970) Antiparkinson drug overuse. Psychosomatics 11:596–601

Gunne LM, Barany S (1976) Haloperidol-induced tardive dyskinesia in monkeys. Psychopharmacology (Berlin) 50:237–240

Keepers GA, Casey DE (1985) Clinical management of acute neuroleptic-induced extrapyramidal syndromes. In: Masserman JH (ed) Current psychiatric therapies. Grune and Stratton, New York

Keepers GA, Clappison VJ, Casey DE (1983) Initial anticholinergic prophylaxis for neuroleptic-induced extrapyramidal syndromes. Arch Gen Psychiatry 40:1113–1117

Klett CJ, Caffey E (1972) Evaluating the long-term need for antiparkinson drugs by chronic schizophrenics. Arch Gen Psychiatry 26:374–379

Kovacic B, Domino EF (1984) Fluphenazine-induced acute and tardive dyskinesias in monkeys. Psychopharmacology (Berlin) 84:310–314
Neale R, Gerhardt S, Fallon S, Liebman JM (1982) Progressive changes in the acute dyskinetic syndrome as a function of repeated elicitation in squirrel monkeys. Psychopharmacology (Berlin) 77:223–228
Paulson GW (1973) Dyskinesias in monkeys. In: Chase TN, Paulson GW (eds) Advances in neurology, vol 1. Raven, New York, pp 647–650
Porsolt R (1984) Lack of tolerance to haloperidol-induced acute dyskinesias in rhesus monkeys. Psychopharmacology (Berlin) 82:145–146
Rifkin A, Quitkin F, Klein DF (1975) Akinesia: a poorly recognized drug-induced extrapyramidal behavioral disorder. Arch Gen Psychiatry 32:672–674
Simpson GM, Laska E (1968) Sensitivity to a phenothiazine (butaperazine). Can Psychiatr Assoc J 13:499–505
Sovner R, DiMascio A (1978) Extrapyramidal syndromes and other neurological side effects of psychotropic drugs. In: Lipton MA, DiMascio A, Killam KF (eds) Psychopharmacology: a generation of progress. Raven, New York, pp 1021–1032
Weiss B, Santelli S, Lusink G (1977) Movement disorders induced in monkeys by chronic haloperidol treatment. Psychopharmacology (Berlin) 53:289–293

Biochemical Alterations Produced by Neuroleptics in Man: Studies of Plasma Homovanillic Acid in Schizophrenic Patients

D. Pickar, O. M. Wolkowitz, R. Labarca, A. R. Doran, A. Breier, and S. M. Paul

1 Introduction

Despite the enormous growth of neuroscience over recent decades, neuroleptic drugs remain overwhelmingly the most important pharmacological treatment for schizophrenia and psychosis in general. The understanding that these antipsychotic agents block dopamine neurotransmission was first suggested by the observation by Carlsson and Lindqvist (1963) that dopamine (DA) metabolites markedly increase in the brain following the acute administration of neuroleptic. The hypothesis that the antipsychotic actions of neuroleptics are linked to this inhibition of dopamine neurotransmission is most strongly supported by the close correlations observed between the binding affinities of a series of neuroleptic drugs for non-adenylcyclase-linked DA (D_2) receptors in rat (Creese et al. 1976; Seeman et al. 1976) and human brains (Richelson and Nelson 1984) and their antipsychotic potencies. An apparent weakness of this hypothesis, however, is the discrepancy between the rapid onset of DA receptor blockade, which occurs within hours following neuroleptic administration, and the delay, usually weeks, necessary to achieve maximum therapeutic effects (Baldessarini 1980). It has now been shown by means of biochemical and electrophysiological techniques that the enhancement of DA turnover which follows acute neuroleptic administration is reversed during chronic administration in nigrostriatal and mesolimbic DA neurons (Roth 1983; Bunney 1984). Mesocortical DA neurons, however, differ as they show diminished responsivity to both DA agonists and antagonists, a phenomenon it is thought may be related to a lack of autoreceptors (Bannon and Roth 1983).

In vivo correlates of DA receptor blockade, including neuroleptic-induced increases in plasma levels of prolactin or in circulating levels of neuroleptics measured by their affinity for the DA receptor using a radioreceptor assay, have been only weak predictors of neuroleptic response (Meltzer et al. 1983). Levels of CSF homovanillic acid (HVA) have been shown to increase during neuroleptic treatment (Bowers 1973; Sedvall et al. 1974) with time-dependent decreases toward baseline (Post and Goodwin 1975), an inconsistent correlate of neuroleptic response (Bowers and Heninger 1981). The potential use of plasma HVA to monitor changes in brain HVA has been suggested by a series of animal indicating that a portion of circulating levels of HVA are derived from brain pools (Bacopoulos

Section on Clinical Studies, Clinical Neuroscience Branch, National Institute of Mental Health, NIH Bldg 10, Rm 4N214, 9000 Rockville Pike, Bethesda, MD 20892, USA.

Clinical Pharmacology in Psychiatry
Editors: Dahl, Gram, Paul, Potter
(Psychopharmacology Series 3)

et al. 1979; Sternberg et al. 1983; Kendler et al. 1982). The contribution of brain HVA to levels in plasma has been suggested to be in the range of 30%–40% in rodents (Bacopoulos et al. 1979; Sternberg et al. 1983). Similar estimates have been made for humans in studies using debrisoquin, a peripherally acting MAO inhibitor which diminishes the peripheral and enhances the brain contribution to circulating levels of HVA (Swann et al. 1980). The notion that longitudinal measurement of levels of plasma HVA may provide clues to neuroleptic-DA interactions is further suggested by animal experiments in which plasma levels of HVA change in parallel with HVA in brain following pharmacological interventions including neuroleptic administration (Kendler et al. 1982).

In an initial report (Pickar et al. 1984) we observed that the neuroleptic, fluphenazine, produced a time-dependent decrease in levels of plasma HVA in eight schizophrenic patients. Our observation that the course of this decrease closely paralleled the development of antipsychotic effects suggested the possibility that this time-delayed decrease in DA "turnover" might be related to the antipsychotic properties of these drugs. In subsequent studies (Pickar et al. 1985), presented in an abbreviated form in this chapter, we have examined the effects of neuroleptic discontinuation and neuroleptic treatment on plasma levels of HVA in a larger group of schizophrenic patients and have examined neuroleptic-induced changes in levels of plasma HVA as predictors of clinical response to treatment.

2 Methods

17 patients (8 males, 9 females; mean ± SEM age: 25 ± 2.5 years) meeting DSM-III (1980) criteria for schizophrenia, and free from any medical illness, granted written informed consent to participate in this study. All subjects were hospitalized on the 4-East research unit of the NIH Clinical Center and were maintained on a low-monoamine, caffeine-restricted diet beginning at least 2 weeks before and extending throughout this study. Blood was collected three times per week by venipuncture in EDTA-containing tubes between 0730 and 0930 h following an overnight fast, and all patients were at restricted activity until collection was complete. Plasma, obtained within 30 min of collection by centrifuging whole blood, was stored at −20 °C until assay. Plasma-free HVA was assayed by high-pressure liquid chromatography with electrochemical detection (Chang et al. 1983); inter-assay and intra-assay variability were 6.3% and 2.2%, respectively. Physicians blind to treatment conditions performed weekly ratings of psychopathology using the Brief Psychiatric Rating Scale (BPRS) (Overall and Gorham 1961) (including positive and negative symptom clusters), Bunney Hamburg Global Psychosis Ratings (Bunney and Hamburg 1963), and the Abrams and Taylor Scale for Emotional Blunting (ATRS) (Abrams and Taylor 1978). A mean of nurses' daily psychosis ratings from the day prior to and the day of blood collection was used for analysis when levels of plasma HVA for individual blood collections were analyzed; when mean weekly levels of plasma HVA were examined, physicians' weekly ratings were used.

There were two phases of this study, a neuroleptic withdrawal phase in 11 subjects and a neuroleptic treatment phase in 16 patients. In the former phase a neuroleptic which had been administered continuously for at least 6 months prior to study was first substituted by fluphenazine upon hospital admission; after at least 3 weeks at a stable dose of fluphenazine (mean ± SEM 29.5 ± 3.6 mg per day) placebo was substituted and maintained for 5 weeks. In the neuroleptic treatment phase fluphenazine was administered after an extended drug-free period (mean ± SEM drug-free days 34 ± 6). The dosage of fluphenazine was adjusted on a clinical basis and maximum doses (30.3 ± 5 mg per day) were achieved within the first 10 days of treatment and continued throughout the study. Benztropine (1.0–3.0 mg per day) was added as required to treat extrapyramidal effects.

3 Results

3.1 Group Effects

As shown in Fig. 1 both neuroleptic withdrawal and neuroleptic treatment produced time-dependent changes in levels of plasma HVA ($F=4.31$, $P<0.01$, $df=5{,}50$; $F=6.59$, $P<0.001$, $df=15{,}75$, respectively), neuroleptic withdrawal being associated with gradual increases and neuroleptic treatment with decreased levels of plasma HVA. Levels of plasma HVA for all data points (3 per week) and corresponding daily nurses' psychosis ratings during neuroleptic treatment are highly correlated ($r=0.89$, $P<0.001$), as shown in Fig. 2. A similar correlation is seen between levels of plasma HVA and nurses' ratings from all data points during neuroleptic withdrawal ($r=0.81$, $P<0.001$) (data not shown).

3.2 Individual Differences

Good correlations were observed between mean weekly levels of plasma HVA in individual patients and their psychosis ratings during both placebo treatment and

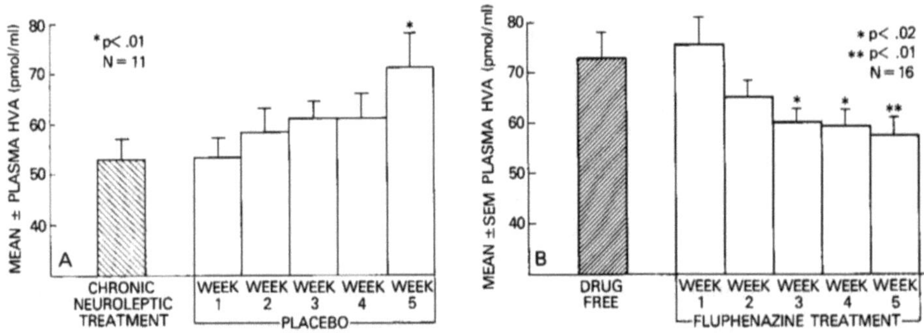

Fig. 1. A Time-dependent increases in mean weekly levels of plasma HVA following discontinuation of chronic neuroleptic treatment; value during 5th week of placebo was significantly greater than baseline ($P<0.01$). **B** Fluphenazine-induced time-dependent decrease in mean weekly levels of plasma HVA; levels at weeks 3, 4, and 5 of fluphenazine-treatment were significantly below baseline ($P<0.02$; $P<0.01$, respectively) and below those at 1st week of fluphenazine treatment ($P<0.01$; $P<0.01$; $P<0.01$). (Pickar et al. 1985)

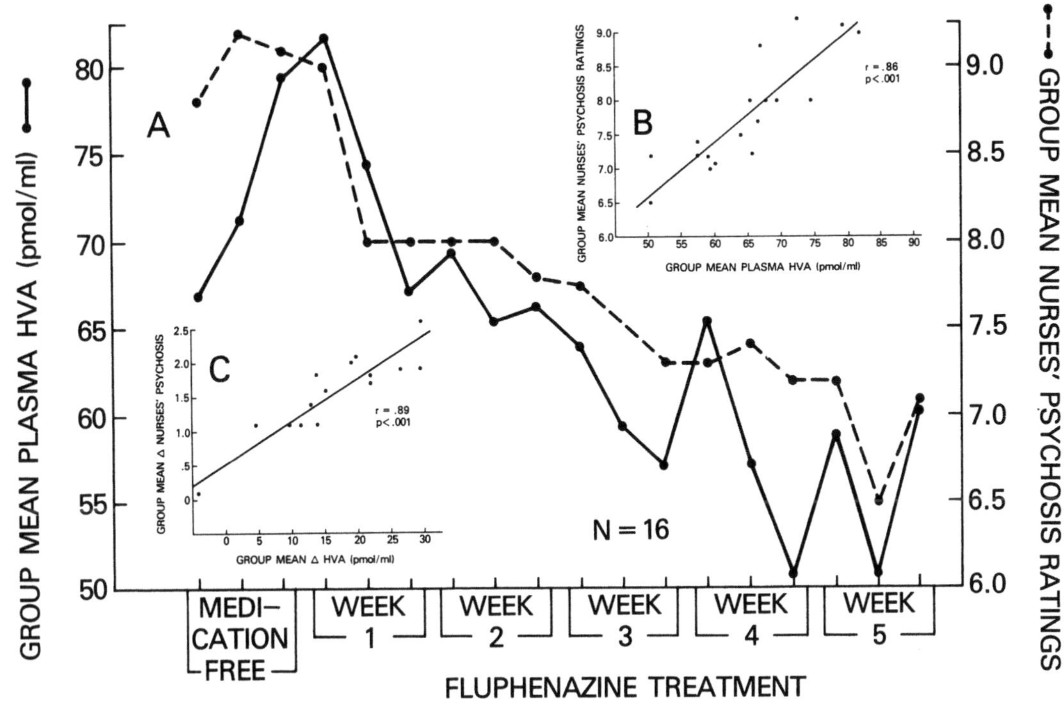

Fig. 2 A–C. Levels of plasma HVA and nurses' psychosis ratings (**A**) and their correlations (**B** and C) during fluphenazine treatment

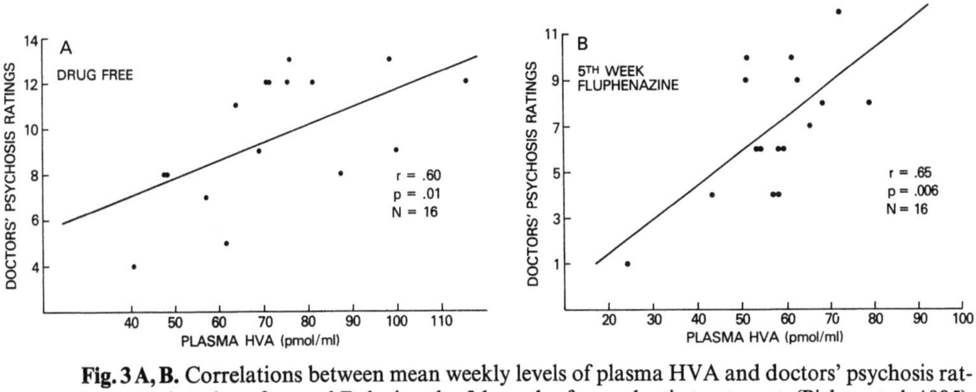

Fig. 3 A, B. Correlations between mean weekly levels of plasma HVA and doctors' psychosis ratings: **A** when drug-free and **B** during the 5th week of neuroleptic treatment. (Pickar et al. 1985)

the 5th week of neuroleptic treatment (Fig. 3 a, b). Moreover, increases in levels of plasma HVA associated with neuroleptic withdrawal (chronic neuroleptic treatment baseline minus value at 5th drug-free week) and neuroleptic-induced decreases (drug-free baseline minus value at 5th week of fluphenazine treatment) were correlated with corresponding changes in ratings of psychopathology, including changes in negative symptoms (Table 1). Thus, the greater the increase in levels of plasma HVA after withdrawal of the neuroleptic, the more severe was

Table 1. Correlation between change in mean weekly levels of plasma *HVA* and change in clinical ratings[a]

	Neuroleptic withdrawal ($n=11$)		Neuroleptic treatment ($n=16$)	
	r	P^b	r	P^b
Doctors' global psychosis	0.77	0.005	0.49	0.05
BPRS				
Total	0.76	0.007	0.44	0.09
Positive symptoms	0.61	0.05	0.40	NS
Negative symptoms	0.44	NS	0.33	NS
ATRS emotional blunting				
Total	0.84	0.001	0.68	0.003

[a] Change for plasma *HVA* and clinical variables obtained by subtracting values at week 5 from those at baseline week for both conditions.
[b] Two-tailed probability.

the exacerbation of symptoms. Similarly, the greater the decrease in plasma HVA levels associated with neuroleptic treatment the better was the clinical response.

Age, sex, and dose of neuroleptic (prior to discontinuation or at 5 weeks of treatment) were all unrelated to baseline levels of plasma HVA and to the change in plasma HVA associated with either neuroleptic administration or withdrawal. BPRS items, "motor retardation," and "motor hyperactivity" were not significantly correlated with levels of plasma HVA, whether drug-free or during the 5th week of fluphenazine treatment, suggesting that, in contrast to studies of enhanced physical activity in normal subjects (Kendler et al. 1983), ambient motor activity did not appear to be a major determinant of plasma HVA levels.

4 Comments

Results from this study support our earlier finding of neuroleptic-induced time-dependent decreases in levels of plasma HVA in schizophrenic patients. These data also extend our observations to include time-dependent increases in levels of plasma HVA following discontinuation of chronic neuroleptic treatment. The good group correlations between levels of plasma HVA and corresponding psychosis ratings during both treatment condition changes are consistent with the hypothesis that the antipsychotic effects of neuroleptics may be related to slow-to-develop changes in DA turnover. The correlations between absolute levels of plasma HVA and psychotic symptoms, both when patients were drug-free and during neuroleptic treatment, are similar to some findings reported by Davis et al. (1985) and support the postulate that higher dopaminergic function is related to greater psychotic symptoms in schizophrenic patients. These data, however, do not necessarily indicate an overall hyper-dopaminergic state in schizophrenia.

Our observation that patients with greater decreases and increases in levels of plasma HVA, respectively, experienced better antipsychotic response to neuroleptic administration and more severe exacerbation of symptoms following neuroleptic discontinuation, suggests the possibility that the monitoring of changes in plasma HVA may prove to be a clinically useful marker for neuroleptic effects. Consistent with these findings, Bowers et al. (1984) have reported that psychotic patients in a general hospital setting who experienced a better short-term response to haloperidol treatment were those in whom levels of plasma HVA were elevated at baseline and showed marked decreases during treatment.

Fluphenazine-induced time-dependent decreases in levels of plasma HVA in schizophrenic patients share some similarities with the effects of chronic neuroleptic treatment on CNS DA system activity in preclinical studies. In contrast to studies of DA metabolism in animal brain, however, we observed that chronic neuroleptic treatment reduced levels of plasma HVA below pretreatment baseline. It is unknown whether this pattern is unique to schizophrenic patients and, thus, linked to psychosis and/or the antipsychotic response, or rather is a pharmacological response observable in non-psychotic psychiatric patients or in normal controls. Moreover, plasma levels of HVA comprise both CNS and peripheral contributions, with the origins of the latter including the sympathetic nervous system, adrenal medulla, carotid body and kidney. It is not known whether peripherally- or centrally-derived HVA (or both) account for the good correlations between plasma HVA and symptomatology observed in our patients. Debrisoquine administration to enhance the CNS HVA "signal" may help to address this issue. In contrast to plasma HVA, levels of CSF HVA are markedly increased following short-term neuroleptic treatment with return to baseline during chronic administration in some, but not all, patients (Bowers and Heninger 1981). The reasons for the differences between plasma and CSF HVA response to neuroleptic treatment are unexplained, although unequal contributions of the different CNS DA systems to levels of HVA in the CSF may be involved.

In summary, our data suggest that the longitudinal measurement of plasma HVA may represent a promising biochemical correlate of psychosis and neuroleptic response in schizophrenia. Ongoing studies including larger numbers of subjects, different neuroleptics and controlled dose changes will be important to evaluate the clinical applicability of this methodology.

References

Abrams R, Taylor MA (1978) A rating scale for emotional blunting. Am J Psychiatry 135:226–229

Bacopoulos NG, Hattox SE, Roth RH (1979) 3,4-dihydroxyphenylacetic acid and homovanillic acid in rat plasma: possible indicators of central dopaminergic activity. Eur J Pharmacol 56:225–236

Baldessarini RJ (1980) Drugs and the treatment of psychiatric disorders. In: Gilman AG, Goodman LS, Gilman A (eds) The pharmacologic basis of therapeutics. McMillan, New York, pp 391–447

Bannon MJ, Roth RH (1983) Pharmacology of mesocortical dopamine neurons. Pharmacol Rev 35:53–68

Bowers MB Jr (1973) 5-HIAA and HVA following probenecid in acute psychotic patients treated with phenothiazines. Psychopharmacologia 28:309–312

Bowers MB, Heninger GR (1981) Cerebrospinal fluid homovanillic acid patterns during neuroleptic treatment. Psychiatry Res 4:285–290
Bowers MB, Swigar ME, Jatlow PI, Goicoecha N (1984) Plasma catecholamine metabolites and early response to haloperidol. J Clin Psychiatry 6:284–251
Bunney BS (1984) Antipsychotic drug effects on the electrical activity of dopaminergic neurons. Trends Neurosci 7:212–215
Bunney WE Jr, Hamburg DA (1963) Methods for reliable longitudinal observation of behavior. Arch Gen Psychiatry 9:280–294
Carlsson A, Lindqvist M (1963) Effect of chlorpromazine or haloperidol on formation of 3-methoxytyramine and normetanephrine in mouse brain. Acta Pharmacol Toxicol 20:140–144
Chang WH, Sheinin M, Burns RS, Linnoila M (1983) Rapid and simple determination of homovanillic acid in plasma using high performance liquid chromatography with electrochemical detection. Acta Pharmacol Toxicol 53:275–279
Creese I, Burt DR, Snyder SH (1976) Dopamine receptor binding predicts clinical and pharmacologic potencies of antischizophrenic drugs. Science 192:481–483
Davis KL, Davidson M, Mohs RC, Kendler KS, Davis BM, Johns CA, DeNegris Y, Horvath TG (1985) Plasma homovanillic acid concentrations and the severity of schizophrenic illness. Science 227:1601–1602
Diagnostic and Statistical Manual of Mental Disorders, 3rd edn (1980) American Psychiatric Association, Washington, DC
Kendler KS, Heninger GR, Roth RH (1982) Influence of dopamine agonists on plasma and brain levels of homovanillic acid. Life Sci 30:2063–2069
Kendler KS, Mohs RC, Davis KL (1983) The effects of diet and physical activity on plasma homovanillic acid in normal human subjects. Psychiatry Res 8:215–223
Meltzer HY, Kane JM, Kalakowska T (1983) Plasma levels of neuroleptics, prolactin levels, and clinical response. In: Coyle JT, Enna SJ (eds) Neuroleptics, neurochemical, behavioral and clinical perspectives. Raven, New York, pp 255–279
Overall JE, Gorham DE (1961) The brief psychiatric rating scale. Psychol Rep 10:799–812
Pickar D, Labarca R, Linnoila M, Roy A, Hommer D, Everett D, Paul SM (1984) Neuroleptic-induced decrease in plasma homovanillic acid and antipsychotic activity in schizophrenic patients. Science 225:957–957
Pickar D, Labarca R, Doran AR, Wolkowitz OM, Roy A, Breier A, Linnoila M, Paul SM (1985) Longitudinal measurement of plasma homovanillic acid levels in schizophrenic patients: correlation with psychosis and response to neuroleptic treatment. Arch Gen Psychiatry 43:669–676
Post RM, Goodwin FK (1975) Time-dependent effects of phenothiazines on dopamine turnover in psychiatric patients. Science 190:488–499
Richelson E, Nelson A (1984) Antagonism by neuroleptics of neurotransmitter receptors of normal human brain in vitro. Eur J Pharmacol 103:197–204
Roth RH (1983) Neuroleptics: functional neurochemistry. In: Coyle JT, Enna SJ (eds) Neuroleptics: neurochemical, behavioral and clinical perspectives. Raven, New York, pp 119–156
Sedvall G, Fyro B, Nyback H, Wiesel FH, Wode-Helgodt B (1974) Mass fragmentographic determinations of HVA in lumbar CSF of schizophrenic patients during treatment with antipsychotic drugs. J Psychiatry Res 11:75–80
Seeman P, Lee T, Chau-Wong M, Wong K (1976) Antipsychotic drug doses and neuroleptic/dopamine receptors. Nature 261:717–719
Sternberg DE, Heninger GR, Roth RH (1983) Plasma homovanillic acid as an index of brain dopamine metabolism: enhancement with debrisoquin. Life Sci 32:2447–2452
Swann AC, Maas JW, Hattox SE, Landis H (1980) Catecholamine metabolites in human plasma as indices of brain function: effects of debrisoquin. Life Sci 27:1857–1862

Effect of Neuroleptics on the Schizophrenic Syndrome

H. Y. Meltzer

1 Introduction

Neuroleptics have been the main form of treatment of schizophrenia since their introduction three decades ago. Their use in thousands of clinical studies has provided extensive data with which to evaluate their contribution to the treatment of the schizophrenic syndrome. The evidence for their effectiveness in treating some aspects of the schizophrenic syndrome, e.g., positive symptoms such as delusions and hallucinations, and prevention of relapse and rehospitalization in a large percentage of schizophrenics is unequivocal (Lipton and Burnett 1979). It is also clear that these agents do not completely alleviate delusions and hallucinations in many schizophrenics or have any effect on them in others, and that many aspects of the schizophrenic syndrome, e.g., negative symptoms such as withdrawal, flat affect and avolition are not as effectively treated by neuroleptics as are positive symptoms (Meltzer 1985).

1.1 The Two-Syndrome Model Versus Psychosocial Factors

Crow (1980a, b) has suggested that negative symptomatology, embracing the essential characteristics of what he refers to as the type II syndrome of schizophrenia "predicts poor long-term outcome irrespective of drug treatment." Crow believes that negative symptoms result mainly from irreversible structural changes in the nervous system, the evidence for which is supplied by the dilated ventricles and cerebral atrophy apparent in some computed tomography (CT) scan studies (Johnstone et al. 1976). This view has been challenged (Meltzer 1985) on the basis of nonspecificity of enlarged ventricles for schizophrenia (Pearlson and Veroff 1981) and lack of relationship to negative symptoms (Nasrallah et al. 1982).

In contrast with Crow's view of the etiology of negative symptoms, social psychiatrists have long attributed aspects of this behavioral pattern to chronic institutionalization or its equivalent. This position has recently been articulated by Ciompi (1984), who proposed that the residual states, characterized by negative-unproductive symptoms, depend more on psychosocial influences than on biological factors. According to Ciompi, the need to limit stress with which the schizophrenic individual cannot cope leads to negative symptomatology. Ciompi (1984)

Case Westen Reserve University School of Medicine, 2040 Abington Road, Cleveland, OH 44106, USA.

Clinical Pharmacology in Psychiatry
Editors: Dahl, Gram, Paul, Potter
(Psychopharmacology Series 3)

reported that the defect state only affects about 20% of the schizophrenic cases he studied (Ciompi and Mueller 1976) and that marked improvement may occur in some cases, irrespective of drug treatment, presumably due to optimal psychosocial conditions. Huber et al. (1980), Bleuler (1974), Nyman and Jonsson (1983), Johnstone et al. (1984), Kolakowska et al. (1985), and Watts (1985) have also examined the long-term outcome of schizophrenia and noted that in as many as 30% of a large series of schizophrenic patients the outcome can be good, without negative or regressive symptoms. It is impossible, however, to conclude from these studies that neuroleptic treatment is of any importance in the prevention of the defect state. Most of the patients in these studies were probably administered neuroleptics during the acute psychotic phases of their illness as well as intermittently between episodes. In the absence of placebo control and random assignment, we cannot conclude that good (or poor) outcome occurred because of neuroleptics. We can with some certainty conclude that 70%–80% of schizophrenics have a fair to poor outcome or worse despite neuroleptic treatment.

1.2 Interaction Between Neuroleptics and Psychosocial Factors

In between the view of strict biological determinism and neuroleptic-insensitivity of the defect state on the one hand, and psychosocial factors as the sole determinant of the defect state on the other, stands the evidence of an interaction between neuroleptic drugs and psychosocial factors. The NIMH-PSC Collaborative Study Group demonstrated a potent interaction between neuroleptic efficacy and ward environment, specifying such factors as type of hospital, patient-to-staff ratio, and ward clinical policy as important determinants of neuroleptic efficacy (Kellam et al. 1967; Moos and Schwartz 1972). Other investigators have questioned these findings, however (Erickson 1975; Lehman et al. 1982). More recently, studies of "expressed emotion," i.e., critical comments and overinvolvement by family members, have shown strong interactions with neuroleptic action (Brown et al. 1972; Leff et al. 1983). Wing (1982) has aptly summarized this field in the following way: "The better the environmental conditions, the less the need for (neuroleptic) medication. The poorer the social milieu, the greater the need (or at least the use) of drugs." This dictum related to long-stay schizophrenics, the patients most likely to manifest the defect state. Wing (1978) also proposed that the same relationship held for acute psychotic phases of schizophrenia. This concept rests on the notion that schizophrenia is due to a condition of overstimulation, perhaps due to a defect in the ability to limit sensory input or to "gate" it to appropriate brain regions at appropriate intensities.

Other evidence supporting the thesis that the interaction of psychosocial factors and neuroleptic drugs is of importance in considering the effect of neuroleptic drugs is available from studies which compare treatment response or relapse rate in various environments. Thus, the International Pilot Study of Schizophrenia (World Helath Organization 1979) demonstrated that the outcome for schizophrenics was better in developing countries than in developed countries and that the predictors of outcome for developed countries were less effective for developing than developed countries. On the other hand, Pietzcker and Gaebel (1983) demonstrated that the relapse rates for neuroleptic-treated schizophrenics were not significantly different in a rural German area than in Berlin. However, the rehospitalization rate in Berlin was 40%, as against 14% in the rural areas, no doubt reflecting the greater availability of beds in Berlin as well as differences in family support.

It is apparent from the literature already reviewed in this article that not all schizophrenics have a deteriorating course and that schizophrenia may show considerable remission, either spontaneously or in response to neuroleptic medication. However, the assertion by Crow (1980 a, b) that the defect state is not sensitive to neuroleptic drug treatment requires closer scrutiny because it has major theoretical and practical effects. Firstly, it is a major piece of evidence for his two-syndrome theory of schizophrenia which has had great influence on current research approaches. It is now fairly routine to characterize patients as type I or II in research reports. There is evidence from twin studies that the presence of negative symptoms is more characteristic of schizophrenia in which there is a genetic influence (Dworkin and Lenzenweger 1984). If so, neuroleptic-non-responsiveness would indicate that the dopaminergic component of schizophrenia is not what is inherited. Secondly, the belief in neuroleptic-insensitivity of the defect state has led to therapeutic nihilism with regard to the treatment of negative symptoms with currently available neuroleptics. The evidence for and against the view that neuroleptics do not affect negative symptoms will be reviewed, and some of our own data bearing on this issue will presented.

2 Responsiveness to Neuroleptic Treatment

2.1 Evidence Against Negative Symptom Responsiveness to Neuroleptic Treatment

The evidence cited by Crow (1980 a) for the unresponsiveness of negative symptoms to neuroleptics was: (a) the ineffectiveness of *cis*-flupenthixol for the treatment of negative compared to positive symptoms (Johnstone et al. 1978); and (b) the study of Angrist et al. (1980), in which negative symptoms were less affected by neuroleptic treatment for 1–6 weeks, or by the administration of 0.5 mg/kg D-amphetamine in a drug-free state, than were positive symptoms. On close examination this evidence does not appear persuasive (see also Mackay 1980; Ashcroft et al. 1981). Firstly, in the study from Crow's group (Johnstone et al. 1978), 45 patients were randomly assigned to one of three treatments: *cis*-flupenthixol, *trans*-flupenthixol (which lacks significant DA receptor blocking properties at the dose used) and placebo. Thus, there were only 15 patients in each group. This may be an insufficient number of subjects to detect a drug effect. Secondly, virtually no information was given as to the subject's age, duration of illness or number of previous episodes. These factors can strongly influence the response of negative symptoms to neuroleptic treatment (Meltzer, unpublished data). Thirdly, the dose of *cis*-flupenthixol, 6–9 mg/day, is relatively low. Fourthly, patients were evaluated after only 28 days. Negative symptoms may require longer periods of treatment (Goldberg et al. 1965). A fifth, and perhaps the most important, critique of this study is that the mean initial rating of negative symptoms in the three groups of subjects was approximately 1, out of a maximum of 4. In addition, only two negative symptoms were examined and these were examined separately rather than as part of a subscale. By contrast, positive symptoms were near maximal for the scale used, suggesting that the sample included a number of patients experiencing severe acute exacerbations, with few negative symptoms.

The other study cited by Crow (1980 b), that of Angrist et al. (1980), utilized the withdrawal-retardation factor of the BPRS (Overall and Gorham 1962) to assess change in negative symptoms. Neither neuroleptic treatment nor D-amphetamine had any effect on its components, motor retardation and blunted affect; however, the emotional withdrawal item did improve with neuroleptic treatment, while it worsened with D-amphetamine, suggesting it might be affected by changes in dopaminergic activity.

2.2 Evidence for Negative Symptom Responsiveness to Neuroleptic Treatment

Review of the literature on negative symptoms and neuroleptic treatment in schizophrenia reveals considerable evidence indicating that such clinical symptoms as: (a) flat affect; poverty of thought and speech content; (b) indifference to environment; (c) impaired social participation; and (d) slowed speech and movements, do respond to neuroleptic treatment in a significant proportion of schizophrenic patients at various phases of their illness (Meltzer 1985). Four types of evidence support the above conclusions: (a) the NIMH Collaborative Study of the effect of phenothiazines (Golberg et al. 1965); (b) the effect of pimozide and other diphenylbutylpiperidine (DPBP) neuroleptics on negative symptoms; (c) the effect of clozapine on negative symptoms; and (d) the effect of sulpiride on negative symptoms. This will be briefly reviewed.

2.2.1 The NIMH Collaborative Study

Goldberg et al. (1965) randomly assigned 340 acute schizophrenic patients to placebo, chlorpromazine (CPZ), thioridazine or fluphenazine. The duration of treatment was 6 weeks and the dose was equivalent to 650 mg per day CPZ. The major rating instrument was the Ward Behavior Rating Scale (WBRS; Burdock et al. 1960) and the Inpatient Multidimensional Psychiatric Rating Scale (IMPS; Lorr et al. 1963). Ratings were done blindly. Drug-treated patients showed significantly more improvement than placebo-treated patients in such prima facie negative symptoms as hebephrenic symptoms, social participation, indifference to environment, and slowed speech and movement. It must be noted that 50% of the patients in the NIMH Collaborative study were experiencing their first psychotic episode, 60% were experiencing their first hospitalization, and a high proportion had an acute onset following a precipitating event. Thus, this study does not specifically bear upon the issue of the responsiveness of negative symptoms to neuroleptic treatment in the most chronic patients.

2.2.2 Diphenylbutylpiperidine (DPBP) Neuroleptic Drugs

There have been a variety of controlled and uncontrolled comparisons involving in the aggregate large numbers of schizophrenic patients, in which pimozide, clopimozide, fluspiriline, and penfluridol, all of which are DPBP-type drugs, have been compared to phenothiazines or butyrophenones with regard to the overall efficacy as antipsychotic drugs and the ability to diminish negative and positive symptoms (Kudo 1972; Singh 1973; Gallant et al. 1974; Lapierre and Lavalle 1975; Shopsin et al. 1977; Lapierre 1978; Frangos et al. 1978; Haas and Beckmann 1982). A large proportion of these studies revealed significant advantages, or trends, suggesting that the DPBP drugs produce greater improvement than other types of neuroleptics in emotional withdrawal, anergia, blunted affect and social interaction, while having equivalent efficacy in treating positive symptoms. For example, Haas and Beckmann (1982) treated 15 schizophrenics with haloperidol (40–60 mg per day) or pimozide (40–60 mg per day) for 30 days. Two-thirds of the patients in both groups had a good or very good response but only the pimozide-treated patients had a significant decrease in emotional withdrawal and blunted affect on the BPRS. Further controlled study of pimozide vs non-DPBP neuroleptics with more sophisticated means of assessing negative symptoms would be of interest. Gould et al. (1983) recently proposed that the greater ability of DPBP drugs to diminish negative symptoms might be related to their greater potency in blocking calcium channels. This is an intriguing suggestion but there is no direct evidence to support this as yet.

2.2.3 Clozapine

Clozapine, a dibenzodiazepine, is another antipsychotic drug for which there is some evidence for its superiority to standard neuroleptics in treating negative symptoms. In a multicenter, double-blind, collaborative study 150 schizophrenic patients were randomly assigned to clozapine or CPZ at median doses of clozapine, 300–450 mg per day or CPZ, 450–900 mg per day, for an 8-week period. Clozapine was superior to CPZ for the treatment of nearly all categories of symptoms, but particularly in diminishing emotional withdrawal and blunted affect as rated with the BPRS at the end of both 2 and 8 weeks of treatment (Fischer-Cornelssen and Ferner 1975; Honigfeld et al. 1983). Clozapine was also superior to CPZ in decreasing anergia in the European collaborative study (Fischer-Cornellssen and Ferner 1975). Similar results were reported by Gelenberg and Doller (1979). There was a trend for clozapine to be superior to CPZ in the reduction of BPRS withdrawal in the study of Gerlach et al. (1974). However, both Niskanen et al. (1974) and Guirguis et al. (1977) reported that clozapine and CPZ had similar, appreciable efficacy in treating negative symptoms. Further investigation of the effect of clozapine vs standard neuroleptics on negative symptoms is clearly necessary.

2.2.4 Sulpiride

Sulpiride is a substituted benzamide which, like clozapine, has a profile of low extrapyramidal side effects and has been claimed to be especially effective in defect stage schizophrenics (Haase et al. 1974; Nishiura 1976; Elizure et al. 1975; Härnryd et al. 1984). For example, Härnryd et al. (1984) compared the effect of CPZ vs sulpiride on 50 schizophrenics on an "autism" scale which consisted of (a) inability to feel; (b) lassitude; (c) withdrawal; (d) reduced speech; and

(e) slowness of movement. Sulpiride produced significantly greater improvement than CPZ at 1–8 weeks in this subscale although there was no overall difference in the change in positive symptoms or global ratings.

2.3 Long-Term Responsiveness of Neuroleptic Treatment

Kolakowska et al. (1985) recently studied the response to neuroleptics in 62 schizophrenics and 15 schizoaffective patients, focusing on consistency of response throughout the course of the illness and various predictors of outcome, including negative symptoms. Subjects were divided into groups according to whether they had good, intermediate, or poor outcome. Treatment response during the current episode was based on at least 4 weeks of treatment with CPZ or its equivalent at 400 mg per day or more. They reported that outcome was good in 25 cases, poor in 20, and intermediate in 32. Response to neuroleptics was closely related to long-term outcome. Good responders (29) had fewer negative symptoms during their first episode (established retrospectively) than partial or poor responders. However, 5 of 25 (20%) good outcome patients had negative symptoms during their first episode. Clinical response to neuroleptics appeared to be consistent across episodes for most patients. These interesting results, all of which were derived from case records and ordinary clinical assessment, must be replicated with more rigorous methods. If replicated, they suggest that the long-term effect of neuroleptics on the schizophrenic syndrome could be related to the type of schizophrenia as determined by the presence of negative symptoms. However, no evidence was presented as to the effect of negative symptoms on response to neuroleptics in the current episode.

3 Effect of Neuroleptic Treatment on Negative Symptoms: A Preliminary Report

Meltzer (1985) previously reported the effect of treatment with neuroleptics, including in some cases periods of treatment with agents such as lithium, ECT, antidepressants, Des-Tyr γ-endorphin, alpha methylparatyrosine, and L-dopa, in 169 schizophrenic or schizoaffective mainly schizophrenic patients diagnosed according to RDC (Research Diagnostic Criteria; Spitzer et al. 1978). Negative and positive symptoms were assessed by means of scales derived from the Schedule for Affective Disorders and Schizophrenia – Change (SADS-C). The Negative Symptom Scale (NSS) consisted of 11 items: blunted affect, inappropriate affect, incoherence, loose associations, poverty of content, loss of interest, loss of sexual interest, slowed speech, slowed body movements, fatigue, and depressed appearance. The Positive Symptom Scale (PSS) consisted of various types of delusions and hallucinations. The duration of treatment was 10.1 ± 5.1 weeks. The mean peak dose of neuroleptics in chlorpromazine equivalents was 727 ± 432 mg per day. Analysis of covariance demonstrated greater improvement in female than in male patients, with overall improvement in positive and negative symptoms. Of 55 patients with NSS scale scores ≥ 5, 21 (38.2%) had an improvement of 5 or more on the NSS, as against 44/78 (56.4%) with an improvement of ≧5 on the PSS in patients with PSS ≧5 at the start of treatment.

We have now examined data from 73 patients who received only standard neuroleptic treatment throughout hospitalization for at least 3 weeks. Patients admitted to the Mental Health Clinical Research Center of The University of Chicago – Illinois State Psychiatric Institute were diagnosed according to RDC based on the Present State Examination (Wing et al. 1974), plus additional questions to obtain the information needed to assess the RDC. Patients were rated weekly with the Schedule for Affective Disorders – Change (Endicott and Spitzer 1978). There were 60 schizophrenics (26 paranoid, 30 undifferentiated, 4 disorganized) and 13 schizoaffective, mainly schizophrenic, patients. The mean age was 26.3 ± 6.7 (SD) years; there were 40 male and 33 female patients. The duration of illness was 4.4 ± 1.8 years. Patients were given placebo for 1–3 weeks, followed by neuroleptic treatment for 3–25 weeks (mean 11.2 ± 4.9 weeks) until discharge. Only two of the subjects were treated for 3 weeks only. The dosage was 400–2000 mg per day chlorpromazine equivalent. We divided each patient's stay in half and determined through an analysis of variance the significance of changes in ratings from admission to mid-hospitalization and discharge. We will report here the changes in PSS, NSS, and two factors of the NSS: a hebephrenic factor consisting of poverty of content, looseness of association, inappropriate affect, and incoherence, and an anergia-anhedonia factor consisting of fatigue, slowed speech, slowed body movements, depressed appearance, blunted affect, loss of interest, and loss of interest in sex. These factors were identified in a principal components factor analysis of the original sample. We also examined the change in negative symptoms, and the hebephrenic and anergia-anhedonia subscales after covarying out the change in positive symptoms, and the change in positive symptoms after covarying out the change in negative symptoms.

The results of the repeated measures analyses of variance are shown in Table 1. There was a significant decrease in positive ($F = 29.27$; $df = 2{,}144$; $P = 0.000$) and negative ($F = 12.18$; $df = 2{,}146$; $P = 0.000$) symptom scale scores as well as the hebephrenic ($F = 18.45$; $df = 2{,}143$; $P = 0.000$) and anergia-anhedonia ($F = 2.98$; $df = 2{,}146$; $P = 0.05$) ratings between admission and discharge. All ratings showed as much improvement between admission and mid-treatment as between mid-treatment and discharge, but these latter changes were not statistically signif-

Table 1. Admission, mid-treatment and discharge ratings[a] in neuroleptic-treated schizophrenic and schizoaffective patients

Time period	Positive Sx	Negative Sx	Hebephrenia	Anergia-anhedonia
Admission	4.9 ± 3.7	4.1 ± 2.2	1.5 ± 1.2	2.7 ± 1.8
Mid-treatment	3.4 ± 3.8	3.3 ± 2.1	1.0 ± 1.1	2.3 ± 1.7
Discharge	1.5 ± 2.2*	2.7 ± 2.1*	0.6 ± 1.0*	2.1 ± 1.8*

[a] Mean ± SD
* $P < 0.01$ compared with to admission ratings.
Sx, symptom scale scores.

icant. However, they suggest that the rate of improvement of positive and negative symptoms is approximately linear rather than having a long latent period. Moreover, these results suggest that the rate of improvement of positive and negative symptoms is not significantly different. In this sample there was a tendency for female patients to show more improvement on negative symptoms than male patients, but it failed to achieve statistical significance. An analysis of covariance showed that improvement in negative symptoms was independent of changes in positive symptoms ($F=7.98$; $df=2{,}143$; $P=0.001$). Similarly, there was a significant improvement in hebephrenic symptoms ($F=9.51$; $df=2{,}139$; $P=0.001$) as well as a nearly significant improvement in nonhebephrenic symptoms ($F=2.84$; $df=2{,}143$; $P=0.06$) after covarying out the improvement in positive symptoms. The improvement in positive symptoms was significant after covarying for change in negative symptoms as indicated by the ANCOVA ($F=23.9$; $df=2{,}143$; $P=0.000$).

4 Conclusions

These results confirm our previous conclusion (Meltzer 1985) that a treatment effect on negative symptoms is discernible over a brief period of time in chronic schizophrenic patients, at least in the relatively young patients included in this study. Our study was not placebo-controlled, however, and the measures of negative symptoms were not as detailed as desirable. It is possible that the improvement in negative symptoms were not drug-related and were due to psychosocial interactions, spontaneous improvement etc., but this seems unlikely because of the stability of the psychopathology during the preneuroleptic treatment period. Further studies to correct these deficiencies are warranted. Nevertheless, the cumulative data available from this study and those previously cited suggest that both the positive and the negative symptoms of schizophrenia are responsive to neuroleptic treatment in many, but not all, patients. Neuroleptic responsivity may be already programmed at the time of the first hospitalization if the results of Kolakowska et al. (1985) are valid, but clinical experience suggests otherwise, that is, that many patients show an initial response, followed by progressively developing resistance to drug treatment. Neuroleptic treatment appears to retard the rate of development of deterioration by preventing the effect of maximal positive and negative symptoms on functioning, including work and interpersonal function and the often deleterious effect of prolonged or repeated institutionalization. Whether neuroleptic treatment may prevent the organic changes which presumably underly the evolution of neuropsychological and psychosocial impairment in schizophrenia, or whether these drugs may actually exacerbate such organic impairment in some patients by neurotoxic mechanism, remains to be determined.

Acknowledgment. The work reported in this paper was supported, in part, by the Cleveland Foundation, USPHS MH 30938 and by Research Scientist Award MH 47008.

References

Angrist B, Rotrosen H, Gershon S (1980) Differential effects of amphetamine and neuroleptics on negative vs positive symptoms in schizophrenia. Psychopharmacology (Berlin) 72:12–19
Ashcroft GW, Blackwood GW, Besson JAO, Palomo T, Waring HL (1981) Positive and negative symptoms and the role of dopamine. Br J Psychiatry 138:268–269
Bleuler M (1974) The long-term course of the schizophrenic psychoses. Psychological Med 4:244–254
Brown GW, Birley JLT, Wing JK (1972) Influence of family life on the course of schizophrenic disorders: a replication. Br J Psychiatry 121:241–258
Burdock EI, Hakerem G, Hardesty AS, Zubin J (1960) A ward behavior rating scale for mental patients. J Clin Psychol 16:246–247
Ciompi L (1984) Is there really a schizophrenia? The long-term course of psychotic phenomena. Br J Psychiatry 145:636–640
Ciompi L, Mueller C (1976) Lebensweg und Alter der Schizophrenen. Eine katamnestische Langzeitstudie bis ins Senium (The life course and aging of schizophrenics. A long-term follow up study into old age). Springer, Berlin Heidelberg New York
Crow TJ (1980a) Molecular pathology of schizophrenia: more than one disease process. Br Med J 280:66–68
Crow TJ (1980b) Positive and negative schizophrenic symptoms and the role of dopamine. Br J Psychiatry 139:379–386
Dworkin RH, Lenzenweger MP (1984) Symptoms and the genetics of schizophrenia: implications for schizophrenia. Am J Psychiatry 141:1541–1546
Elizur A, Davidson S, Psych FRC (1975) The evaluation of the antibiotic activity of sulpiride. Curr Therapeutic Res 18:578–584
Endicott J, Spitzer R (1978) A diagnostic interview. A schedule for affective disorders and schizophrenia. Arch Gen Psychiatry 35:837–844
Erickson RC (1975) Outcome studies in mental hospitals: a review. Psychol Bull 82:519–540
Fischer-Cornellssen K, Ferner J (1976) An example of European multicenter trials: multispectral analysis of clozapine. Psychopharmacol Bull 12:34–39
Frango H, Zissis NP, Leontopoulos I, Diamantas N, Tsitouridis S, Gavriel I, Tsolis K (1978) Double-blind therapeutic evaluation of fluspirilene compared with fluphenazine decanoate in chronic schizophrenics. Acta Psychiatr Scand 57:436–446
Gallant DM, Mielke DH, Spirtes MA, Swanson WC, Bost R (1974) Penfluridol: an efficacious long-acting oral antipsychotic compound. Am J Psychiatry 131:699–702
Gelenberg AJ, Doller JC (1979) Clozapine versus chlorpromazine for the treatment of schizophrenia: Preliminary results from a double-blind study. J Clin Psychiatry 40:238–240
Gerlach J, Koppelhus P, Helweg E, Monrad A (1974) Clozapine and haloperidol in a single-blind cross-over trial: therapeutic and biochemical aspects in the treatment of schizophrenia. Acta Psychiatr Scand 50:410–424
Goldberg SC, Klerman GL, Cole JO (1965) Changes in schizophrenic psychopathology and ward behavior as a function of phenothiazine treatment. Br J Psychiatry 111:120–135
Gould RJ, Murphy KMM, Reynolds IJ, Snyder SH (1983) Antischizophrenic drugs of the diphenylbutylpiperidine type act as calcium channel antagonists. Proc Natl Acad Sci USA 80:5122–5125
Guirguis E, Voinesko G, Gray J, Schlieman E (1977) Clozapine (Leponex) vs chlorpromazine (Largactil) in acute schizophrenia. (A double-blind controlled study.) Curr Therapeutic Res 21:707–719
Haas S, Beckmann H (1982) Pimozide versus haloperidol in acute schizophrenia. A double-blind controlled study. Pharmacopsychiatry 15:70–74
Haase HJ, Floru L, Ulrich F (1974) Klinisch neuroleptische Untersuchung des *N*-(1-Äthyl-pyrrolidin-2-YL)-methyl-2 methoxy-5-sulfamoyl-benzamide-neurolepticums Sulprid (Dogmatil) an akut erkrankten Schizophrenen. Int Pharmacopsychiatry 9:77–94
Härnryd C, Bjerkenstedt L, Bjork, Gullberg B, Oxenstierna G, Sedvall G, Wiesel FA, Wik G, Asberg-Wistedt A (1984) Clinical evaluation of sulpiride in schizophrenic patients – a double-blind comparison with chlorpromazine. Acta Psychiatr Scand 69:7–30

Honigfeld G, Patin J, Belendiuk G, Singer J (1983) Efficacy. In the clozapine monograph: a summary of safety and antipsychotic efficacy findings. Sandoz Pharmaceuticals, East Hanover, NJ
Huber G, Gross G, Schuttler R, Linz M (1980) Longitudinal studies of schizophrenic patient. Schizophr Bull 6:592–605
Johnstone EC, Crow TJ, Frith CD, Husband J, Kreel J (1976) Cerebral ventricular size and cognitive impairment in chronic schizophrenia. Lancet 2:924–926
Johnstone EC, Frith CD, Crow TJ, Carney MWP, Price JS (1978) Mechanism of the antipsychotic effect in the treatment of acute shizophrenia. Lancet 1:848–851
Johnstone EC, Owens DGC, Gold A, Crow TJ, Macmillan JF (1984) Schizophrenic patients discharged from hospital: a follow up study. Br J Psychiatry 145:586–590
Kellam S, Goldberg SC, Schooler NR et al. (1967) Ward atmosphere and outcome of treatment of acute schizophrenia. J Psychiatr Res 5:145–163
Kolakowska T, Williams AO, Ardern M, Reveley MA, Jambor K, Gelder MG, Mandelbrote BM (1985) Schizophrenia with good and poor outcome: I. early clinical features, response to neuroleptics and signs of organic dysfunction. Br J Psychiatr 146:229–246
Kudo T (1972) A double-blind comparison of pimozide with carpipramine in schizophrenic patients. Acta Psychiatr Belg 72:685–697
Lapierre YD (1978) A controlled study of penfluridol in the treatment of chronic schizophrenia. Am J Psychiatry 135:956–959
Lapierre YD, Lavallee J (1975) Pimozide and the social behaviors of schizophrenics. Curr Therapeutic Res 18:181–188
Leff J, Kuipers L, Berkowitz R, Vaughn C, Sturgeon D (1983) Life events, relatives: expressed emotion and maintenance neuroleptic in schizophrenic relapse. Psychol Med 13:799–806
Lehman AF, Strauss JS, Ritzler BA, Kokes RF, Harder DW, Gift TE (1982) First-admission psychiatric ward milieu: treatment process and outcome. Arch Gen Psychiatry 39:1293–1298
Lewine RJ, Fogg L, Meltzer HY (1983) Assessment of negative and positive symptoms in schizophrenia. Schizophrenia Bull 9:368–376
Lipton MA, Burnett GB (1979) Pharmacological treatment of schizophrenia. In: Bella KL (ed) Disorders of the schizophrenic syndrome. Basic Books, New York, pp 320–352
Lorr M, Klett CJ, McNair DM, Laskey JJ (1963) Inpatient multidimensional psychiatric scale (IMPS) Manual. Consulting Psychologists Press, Palo Alto
Mackay A (1980) Positive and negative schizophrenic symptoms and the role of dopamine. Br J Psychiatry 137:379–383
Meltzer HY (1985) Dopamine and negative symptoms in schizophrenia: critique of type I–II hypothesis. In: Alpert M (ed) Controversies in schizophrenia, chap 7. Guilford, New York, pp 110–136
Moos R, Schwartz J (1972) Treatment environment and treatment outcome. J Nerv Ment Dis 154:264–275
Nasrallah HA, Jacoby CG, McCalley-Whitters M, Kuperman S (1982) Cerebral ventricular enlargement in subtypes of chronic schizophrenia. Arch Gen Psychiatry 39:774–777
NIMH-PSC Collaborative Study Group (1964) Phenothiazine treatment in acute schizophrenia. Arch Gen Psychiatry 10:246–261
Nishiura M (1976) Clinico-pharmacological studies in sulpiride. Curr Therapeutic Res 20:164–172
Niskanen P, Achte K, Jaskari M, Karesoja M, Meisted B, Nilsson LB, Routavaara M, Tamminen T, Tienari P, Vogel G (1974) Results of a comparitive double-blind study with clozapine and chlorpromazine in the treatment of schizophrenic patients. Psychiatria Fennica 1974:307–313
Nyman AK, Jonsson H (1983) Differential evaluation of outcome in schizophrenia. Acta Psychiatr Scand 68:458–475
Overall JE, Gorham DR (1962) Brief psychiatric rating scale (BPRS). Psychological Rep 10:799–812
Pearlson GH, Veroff AE (1981) Computerized tomographic scan changes in manic-depressive illness. Lancet 2:470

Pietzcker A, Gaebel W (1983) Prediction of "natural" course, relapse and prophylactic response in schizophrenic patients. Pharmacopsychiatria 16:206–211

Shopsin B, Klein H, Gerbino L, Selzer G (1977) Penfluridol: An open phase III study in acute newly admitted hospitalized schizophrenic patients. Psychopharmacology (Berlin) 55:157–164

Singh AN (1973) Clinical evaluation of fluspirilene as a maintenance therapy in chronic schizophrenic patients. Can Psychiatric Assoc J 18:415–419

Spitzer RL, Endicott J, Robins E (1978) Research diagnostic criteria: rationality and reliability. Arch Gen Psychiatr 35:773–782

Watts CAH (1985) A long-term follow-up of schizophrenic patients: 1946–1983. J Clin Psychiatr 46:210–216

Wing JK (1978) The social context of schizophrenia. Am J Psychiatry 135:1333–1338

Wing JK, Cooper JE, Sartorius N (1974) The measurement and classification of psychiatric symptoms. Cambridge University Press, London

World Health Organization (1979) Schizophrenia. An International Follow-up study. Wiley, New York

Pharmacokinetic and Pharmacodynamic Factors Causing Variability in Response to Neuroleptic Drugs

S. G. DAHL and P.-A. HALS

1 Clinical Variability in Neuroleptic Drug Treatment

When a new psychotropic drug is introduced on the market with claims that it acts more specifically than the previous ones this has to be proven – not just in in vitro receptor binding systems and animal experiments – but also in patients. That can only be done by properly designed clinical studies.

Certainly one of the main problems in neuroleptic drug treatment is the variability in the outcome of the treatment in individual patients, both in terms of therapeutic response and side effects. The main reasons for interpatient variability in response to drug treatment can be divided into three groups: (a) Variable compliance; (b) pharmacokinetic variations; and (c) variations in concentration-response relationships.

Multidrug therapy, which is frequently used in the treatment of psychotic disorders, may generally reduce the degree of patient compliance in taking the prescribed drugs (Hulka et al. 1976). Interpatient variability both in the pharmacokinetics and in the concentration-response relationships of a drug may be caused by disease, diet, physical excercise, and advanced age, and by genetic factors influencing both the disposition of the drug in the body and how the organism responds to a certain time-course of drug concentrations.

Interindividual variations in the pharmacokinetics of a drug may in some cases be compensated for by dosage adjustments based on measurements of plasma drug concentrations. Inherent variations in concentration-response relationships at the receptor level, on the other hand, can only be compensated for by dosage adjustment after clinical evaluation. The clinical value of monitoring plasma drug levels therefore depends, among other factors, on the relative contributions from the pharmacodynamic and pharmacokinetic factors to the overall variance in therapeutic response.

2 Pharmacokinetic Factors of Variance

Most neuroleptic drugs are characterized by substantial interpatient variations in steady-state plasma levels relative to the administered daily dose. A number of different studies have reported 10- to 30-fold interpatient variations in plasma

Department of Pharmacology, Institute of Medical Biology, University of Tromsö, N-9001 Tromsö,Norway.

Clinical Pharmacology in Psychiatry
Editors: Dahl, Gram, Paul, Potter
(Psychopharmacology Series 3)

level-to-dose ratios after repeated oral doses of neuroleptics of the butyrophenone, dibenzoxazepine, phenothiazine and thioxanthene classes (for review see Dahl 1981, 1986). Significantly smaller interpatient variations in the steady-state plasma level-to-dose ratios, generally of a 3- to 5-fold order, have been reported for benzamides, which are the most highly water-soluble compounds among the neuroleptics, having elimination half-lives in the order of 3–10 h, and for the extremely lipid-soluble diphenylbutylpiperidines, which have elimination half-lives in the order of 50–200 h (Dahl 1981; Jorgensen 1986).

In hospitalized patients significantly less day-to-day variance in the plasma levels of neuroleptic drugs has been found within individual patients than between different patients (Dahl 1986). Also, much less variation in plasma level-to-dose ratios was observed after i.m. than after p.o. doses of levomepromazine (Dahl 1976), chlorpromazine (Dahl and Strandjord 1977), haloperidol (Balant-Gorgia et al. 1984) and perphenazine (Larsson et al. 1984), indicating that variation in presystemic metabolism may be important after oral doses.

3 Plasma Drug Levels and Therapeutic Response

While the pharmacokinetics have been fairly well documented for most of the commonly used neuroleptic drugs (Jørgensen 1986), relatively few well-designed studies of the possible relationships between plasma levels and therapeutic response of neuroleptic drugs have been reported. The clinical consequences of their pronounced pharmacokinetic variance is, therefore, far from clear.

As discussed in many other reviews and original articles, studies of plasma drug levels and therapeutic response to neuroleptic drugs are of very limited value if the drug doses are determined individually by clinical judgement. Studies of plasma drug concentration-therapeutic effect relationships using specific chemical assay methods, and randomly allocated, fixed drug doses, have been reported for chlorpromazine, fluphenazine, haloperidol, perphenazine, sulpiride, thioridazine and thiothixene. The results of these studies are summarized in Table 1.

All three studies with chlorpromazine referred to in Table 1 reported that responders and nonresponders had plasma drug levels within the same ranges after 4 weeks of treatment. However, Van Putten et al. (1981) observed some cases of apparent drug-induced toxicity related to plasma chlorpromazine levels above 100 ng/ml. Most patients who responded well to chlorpromazine treatment had plasma drug levels within a range of 30–100 ng/ml, and there seems to be no advantage in obtaining plasma chlorpromazine levels above 100 ng/ml.

Both the studies with fluphenazine referred to in Table 1 concluded that there seems to be a therapeutic plasma level "window" somewhere around 0.5–2.5 ng/ml after 2 weeks of treatment with oral doses of fluphenazine.

About half the studies of plasma levels and therapeutic response to haloperidol using a fixed-dose design revealed no relationship (Table 1). The other four studies reported apparent therapeutic plasma level windows in the range of 3–20 ng/ml. However, the relationships between clinical response and plasma haloperidol levels were generally far from clear-cut, and the conclusions from some of these studies have since been challenged by others (Van Putten et al. 1985b;

Table 1. Fixed-dose studies of clinical response and plasma levels of neuroleptic drugs

Compound	Authors	Number of patients	Duration weeks	Concentration-response relationship	
				Yes	No
Chlorpromazine	Wode-Helgodt et al. (1978)	44	2–4	× (2 weeks)	× (4 weeks)
Chlorpromazine	Alfredsson et al. (1984, 1985)	19	2–4	× (2 weeks)	× (4 weeks)
Chlorpromazine	Van Putten et al. (1981)	34	4		×
Fluphenazine	Dysken et al. (1981)	29	2	×	
Fluphenazine	Mavroidis et al. (1984a, b)	19	2	×	
Haloperidol	Smith et al. (1984a, 1985)	34	3	×	
Haloperidol	Garver et al. (1984)	14	2	×	
Haloperidol	Linkowski et al. (1984)	20	6		×
Haloperidol	Davis et al. (1985)	35	3	×	
Haloperidol	Mavroidis et al. (1983, 1985)	14	2	×	
Haloperidol	Potkin et al. (1985)	43	6		×
Haloperidol	Van Putten et al. (1985a)	47	4		×
Haloperidol	Bigelow et al. (1985)	19	6		×
Perphenazine	Bolvig Hansen et al. (1982)	26	5	×	
Sulpiride	Alfredsson et al. (1984, 1985)	25	4	×	
Thioridazine	Smith et al. (1984b, 1985)	35	3		×
Thiothixene	Mavroidis et al. (1984c)	19	2	×	

Kirch et al. 1985). In two of these studies (Garver et al. 1984; Mavroidis et al. 1983, 1985), the pre-drug washout periods were only 2–3 days, which is usually assumed to be shorter than necessary to avoid carryover effects from previous treatment. From all these studies it must be concluded that a therapeutic or toxic plasma level range has not been demonstrated for haloperidol. On the other hand, plasma haloperidol levels above 20–30 ng/ml, although well tolerated by some patients, generally seem to offer no therapeutic advantage and probably produce an increased risk of drug toxicity.

Bolvig Hansen et al. (1982) reported that optimal therapeutic response to perphenazine treatment and a low risk of extrapyramidal side effects could be obtained by careful monitoring of plasma perphenazine levels in psychotic patients. This was later confirmed in a second study including 228 acutely psychotic patients (Bolvig Hansen and Larsen 1985).

Alfredsson et al. (1984) reported that a favorable response to treatment with sulpiride in patients with "negative" schizophrenic symptoms was associated with plasma drug levels below 500 ng/ml. However, only a 4-fold variation in plasma drug level-to-dose ratios was observed in 25 patients, and these relatively small

Table 2. Suggested therapeutic and toxic plasma levels of neuroleptic drugs (ng/ml), measured 8–12 h after oral dose

Compound	Suggested therapeutic range	Suggested toxic range
Chlorpromazine	30–100 (?)	>100–150
Fluphenazine	0.2–2.0	>2.0
Haloperidol	5–20 (?)	>20–30
Perphenazine	>0.8	>2.4
Thiothixene	2–15	>15
Sulpiride	<500	

interpatient variations in plasma levels may diminish the clinical utility of monitoring plasma sulpiride levels.

A study of therapeutic response and plasma levels of thioridazine and one of its main metabolites concluded that no relationship was found (Smith et al. 1984b, 1985). Another study revealed an apparent therapeutic plasma level window between 2 and 15 ng/ml for thiothixene (Mavroidis et al. 1984c).

The possible therapeutic and toxic plasma level ranges that can be inferred from these studies are summarized in Table 2. It must be emphasized that these values must still be regarded as preliminary, and that they may have some validity only for patients who are not concomitantly being treated with other neuroleptic drugs.

4 Free Drug Concentrations and Variations in "Receptor Sensitivity"

Cross et al. (1981) found an increased number of dopamine D_2 receptors in the brains of drug-free schizophrenic patients compared to controls. Others have examined the binding affinities of a series of neuroleptic drugs to dopamine D_2 and other neurotransmitter receptors in the human brain (Richelson and Nelson 1984). However, there is little information in the literature concerning interindividual variations in neurotransmitter receptor binding and functioning. Some of the currently used receptor binding assays yield considerable day-to-day variation in the results (Hals et al. 1986), and it is questionable whether they are sufficiently precise to detect interindividual variations in postmortem brain tissue receptor binding.

Some neuroleptic drugs have active metabolites which may contribute to their therapeutic and toxic effects (Dahl 1982). In addition to interindividual variations in drug concentrations and concentration-response relationships, it is possible that variations in metabolite concentrations may also add to the interindividual variations in therapeutic effects and side effects of these drugs.

Table 3 shows estimated CSF concentrations and measured neurotransmitter binding affinities of two "high-dose" neuroleptics, chlorpromazine and levomepromazine, two "low-dose" neuroleptics, fluphenazine and perphenazine, and

Table 3. Phenothiazine drugs and metabolites: Binding affinities (K_i) to rat brain receptors and estimated CSF concentration ranges after therapeutic doses

Compound	CSF concentration range (n*M*)	Ki (n*M*)		
		Dopamine D_2	α_1-Adrenergic	Cholinergic M_1
Chlorpromazine (CPZ)	1–15	20	8	220
7-Hydroxy CPZ	1–15	40	14	1000
N-Desmethyl CPZ	1–15	60	20	1300
Levomepromazine (LM)	1–15	30	3	170
3-Hydroxy LM	1–15	45	70	1300
N-Desmethyl LM	1–15	70	12	500
Fluphenazine	0.02–0.2	5	40	4500
7-Hydroxy FPZ		6	120	16000
Perphenazine	0.02–0.2	6	25	6000
7-Hydroxy PPZ		9	45	12000

Table 4. Studies of clinical response and "neuroleptic plasma levels" measured by radioreceptor assay

Authors	Fixed-dose design		Concentration-response relationship	
	Yes	No	Yes	No
Calil et al. (1979)		×	×	
Cohen et al. (1980a, b)		×	×	
Tune et al. (1980, 1981)		×	×	
Smith et al. (1980)	×			×
Csernansky et al. (1983)		×		×
Meltzer et al. (1983)	×			×
Van Putten et al. (1983)	×			×
Newman et al. (1984)		×		×
Lindenmayer et al. (1984)		×		×
Silverstone et al. (1984)		×		×
Kucharski et al. (1984)		×	×	
Tang et al. (1984)	×			×
Smith et al. (1984a, 1985)	×			×
Brown and Silver (1985)		×		×

some of their main metabolites. The CSF concentration ranges were estimated from the plasma levels usually obtained after therapeutic doses, and information about plasma protein binding of phenothiazine drugs and drug metabolites (Ahte et al. 1967; Krieglstein et al. 1972; Freedberg et al. 1979) or from measured CSF concentrations (Wode-Helgodt and Alfredsson 1981; Alfredsson et al. 1982). Receptor binding affinities, expressed as K_i values, were obtained by essentially the same techniques as in a previous study (Dahl and Hall 1981), using rat brain and tritiated spiroperidol, WB-4101 and QNB for dopamine D_2, α_1-adrenergic and muscarinic cholinergic M_1 receptors, respectively. For experimental details see Hals et al. 1986.

The results shown in Table 3 indicate that some of the metabolites which were examined may contribute both to antidopaminergic effects and to side effects caused by blockade of α_1-adrenergic or muscarinic cholinergic M_1 receptors. Since the metabolite-to-parent drug concentration ratios of such compounds may show substantial interindividual variation (Dahl 1982), it appears from these results that the metabolites may also contribute to the variability in therapeutic response to the drugs.

The radioreceptor assay, based on binding to dopamine D_2 receptors, measures the total activity of drugs and metabolites in a sample. This assay method has been used in several studies of the relationship between therapeutic response to neuroleptic drugs and "neuroleptic serum levels," which are summarized in Table 4. As evident from this table, most of these studies found no such relationship, although some of the initial studies came out with a positive conclusion. One reason for the apparent lack of such a relationship may be that different drugs, which were often included in the same study, and their metabolites may have different blood-brain distribution. Therefore, the total brain levels of drug-induced receptor blocking activity may not be directly reflected by the "neuroleptic serum levels."

5 Conclusions

The interpatient variability in response to antipsychotic drug treatment may be caused by variability both in pharmacokinetic factors and in the concentration-effect relationships at the receptor level. The pharmacokinetic variation may be assessed in some cases by measuring plasma drug and metabolite levels by specific chemical methods, and compensated for by dose adjustments. The inherent variability in how each patient responds to a certain time-course of drug and metabolite concentrations at the receptor site is much more difficult to assess, and can only be compensated for by dose adjustments based on clinical judgement.

It has been demonstrated for a few neuroleptic drugs (Table 2) that monitoring of plasma drug levels by chemical methods may be clinically useful. This indicates that variability in pharmacokinetic factors is important for the patient-to-patient variability in therapeutic response to these drugs.

Although no definite therapeutic plasma level ranges have been established for chlorpromazine and haloperidol, monitoring plasma levels of these drugs may still be of value in some patients when there is reason to suspect drug-induced toxicity.

References

Ahtee L, Mattila MJ, Vapaatalo HI (1967) The binding of some phenothiazines to human serum in vitro. Biochem Pharmacol 16:2432–2435
Alfredsson G, Lindberg M, Sedvall G (1982) The presence of 7-hydroxychlorpromazine in CSF of chlorpromazine-treated patients. Psychopharmacology (Berlin) 77:376–378
Alfredsson G, Härnryd C, Wiesel F-A (1984) Effects of sulpiride and chlorpromazine on depressive symptoms in schizophrenic patients – relationship to drug concentrations. Psychopharmacology (Berlin) 84:237–241
Alfredsson G, Härnryd C, Wiesel FA (1985) Effects of sulpiride and chlorpromazine on autistic and positive symptoms in schizophrenic patients – relationship to drug concentrations. Psychopharmacology (Berlin) 85:8–13
Balant-Gorgia AE, Eisele R, Balant L, Garrone G (1984) Plasma haloperidol levels and therapeutic response in acute mania and schizophrenia. Eur Arch Psychiatr Neurol Sci 234:1–4
Bigelow LB, Kirch DG, Braun T, Korpi ER, Wagner RL, Zalcman S, Wyatt RJ (1985) Absence of relationship of serum haloperidol concentration and clinical response in chronic schizophrenia: a fixed-dose study. Psychopharmacol Bull 21:66–68
Bolvig Hansen L, Larsen N-E (1985) Therapeutic advantages of monitoring plasma concentrations of perphenazine in clinical practice. Psychopharmacology (Berlin) 87:16–19
Bolvig Hansen L, Larsen NE, Gulmann N (1982) Dose-response relationships of perphenazine in the treatment of acute psychoses. Psychopharmacology (Berlin) 78:112–115
Brown WA, Silver MA (1985) Serum neuroleptic levels and clinical outcome in schizophrenic patients treated with fluphenazine decanoate. J Clin Psychopharmacol 5:143–147
Calil HM, Avery DH, Hollister LE, Creese I, Snyder SH (1979) Serum levels of neuroleptics measured by dopamine radio receptor assay and some clinical observations. Psychiatry Res 1:39–44
Cohen BM, Lipinski JF, Harris PQ, Pope HG, Friedman M (1980a) Clinical use of the radioreceptor asssay for neuroleptics. Psychiatry Res 1:173–178
Cohen BM, Lipinski JF, Pope HG, Harris PQ, Altesman RI (1980b) Neuroleptic blood levels and therapeutic effect. Psychopharmacology (Berlin) 70:191–193
Cross AJ, Crow TJ, Owen F (1981) ^{3}H-Flupenthixol binding in post-mortem brains of schizophrenics: Evidence for a selective increase in dopamine D2 receptors. Psychopharmacology (Berlin) 74:122–124
Csernansky JG, Kaplan J, Holman CA, Hollister LE (1983) Serum neuroleptic activity, prolactin, and tardive dyskinesia in schizophrenic outpatients. Psychopharmacology (Berlin) 81:115–118
Dahl SG (1976) Pharmacokinetics of methotrimeprazine after single and multiple doses. Clin Pharmacol Ther 19:435–442
Dahl SG (1981) Pharmacokinetic aspects of new antipsychotic drugs. Neuropharmacology 20:1299–1302
Dahl SG (1982) Active metabolites of neuroleptic drugs: possible contribution to therapeutic and toxic effects. Ther Drug Monit 4:33–40
Dahl SG (1986) Plasma level monitoring of antipsychotic drugs: clinical utility. Clin Pharmacokinet 11:36–61
Dahl SG, Hall H (1981) Binding affinity of levomepromazine and two of its major metabolites to central dopamine and adrenergic receptors in the rat. Psychopharmacology (Berlin) 74:101–104
Dahl SG, Strandjord RE (1977) Pharmacokinetics of chlorpromazine after single and chronic dosage. Clin Pharmacol Ther 21:437–448
Davis JM, Ericksen SE, Hurt S, Chang SS, Javaid JI, Dekirmenjian H, Casper R (1985) Haloperidol plasma levels and clinical response: basic concepts and clinical data. Psychopharmacol Bull 21:48–51
Dysken MW, Javaid JI, Chang SS, Schaffer C, Shahid A, Davis JM (1981) Fluphenazine pharmacokinetics and therapeutic response. Psychopharmacology (Berlin) 73:205–210
Freedberg KA, Innis RB, Creese I, Snyder SH (1979) Antipsychotic drugs: differential plasma protein binding and therapeutic activity. Life Sci 24:2467–2474

Garver DL, Hirschowitz J, Glicksteen GA, Kanter DR, Mavroidis ML (1984) Haloperidol plasma and red blood cell levels and clinical antipsychotic response. J Clin Psychopharmacol 4:133–137

Hals PA, Hall H, Dahl SG (1986) Phenothiazine drug metabolites: Dopamine D2 receptor, α_1- and α_2-adrenoceptor binding. Eur J Pharmacol 125:373–381

Hulka BS, Cassel JC, Kupper LL (1976) Disparities between medications prescribed and consumed among chronic disease patients. In: Lasagna L (ed) Patient Compliance. Futura Mount Kisco, New York, pp 123–152

Jørgensen A (1986) Metabolism and pharmacokinetics of antipsychotic drugs. In: Bridges JW, Chasseaud LF (eds) Progress in drug metabolism, vol 9. Taylor and Francis, London, pp 111–174

Kirch DG, Bigelow LB, Wyatt RJ (1985) The interpretation of plasma haloperidol concentrations. Arch Gen Psychiatry 42:838–836

Krieglstein J, Lier F, Michaelis J (1972) Albumin binding and hydrophobic character of promazine and chlorpromazine metabolites. Arch Pharmacol 272:121–130

Kucharski LT, Alexander P, Tune L, Coyle J (1984) Serum neuroleptic concentrations and clinical response: a radioreceptor assay investigation of acutely psychotic patients. Psychopharmacology (Berlin) 82:194–198

Larsson M, Axelsson R, Forsman A (1984) On the pharmacokinetics of perphenazine: a clinical study of perphenazine enanthate and decanoate. Curr Therapeutic Res 36:1071–1088

Lindenmayer JP, Smith D, Katz I (1984) Radioreceptor assay of neuroleptics in refractory chronic schizophrenic patients. J Clin Psychiatry 45:117–119

Linkowski P, Houbain P, Von Frenckell R, Mendlewicz J (1984) Haloperidol plasma levels and clinical response in paranoid schizophrenics. Eur Arch Psychiatr Neurol Sci 234:231–236

Mavroidis ML, Kanter DR, Hirschowitz J, Garver DL (1983) Clinical response and plasma haloperidol levels in schizophrenia. Psychopharmacology (Berlin) 81:354–356

Mavroidis ML, Kanter DR, Hirschowitz J, Garver DL (1984a) Therapeutic blood levels of fluphenazine: Plasma or RBC determinations? Psychopharmacol Bull 20:168–170

Mavroidis ML, Kanter DR, Hirschowitz J, Garver DL (1984b) Fluphenazine plasma levels and clinical response. J Clin Psychiatry 45:370–373

Mavroidis ML, Kanter DR, Hirschowitz J, Garver DL (1984c) Clinical relevance of thiothixene plasma levels. J Clin Psychopharmacol 4:155–157

Mavroidis ML; Garver DL, Kanter DR, Hirschowitz J (1985) Plasma haloperidol levels and clinical response: confounding variables. Psychopharmacol Bull 21:62–65

Meltzer HY, Busch DA, Fang VS (1983) Serum neuroleptic and prolactin levels in schizophrenic patients and clinical response. Psychiatry Res 9:271–283

Newman DC, Epperly M, Sangarasivam S, Maruta T, Homburger HA (1984) Neuroleptic levels in serum: clinical usefulness in schizophrenic patients. Clin Res 32:741A

Richelson E, Nelson A (1984) Antagonism by neuroleptics of neurotransmitter receptors of normal human brain in vitro. Eur J Pharmacol 103:197–204

Potkin SG, Shen Y, Zhou D, Pardes H, Shu L, Phelps B, Poland R (1985) Does a therapeutic window for plasma haloperidol exist? Preliminary Chinese data. Psychopharmacol Bull 21:59–61

Silverstone T, Cookson J, Ball R, Chin CN, Jacobs D, Lader S, Gould S (1984) The relationship of dopamine receptor blockade to clinical response in schizophrenic patients treated with pimozide or haloperidol. J Psychiatry Res 18:255–268

Smith RC, Vroulis G, Misra CH, Schoolar J, De John C, Korivi P, Leelavahti DE, Arzu D (1980) Receptor techniques in the study of plasma levels of neuroleptics and antidepressant drugs. Commun Psychopharmacol 4:451–465

Smith RC, Baumgartner R, Misra CH, Mauldin M, Shvartsburd A, Ho BT, De John C (1984a) Haloperidol. Plasma levels and prolactin response as predictors of clinical improvement in schizophrenia: chemical v radioreceptor plasma level assays. Arch Gen Psychiatry 41:1044–1049

Smith RC, Baumgartner R, Ravichandran GK, Shvartsburd A, Schoolar JC, Allen P, Johnson R (1984b) Plasma and red cell levels of thioridazine and clinical response in schizophrenia. Psychiatry Res 12:287–296

Smith RC, Baumgartner R, Burd A, Ravichandran GK, Mauldin M (1985) Haloperidol and thioridazine drug levels and clinical response in schizophrenia: comparison of gas-liquid chromatography and radioreceptor drug level assays. Psychopharmacol Bull 21:52–58

Tang SW, Glaister J, Davidson L, Toth R, Jeffries JJ, Seeman P (1984) Total and free plasma neuroleptic levels in schizophrenic patients. Psychiatry Res 13:285–293

Tune LE, Creese I, De Paulo JR, Slavney PR, Coyle JT, Snyder SH (1980) Clinical state and serum neuroleptic levels measured by radioreceptor assay in schizophrenia. Am J Psychiatry 137:187–190

Tune LE, Creese I, De Paulo JR, Slavney PR, Snyder SH (1981) Neuroleptic serum levels measured by radioreceptor assay and clinical response in schizophrenia. J Nerv Ment Dis 169:60–63

Van Putten T, May PRA, Jenden DJ (1981) Does a plasma level of chlorpromazine help? Psychol Med 11:729–734

Van Putten T, May PRA, Marder SR, Wilkins JN, Rosenberg BJ (1983) Plasma levels of thiothixene by radioreceptor assay: clinical usefulness. Psychopharmacology (Berlin) 79:40–44

Van Putten T, Marder SR, May PRA, Poland RE, O'Brien RP (1985 a) Plasma levels, haloperidol and clinical response. Psychopharmacol Bull 21:69–72

Van Putten T, Marder SR, Mintz (1985 b) Plasma haloperidol levels: clinical response and fancy mathematics. Arch Gen Psychiatry 42:835

Wode-Helgodt B, Alfredsson G (1981) Concentrations of chlorpromazine and two of its active metabolites in plasma and cerebrospinal fluid of psychotic patients treated with fixed drug doses. Psychopharmacology (Berlin) 73:55–62

Wode-Helgodt B, Borg S, Fyrö B, Sedvall G (1978) Clinical effects and drug concentrations in plasma and cerebrospinal fluid in psychotic patients treated with fixed doses of chlorpromazine. Acta Psychiatr Scand 58:149–173

Acknowledgements. This Fourth International Meeting on Clinical Pharmacology in Psychiatry held in Bethesda, Maryland, Sept. 5–8, 1985, would not have been possible without the generous financial support received from a number of drug companies, which we gratefully acknowledge: American Cyanamid Company, New York, USA; Astra, Södertälje, Sweden; Beecham Pharmaceuticals, Harlow, UK; Boehringer Ingelheim Corporation, Connecticut, USA; Bristoll-Myers, New York, USA; Burroughs Wellcome, North Carolina, USA; Ciba-Geigy Corporation, New Jersey, USA; Ferrosan, Copenhagen, Denmark; Hoffmann-La Roche, New Jersey, USA; Janssen Pharmaceutics, New Jersey, USA; Leo, Hälsingborg, Sweden; H. Lundbeck, Copenhagen, Denmark; Merrell Dow Pharmaceuticals, Ohio, USA; Organon, Oss, The Netherlands; Pfeizer, New York, USA; Rhône-Poulenc Santé, Paris, France; Roche, Copenhagen, Denmark; Sandoz Informasjon, Oslo, Norway; Schering, Berlin, West Germany; Stuart Pharmaceuticals, Delaware, USA; Upjohn, Michigan, USA.

The front page illustration was produced at the Computer Graphics Laboratory, Department of Pharmaceutical Chemistry, University of California, San Francisco. The use of their facilities in producing this illustration, as well as the indexes and lists of contents and contributors, is gratefully acknowledged. This laboratory is supported by the National Institutes of Health, grant RR-1081.

List of Participants

Åsberg, Marie, Dr.
Department of Psychiatry,
Karolinska Hospital,
S-141 01 Stockholm, Sweden

Blier, Pierre, Dr.
Université de Montreal, Faculté de Médecine, Centre de Recherche en Sciences Neurologiques,
C.P. 6128, Succursale A,
Montreal, Quebec H3C 3J7, Canada

Bunney, Benjamin S., Dr.
Neuropsychopharmacology Research Unit, Yale University School of Medicine, 333 Cedar Street,
P.O. Box 3333,
New Haven, CT 06510, USA

Calil, Helena, Dr.
Depto. de Psicobiologia,
Escola Paulista de Medicina,
R. Botucatu, 862, Cx.P.20.399,
04034 Sao Paulo, Brazil

Casey, Daniel E., Dr.
Dept. Psychiatry and Neurology,
Oregon Health Sciences Univ.,
P.O. Box 1034, Portland, OR 97207, USA

Christensen, Anne Vibeke, Dr.
H. Lundbeck A/S, Ottiliavej 7-9,
DK-2500 Valby, Denmark

Christensen, Peder, Dr.
Department of Clinical Pharmacology,
Odense University,
J. B. Winsløwsvej 19,
DK-5000 Odense C, Denmark

Costa, Erminio, Dr.
Laboratory of Preclinical Pharmacology, National Institute of Mental Health, St. Elizabeths Hospital,
William A. White Building,
Washington, DC 20010, USA

Dahl, Svein G., Dr.
Institute of Medical Biology,
University of Tromsø School of Medicine, P.O. Box 977,
N-9001 Tromsø, Norway

De Montigny, Claude, Dr.
Department of Physiology, University of Montreal, CP 6208, Succ A,
Montreal, Quebec, Canada H3C 3T8

De Vane, C. Lindsay, Dr.
Department of Pharmacy Practice,
College of Pharmacy (Box J-4),
University of Florida,
Gainesville, FL 32610, USA

Dorow, Rainer, Dr.
Schering AG, Pharmaceutical Research, Neuroendocrinology and Neuropsychopharmacology,
Postfach 650311,
D-1000 Berlin (West) 65, Germany

ELLINWOOD, EVERETT H., Dr.
Duke University Medical Center,
Department of Psychiatry,
Durham, NC 27710, USA

ETIENNE, PIERRE, Dr.
CIBA/GEIGY Pharmaceutical Div.,
Clinical Biology, TOV 1,
Summit, NJ 07901, USA

FORSMAN, ANDERS, Dr.
Psychiatry Department III,
Lillhagen Hospital,
S-42203 Hisings Backa, Sweden

FREIDINGER, ROGER M., Dr.
Department of Medicinal Chemistry,
Merck, Sharp and Dohme Research
Laboratories,
West Point, PA 19486, USA

GERLACH, JES, Dr.
Sct. Hans Hospital,
DK-4000 Roskilde, Denmark

GLASSMAN, ALEXANDER H., Dr.
Department of Psychiatry, College of
Physicians and Surgeons, Columbia
University, 722 West 168th Street,
New York, NY 10032, USA

GOLDMAN, MARK, Dr.
Clinical Neuroscience Branch,
National Institute of Mental Health,
Bldg. 10, Rm. 4N214,
9000 Rockville Pike,
Bethesda, MD 20892, USA

GOODWIN, FREDERICK K., Dr.
National Institute of Mental Health,
Bldg. 10, Rm. 4N224,
9000 Rockville Pike,
Bethesda, MD 20892, USA

GRAM, LARS F., Dr.
Department of Clinical Pharmacology,
Odense University, 5000 C Odense,
DK-Odense, Denmark

GREENBLATT, DAVID J., Dr.
Division of Clinical Pharmacology,
Box 1007, New England Medical
Center Hospital, 171 Harrison Avenue,
Boston, MA 02111, USA

GRIFFITHS, ROLAND R., Dr.
Department of Psychiatry and
Behavioral Sciences,
Johns Hopkins School of Medicine,
Baltimore, MD 21205, USA

HALS, PETTER-ARNT, Dr.
Institute of Medical Biology,
University of Tromsø,
N-9001 Tromsø, Norway

HOMMER, DANIEL W., Dr.
Clinical Neuroscience Branch,
National Institute of Mental Health,
Bldg. 10, Room 4N214,
9000 Rockville Pike,
Bethesda, MD 20892, USA

HONORÉ, PIERRE LEFEVRE, Dr.
Ferrosan Ltd., Sydmarken 1–5,
DK-2860 Søborg, Denmark

HYTTEL, JOHN, Dr.
Research Laboratories, H. Lundbeck
and Co. A/S, Ottiliavej 7–9,
DK-2500 Valby, Denmark

JOHNSON, ANTHONY M., Dr.
Beecham Pharmaceuticals, Medicinal
Research Centre, Coldharbour Road,
The Pinnacles
GB-Harlow, Essex CM19 5AD,
Great Britain

Kellar, Kenneth, Dr.
Department of Pharmacology,
Georgetown University School of Medicine, 3900 Reservoir Road, N.W.,
Washington, DC 20057, USA

Kragh-Sørensen, Per, Dr.
Department of Psychiatry,
Odense University Hospital,
J.B. Winsløws Vej 20
DK-5000 Odense C, Denmark

Kupfer, David, Dr.
Department of Psychiatry, Western Psychiatric Institute and Clinic,
3811 O'Hara Street,
Pittsburgh, PA 15213, USA

Leber, Paul D., Dr.
Drug Products, HFD 120, Center for Drugs and Biologics, FDA,
5600 Fishers Lane,
Rockville, MD 20857, USA

Leysen, Josée E., Dr.
Department of Biochemical Pharmacology, Janssen Pharmaceutica,
B-2340 Beerse, Belgium

Linnoila, Markku, Dr.
Laboratory of Clinical Studies,
NIAAA, Bldg. 10, Rm. 3B-19,
9000 Rockville Pike,
Bethesda, MD 20205-1000, USA

Lloyd, Kenneth G., Dr.
Laboratoire d'Etudes et de Recherches Synthelabo, 58 Rue de la Glacière,
F-75013 Paris, France

Manniche, Poul, Dr.
Ferrosan Ltd., Sydmarken 1–5,
DK-2860 Søborg, Denmark

Marshall, Garland R., Dr.
Department of Physiology and Biophysics, School of Medicine,
Washington University,
St. Louis, MO 63110, USA

Meltzer, Herbert Y., Dr.
Univ. of Chicago Pritzker School of Medicine and Illinois State Psychiatric Institute, 5841 South Maryland Avenue,
Chicago, IL 60637, USA

Montgomery, Stuart A., Dr.
St. Mary's Hospital, Academic Department of Psychiatry,
Praed Street,
London W2 1NY, Great Britain

Murphy, Dennis, L., Dr.
Laboratory of Clinical Sciences,
National Institute of Mental Health,
Building 10, Room 3D41,
9000 Rockville Pike,
Bethesda, MD 20892, USA

Naranjo, Claudio, Dr.
Addiction Research Foundation,
Clinical Pharmacology Program and Clinical Research Unit,
33 Russell Street,
Toronto, Ontario M5S 2S1 Canada

Nilsson, Maj-Inger, Dr.
Astra Läkemedel AB,
S-151 85 Södertälje, Sweden

Nutt, David, Dr.
Department of Psychiatry, Warneford Hospital, University of Oxford,
Oxford, United Kingdom

Overø, Kerstin Fredricson, Dr.
Research Laboratories, H. Lundbeck and Co. A/S, Ottiliavej 7–9,
DK-2500 Valby, Denmark

PAUL, STEVEN M., Dr.
National Institute of Mental Health,
Building 10, Room 4N214,
9000 Rockville Pike,
Bethesda, MD 20892, USA

PEREL, JAMES M., Dr.
Department of Psychiatry, University of Pittsburgh School of Medicine,
Western Psychiatric Institute and Clinic,
Pittsburgh, PA 15216, USA

PICKAR, DAVID, Dr.
National Institute of Mental Health,
Building 10, Room 4N214,
9000 Rockville Pike,
Bethesda, MD 20982, USA

POLLOCK, BRUCE, Dr.
Department of Psychiatry, University of Pittsburgh School of Medicine,
Western Psychiatric Institute and Clinic,
Pittsburgh, PA 15216, USA

POTTER, WILLIAM Z., Dr.
National Institute of Mental Health,
Building 10, Room 2D46,
9000 Rockville Pike,
Bethesda, MD 20892, USA

REIMANN, INGRID, Dr.
CIBA/GEIGY, Pharmaceutical Div.,
Clinical Biology, TOV 1
Summit, NJ 07901, USA

RICKELS, KARL, Dr.
Piersol Building, Suite 203, Hospital of University of Pennsylvania,
3400 Spruce Street,
Philadelphia, PA 19104, USA

RUDORFER, MATTHEW V., Dr.
Section on Clinical Psychopharmacology, LCS, National Institute of Mental Health, Building 10, Room 2D46,
9000 Rockville Pike,
Bethesda, MD 20892, USA

SHELTON, RICHARD, Dr.
Department of Psychiatry,
Vanderbilt University,
Nashville, TN 37240, USA

SITSEN, JOHANNES, Dr.
Organon Scientific Development Group, The Medical Unit,
Oss, The Netherlands

SKOLNICK, PHIL, Dr.
Laboratory of Bioorganic Chemistry,
NIADDK, Building 4, Room 412,
9000 Rockville Pike,
Bethesda, MD 20892, USA

STULA-DELINI, ALEXANDRA, Dr.
Ciba-Geigy Ltd., PH 2.19,
CH-4002 Basel, Switzerland

TALLMAN, JOHN, Dr.
Department of Psychiatry, Yale University School of Medicine,
CMCHC, Room 304, 34 Park Street,
New Haven, CT 06508, USA

VESTERGAARD, PER, Dr.
Department A, Århus Psychiatric Hospital,
DK-8240 Risskov, Denmark

VOCCI, FRANK, Dr.
Division of Neuropharmacological Drug Products, HFD 120, Center for Drugs and Biologics, FDA,
5600 Fishers Lane,
Rockville, MD 20857, USA

von Bahr, Christer, Dr.
Astra Läkemedel AB,
Strangnäsvägen 44,
S-151 85 Södertälje, Sweden

Wagner, Anna, Dr.
Department of Psychiatry,
Karolinska Hospital,
S-141 01 Stockholm, Sweden

Zarifian, Edouard, Dr.
Centre Esquirol, C.H.U.,
Côte de Nacre,
F-14033 Caen, France

Subject Index

Page numbers given are the first pages of chapters in which the subject listed is discussed

MIX
Papier aus verantwortungsvollen Quellen
Paper from responsible sources
FSC® C105338

If you have any concerns about our products,
you can contact us on
ProductSafety@springernature.com

In case Publisher is established outside the EU,
the EU authorized representative is:
Springer Nature Customer Service Center GmbH
Europaplatz 3, 69115 Heidelberg, Germany

Printed by Libri Plureos GmbH
in Hamburg, Germany